Health Services
Research Methods

Second Edition

Health Services Research Methods

Second Edition

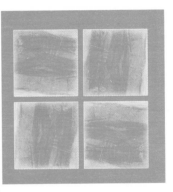

Leiyu Shi, Dr.PH., MBA, MPA

Professor, Johns Hopkins University
Bloomberg School of Public Health
Baltimore, Maryland

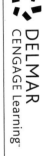

DELMAR
CENGAGE Learning™

Australia   Brazil   Canada   Japan   Korea   Mexico   Singapore   Spain   United Kingdom   United States

DELMAR
CENGAGE Learning™

Health Services Research Methods,
Second Edition
by Leiyu Shi, Dr.PH., MBA, MPA

Vice President,
Health Care Business Unit:
William Brottmiller

Director of Learning Solutions:
Matthew Kane

Acquisitions Editor:
Kalen Conerly

Product Manager:
Natalie Pashoukos

Editorial Assistant:
Meaghan O'Brien

Marketing Director:
Jennifer McAvey

Marketing Manager:
Michele McTighe

Marketing Coordinator:
Chelsey Iaquinta

Production Director:
Carolyn Miller

Senior Art Director:
Jack Pendleton

Content Project Manager:
Brooke Baker

Library of Congress Control Number: 2007040628

ISBN-13: 978-1-4283-5229-2

ISBN-10: 1-4283-5229-5

Delmar Cengage Learning
5 Maxwell Drive
Clifton Park, NY 12065-2919
USA

Cengage Learning products are represented in Canada by Nelson Education, Ltd.

For your lifelong learning solutions, visit **delmar.cengage.com**

Visit our corporate website at **www.cengage.com**

Notice to the Reader

Printed in the United States of America
3 4 5 6 7 11 10 09

CONTENTS

PREFACE

The term *health services research* (HSR) began to be widely used in the 1960s, and the field was developing rapidly by 1981, when the Association for Health Services Research was formed. Since then, HSR has developed into a recognized discipline by merging health-related methods and results from a number of the traditional disciplines of inquiry, ranging from sociology, political science or policy analysis, economics, epidemiology to nursing, medicine, and pharmacology. Typically health services researchers conduct investigations within different disciplinary fields: health policy, health systems research, health outcomes research, clinical epidemiology, technology assessment, clinical decision analysis, operations research, health economics, medical sociology, medical anthropology, to name a few. Indeed, HSR is in part *defined* by its field of interest rather than by a method, although methods—and agreement about methods among researchers—are as central to the creation of this discipline as to any other unique discipline. HSR is also an enterprise that is aimed at improving health services: it therefore seeks practical more than theoretical wisdom.

Despite the extensive literature related to HSR, few textbooks exist that examine the field of HSR and systematically describe the design, methodology, and analysis commonly used in HSR. As a student and later a professor in HSR, I was continually nagged by the lack of a relevant textbook on HSR. The research methods books I have encountered are primarily written by sociologists with little health care applications. Students frequently complain about the lack of relevance of those textbooks. In the course of teaching "Health Services Research Methods," I developed the current textbook that integrates HSR applications in the presentation of research methods and analysis.

AUDIENCE

The major audiences of this book include doctoral- and master-level students in health services administration programs. Students from nursing administration and clinical nursing programs can also benefit from this book. These programs may be offered by schools of public health, nursing, business administration, public administration, public policy, or medical schools. Students in other disciplines with an interest in HSR are also potential targets.

For doctoral programs, a two-semester sequence could be set aside for the research methods course. The course focus may be given to enhance the following areas: knowledge regarding HSR topics and conceptualization; research methodology with emphasis on design; survey research including design, sampling, questionnaire preparation, measurement, interview, pretest, and coding; and statistical analysis with emphasis on the choice of appropriate statistical methods. Sufficient emphasis should be given to the integrated nature of various stages of HSR. If only one semester can be allocated, as in most master's level programs, the emphasis should be given to the conceptual understanding of research stage with particular focus on conceptualization, methods, design, and survey measurement. The remaining content areas of the book may be integrated with other courses (e.g., statistics, health policy).

In addition to students, health services practitioners and researchers can also benefit from the book. They include those working in public health agencies, nonprofit health services organizations, insurance companies, and the like. My private consulting experience in these sectors shows that many of them are involved in HSR and frustrated by the lack of a relevant guidebook.

CHANGES IN THE INDUSTRY

Since the first edition of this textbook in 1997, the field of HSR has flourished. At present, many universities, particularly public health and medical schools, house HSR programs that train graduate students and conduct research related to health services. Private organizations, such as large managed care organizations, pharmaceutical and insurance companies, and think-tanks, also develop their own HSR programs. There has been a steady but growing demand for a textbook like *Health Services Research Methods*.

An important impetus to the rapid development of HSR is the breathtaking advance of the medical enterprises. The growing costs of the medical care systems and the increasing role of government in financing health institutions and services, and in paying for medical education, require the generation of information about the effectiveness, efficiency, and appropriateness of these enterprises. As health care costs continue to escalate and as the nation approaches health care reform, there will be an increasing demand for HSR.

ORGANIZATION OF THIS TEXT

The book is organized into 15 chapters. Chapter 1 lays the groundwork for the chapters that follow by describing the scientific foundations of HSR. Chapter 2 examines the conceptualization of HSR by summarizing major HSR topics. Chapter 3 describes the preparation for HSR including identifying relevant data sources, exploring potential funding sources, developing a research plan or proposal, and getting prepared organizationally and administratively to carry out the research. Chapters 4 through 9 summarize and illustrate the various types of HSR methods including research review, meta-analysis, secondary analysis, research analysis of administrative records, qualitative research, case study, experiment, survey research, longitudinal study, and evaluation research. Chapter 10 looks at research design options. Chapter 11 summarizes sampling procedures in HSR. Chapter 12 presents measurement issues in HSR. Chapter 13 delineates major data collection methods. Chapter 14 focuses on representative statistical analyses carried out in HSR. Chapter 15 explores ways of publicizing and implementing research findings.

FEATURES

There are a number of features of this book. First, the book intends to be a practical guide for those interested in HSR. Steps are delineated and illustrated clearly in the text, tables, and figures. Second, HSR examples are used throughout. Third, the book integrates research design with analysis. While this is not a statistics textbook, commonly used statistics are discussed in terms of their use for different levels of analysis and the nature of the variables. Fourth, the book also provides resources for students and researchers of health services. For example, the book includes current HSR journals, funding sources (public and private), and data sources.

NEW TO THIS EDITION

In addition to retaining the strengths of the first edition, e.g., its overarching framework, clear organization, and simplicity, the current edition has improved on the first edition by providing updates on the references and information throughout the book, including more HSR examples and applications, and significantly expanding several chapters that reflect the latest development of HSR. Specifically, the new edition includes new and expanded passages on important HSR topics, concepts, and theories, such as: the scientific foundations of HSR, social epidemiology and the life course approach to HSR, bio-ethics in HSR, policy analysis as a HSR tool, the importance of evidence-based medicine (EBM) and the role of HSR in promoting EBM, effects of HIPAA on HSR, the translation of HSR to policy and program applications, and training health services researchers through core competencies and necessary skills.

The new edition has also made an effort to provide updated descriptions of established and emerging HSR tools, skills, and methods, including: conceptual framework development, use of quantitative, qualitative, and mixed methods in HSR, use of the Internet in literature searches, secondary data retrieval, and primary data collection, computer-based data collection and analysis, including CATI and CAPI, statistical analysis packages, experimental and quasi-experimental study design, sampling and measurement, power and sample size estimates, multilevel analysis, factor analysis and other scaling procedures, and economic evaluation and modeling, including decision analysis, cost-effectiveness analysis, and cost-benefit analysis.

The current edition also offers new examples of contemporary and salient HSR topics, drawn from the HSR literature, government, and other public and private-sector sources, and updated descriptions of research aids and directories, including funding sources, primary and secondary data sources, Internet search engines, and government agencies involved in HSR.

ACKNOWLEDGMENTS

The preparation of this book, both at the initial and later phase, has been greatly aided by a number of devoted reviewers who themselves are active health services researchers. The author wishes to thank Patricia Collins who served as my research assistant and helped with numerous tasks associated with the revision on the first edition. Similar thanks and gratitudes are extended to all those who have reviewed either the proposal or selected chapters of the manuscripts and provided comments and feedback. Their time and effort spent in reviewing the manuscripts are warmly and graciously appreciated and acknowledged. The author is also grateful to Delmar Cengage Learning and former series editor, Stephen Williams, for encouraging the development and publishing of the original book and the new edition. The direct assistance provided by Delmar Cengage Learning staff Kalen Conerly, Natalie Pashoukos, Brooke Baker, Jack Pendleton, and Meaghan O'Brien is much appreciated. All suggestions concerning any aspects of this second edition of the book are welcome and will be acknowledged and incorporated in future editions.

Leiyu Shi
Johns Hopkins University
Bloomberg School of Public Health

REVIEWERS

ABOUT THE AUTHOR

Dr. Leiyu Shi is Professor of Health Policy and Health Services Research at Johns Hopkins University's Bloomberg School of Public Health Department of Health Policy and Management. He is Co-Director of Johns Hopkins Primary Care Policy Center. He received his doctoral education from University of California Berkeley majoring in health policy and services research. He also has a Masters degree in business administration focusing on finance. Dr. Shi's research focuses on primary care, health disparities, and vulnerable populations. He has conducted extensive studies about the association between primary care and health outcomes, particularly on the role of primary care in mediating the adverse impact of income inequality on health outcomes. Dr. Shi is also well known for his extensive research on the nation's vulnerable populations, in particular community health centers that serve vulnerable populations, including their sustainability, provider recruitment and retention experiences, financial performance, experience under managed care, and quality of care. Dr. Shi is the author of seven textbooks and over 100 journal articles.

Scientific Foundations of Health Services Research

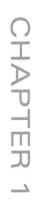

KEY TERMS

anonymity
applied
assumptions
asymmetrical relationship
biomedical research
causal relationship
clinical research
concept
conceptual framework
confidentiality
constant
construct
deductive process
dependent variable
empiricism
environmental health research
epidemiological research
ethical standards
financing
grounded theory

Hawthorne effect
health services research
hypothesis
independent variable
inductive process
informed consent
Institutional Review Board
(IRB)
intervening variable
linear relationship
multidisciplinary
natural science
negative/inverse relationship
nonlinear relationship
objectivity
operationalization
outcomes research
paradigm
peer review
placebo

positive/direct relationship
positivism
process
proposition
randomized clinical trial
reactivity
replication
resources
right to service
scientific inquiry
scientific method
scientific theory
small area analysis
social science
spurious relationship
suppressor variable
symmetrical relationship
variable
voluntary participation

LEARNING OBJECTIVES

- To understand and describe the major characteristics of scientific inquiry.

- To understand and describe the process of generating scientific theory.

- To understand and describe the major types of relationships between variables.

- To understand and describe the major characteristics of health services research.

- To understand and describe the process of health services research.

Chapter 1 lays the groundwork for the chapters that follow. By providing an overview of the scientific foundations of health services research (HSR), the chapter serves as a framework on which specific aspects of HSR are based. The nature of scientific inquiry is discussed, followed by a description of HSR. Since social scientists have made significant contributions to the development of health services research, the discussion of scientific inquiry centers on social science research. The chapter concludes with a summary of the stages of health services research, based on the major components of scientific inquiry. After completing this chapter, readers should be ready to examine some of the more concrete aspects of health services research related to the delineated stages.

THE NATURE OF SCIENTIFIC INQUIRY

The origin of the word *science* is the Latin word *scientia*, which indicates "knowledge." The major purpose of **scientific inquiry** is to create knowledge that clarifies a particular aspect of the world around us (Kaplan and Wolf, 1998). The earliest root of scientific inquiry may be traced to the Edwin Smith papyrus (c. 1600 BC), an ancient surgical textbook, which includes the basic components of the scientific method: examination, diagnosis, treatment, and prognosis. The **scientific method** in its modern form may be traced in early Muslim philosophy (c. AD 800), which embraces experiments to distinguish between competing scientific theories. Over the years, scientific method has been successively refined through the work of a succession of historians, philosophers, and scientists such as Francis Bacon (first controlled experiment, 1590), René Descartes (first scientific method, 1637), Robert Boyle (repeatability established, 1665), Isaac Newton (hypothesis testing, 1687), David Hume (problem of induction, 1710), Ronald Fisher (randomized design, 1930), Karl Popper (falsifiability in evaluating new hypotheses, 1934), and Thomas Kuhn (meta study of scientific method, 1962).

The fundamental assumption of scientific inquiry is that life is not totally chaotic or random but has logical and persistent patterns of regularity (Sjoberg and Nett, 1996). This assumption, labeled **positivism**, is responsible for the two major pillars of scientific inquiry: scientific theory and empiricism. **Scientific theory** is related to the logical aspect of science and is used as a framework to guide the understanding and explanation of patterns of regularity in life (DiRenzo, 1967). **Empiricism** is the approach used in scientific inquiry to discover the patterns of regularity in life (Hempel, 1965, 1967). Scientific inquiry relies on or derives from data that can be observed under specifiable conditions (Selltiz, Wrightsman, and Cook, 1976). A scientific understanding of the world must be logical and correspond with what we observe. Since empirical evidence may be colored by the perspectives of the very individuals conducting the research, it is important that they maintain **objectivity** in their observations, uninfluenced by their personal feelings, conjectures, or preferences. Scientific methodology, properly used, strengthens the objectivity of the observational aspect of the research. Equally important, researchers, particularly in the applied social sciences, should uphold **ethical standards** in conducting research, always considering the interests of the study subjects. This textbook deals primarily with research methods—demonstrating how to conduct empirical health services research. The remainder of this section takes a closer look at these important characteristics of scientific inquiry, namely, positivism, scientific theory, empiricism, objectivity, and ethical standards.

Positivism

Scientific disciplines, whether physical, natural, social, or medical, are typically based on the fundamental assumption that there exists a relatively persistent pattern or regularity in what is being studied. This assumption is particularly upheld in **natural science**, which is the rational study of the universe via rules or laws of natural order. However, the assumption is often challenged in **social science**, which studies human behavior and social phenomena. For example, Wilhelm Dilthey (1988), a 19th-century sociologist, took the extreme position that humans had free will, and thus no one could generalize about their actions. He believed that scientists could only study unique events, not make generalizations.

The opposite view was held by Émile Durkheim (1974), who maintained that social phenomena, just like physical phenomena, are orderly and generalizable. Social scientists could study and explain social phenomena just as well as physical scientists study and explain physical phenomena. Durkheim's study of suicide rates in European countries was an example. His work on suicide began in 1888, and his monumental book *Le Suicide* was published in 1897 (Lester, 1994). Durkheim (1951) noted that although suicide rates changed over time, they were consistently and inversely correlated with the degree of social integration. This finding was later termed "Durkheim's law of suicide."

However, most social scientists favor an intermediate approach as espoused by Max Weber. According to Weber (1949), social phenomena are the product of both social laws and human volitional action. The fact that humans have free will does not mean that their actions are random and totally unpredictable. Rather, human actions are guided by rational decision making and can be predicted by understanding the rationale behind the actions.

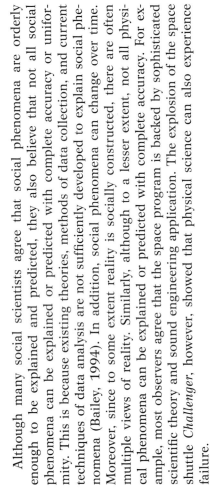

Although many social scientists agree that social phenomena are orderly enough to be explained and predicted, they also believe that not all social phenomena can be explained or predicted with complete accuracy or uniformity. This is because existing theories, methods of data collection, and current techniques of data analysis are not sufficiently developed to explain social phenomena (Bailey, 1994). In addition, social phenomena can change over time. Moreover, since to some extent reality is socially constructed, there are often multiple views of reality. Similarly, although to a lesser extent, not all physical phenomena can be explained or predicted with complete accuracy. For example, most observers agree that the space program is backed by sophisticated scientific theory and sound engineering application. The explosion of the space shuttle *Challenger*, however, showed that physical science can also experience failure.

The fact that there are exceptions to regularity is insufficient evidence to overthrow the assumption that regularity exists in both physical and social phenomena, because scientific inquiry is concerned with the study of patterns rather than exceptions. The pattern that, given the same educational level, men earn more money than women overall is not problematic when a particular woman earns more than a particular man. The trend that women live longer than men overall is not violated when a particular man lives longer than a particular woman. Social scientists primarily study social patterns. Regularities and patterns are probabilistic and do not need to be manifested in every observation.

It is also important to know that a particular pattern may not always persist (Skinner, 1953). In other words, regularity is not certainty. Scientific "truth" is based on observable evidence, but that truth is always subject to change when new evidence is presented that contradicts it. Thus, at some point a scientific proposition is accepted because it describes or interprets a recurring, observable event. But just because an event has occurred on several occasions is no guarantee that it will always recur. Scientific knowledge represents the best understanding that we have been able to produce thus far by means of current empirical evidence.

Scientific Theory

Scientific inquiry generally works within the framework of scientific theories. Scientific theories are based on overwhelming evidence and are used to derive research hypotheses, plan research, make observations, and explain generalizations and patterns of regularity in life (McCain and Segal, 1988; Zetterberg, 1954). They provide a systematic explanation and make predictions for a particular phenomenon. A statement that does not seek to explain or predict something is not a theory. Theories must also be potentially testable. A statement that is too vague to be understandable is not an adequate theory.

In searching for theories, scientists generally do not start out with a completely clean slate. Rather, they are influenced by the paradigms of their discipline. A **paradigm** is normative in that it reflects a general perspective, a fundamental model or scheme that breaks down the complexity of reality and organizes our views. As such, paradigms are deeply embedded in the socialization of researchers and tell them what is important, legitimate, and reasonable (Patton, 2002).

Thomas Kuhn (as cited in Neurath, Carnap, and Morris, 1970) was responsible for popularizing the term *paradigm*, which he described as essentially a collection of beliefs shared by scientists, a set of agreements about how problems are to be understood. According to Kuhn, paradigms are essential to scientific inquiry, for "no natural history can be interpreted in the absence of at least some implicit body of intertwined theoretical and methodological belief that permits selection, evaluation, and criticism." Indeed, a paradigm guides the research efforts of scientific communities, and it is this criterion that most clearly identifies a field as a science. A fundamental theme of Kuhn's argument is that the typical developmental pattern of a mature science is the successive transition from one paradigm to another through a process of revolution. When a paradigm shift takes place, "a scientist's world is qualitatively transformed [and] quantitatively enriched by fundamental novelties of either fact or theory."

Often, a paradigm doesn't readily provide answers to research questions, but it tells researchers where to look for answers and provides them with concepts that are the building blocks of theories. For example, many theories have been suggested to account for the fact that females in the United States and in other modern industrialized societies have higher rates of morbidity than males but live longer than males. One biomedical explanation for this posits a fundamental physiological difference that causes women to experience more morbidity than men but to live longer for reasons not yet clearly understood. A sociological suggestion is that the different roles men and women play in society expose them to different sources of illness or disability. A psychological explanation is that perhaps men and women do not differ in their underlying rates of morbidity. Rather, they have differential perceptions of and tolerance for morbidity, as well as different ways of expressing their feelings about that morbidity. Our social systems might have processed them differently so that it appears, when we count up hospital visits and the like, that women have greater morbidity rates.

Since it is possible to have several theories that explain a given empirical regularity and that make similar predictions, the confirmation of a prediction does not confirm that only one theory is correct (Hempel, 1967). Scientific inquiry is directed toward testing and choosing from alternative theories. One theory is generally judged to be superior to other competing theories if it: (1) involves the fewest number of statements and assumptions, (2) explains the broadest range of phenomena, and (3) predicts with the greatest level of accuracy (Singleton and Straits, 2005). In short, scientific theories should be efficient, comprehensive, and accurate.

There is an intimate connection between theory and research. Theory provides guidance for research. Research, in turn, verifies, modifies, or reconstructs theory. This interactive process between theory and research contributes to the

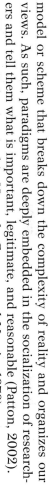

enrichment and development of scientific theories. Specifically, there are two components within this process: the **deductive process**, which emphasizes theory as guidance for research, and the **inductive process**, which stresses research as impetus for theory (Salmon, 1967, 1973). In the deductive process, hypotheses are derived from existing theories to provide guidance for further research. Indeed, scientific research is guided by accumulated scientific knowledge. In the inductive process (more frequently encountered in HSR), propositions are formulated and new theories are developed from research findings. The resulting corroborated, modified, or reconstructed theories guide future research along similar fields of inquiry.

Empiricism

The most critical characteristic of scientific inquiry is that it is based on empiricism. As Thomas Kuhn (as cited in Neurath, Carnap, and Morris, 1970) stated, science is a cognitive empirical investigation of nature. Empirical evidence is the only means by which scientists can corroborate, modify, or construct theories. Whether a question can be studied scientifically depends on whether it can be subjected to verifiable observations (Singleton and Straits, 2005). That is, it must be possible for the scientist to make observations that can answer the question.

The empirical requirement of scientific inquiry has several ramifications. First, it means that nonempirical ways of acquiring knowledge cannot produce scientific evidence. Examples of nonempirical approaches include appeals to authority, tradition, common sense or intuition, and so on.

In general, scientists do not generalize about the world based on what an authority or expert says. An authority or expert may be knowledgeable about the subject matter, but his opinion alone cannot serve as scientific evidence to prove or refute a hypothesis. However, this does not mean experts cannot be studied in research. A representative sample of experts can be surveyed regarding their perceptions of issues of research interest, as in the Delphi method.

Tradition refers to inherited culture that is made up of firmly accepted knowledge about the workings of the world (Babbie, 2004). These are the things that "everyone knows." An example is to consult a doctor when one is sick. The advantage of tradition is that one is spared the task of starting from scratch in searching for understanding. The disadvantage is that tradition keeps us from seeking a fresh and different understanding of something that everyone already knows. Tradition is not always correct. Maybe better diet and exercise are more important to one's health than relying on medical treatment.

Common sense cannot be regarded as scientific evidence. Common sense tends to be unconditional, uncomplicated, and nonsituational, and it does not require systematic testing. It limits people's reliance to the familiar and implies that seeing is believing, although the reverse is often true. When one believes in something, one is more likely to see (notice) it.

Second, empiricism in science also implies that researchers focus on problems and issues that can be observed. Observations may be direct, as in field studies, or indirect, as in surveys and interviews that primarily rely on the empirical experience of research subjects. These observations are then used to form **constructs**, intangible or nonconcrete characteristics or qualities with respect to which individuals or populations differ. Examples of constructs are patient satisfaction with a visit to the doctor, or the American people's impression of the health care system. Constructs are often the building blocks of scientific theories.

Third, empiricism means scientific inquiry cannot settle debates on values or beliefs. Scientific inquiry has to do with what is, not what should be. This means that philosophical questions about righteousness, essence, or morality are beyond the realm of science. For example, the value judgment that people should not use birth control is an opinion, not a testable statement. Science cannot determine whether a market-controlled health care system (a laissez-faire approach) is better or worse than a government-controlled and -financed system (a single-payer approach) except in terms of some set of agreed-on criteria. We could only determine scientifically whether the laissez-faire or single-payer system better supports access to care and/or cost containment, and our conclusion would have no general meaning beyond the measures agreed upon.

The fact that scientific inquiry cannot settle values or beliefs does not mean it is not influenced by them. Rather, personal values and beliefs frequently influence the process of research. Indeed, the challenge for scientists, particularly in the social sciences, is to maintain objectivity and openness as much as possible in their scientific inquiry.

Objectivity

Scientists, like most people, have their own values and often make value judgments. This fact in and of itself is not problematic. But, in terms of research, individual values may affect the validity of the inquiry and make the findings biased. The problem with value judgments in research is that not only are they essentially untestable but they may make a researcher prejudiced in undertaking research. Although it can be difficult, researchers should strive to suppress values and conduct value-free research in order to minimize bias in their findings. They are perfectly free to hold and express their values in a nonresearch environment.

Even though researchers may hold back their personal values while conducting research, they are likely to be influenced by their scientific disciplines or paradigms. Different paradigms tend to espouse different values. They affect the types and scope of problems to be studied, the methods adopted, and the ways to interpret the findings. Biases may enter into the selection of problems for study and the preference for certain research strategies. Often, where and how one investigates largely determines the answers one will find. Since it is very

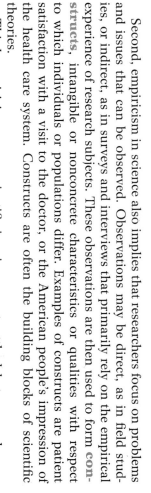

hard to think beyond one's established paradigm and difficult to suppress one's professional values, it is important that researchers state their professional values (i.e., the research paradigm) explicitly so that readers may judge for themselves the limitations of the research when considering other relevant paradigms. Perhaps the worst approach is to deny that one has a value position that has in fact influenced the research. Such a lack of openness will make it difficult for the reader to assess the validity of the research.

Sponsorship and funding can be another source of bias. Large-scale studies are typically beyond the means of researchers and require outside funding support as well as sponsorship. If the study has relevance to the interests of the sponsor or funder and an adverse finding might negatively affect those interests, researchers may be hesitant in being forthright about their conclusions for fear of endangering current or future support and sponsorship.

Sometimes, particularly in social sciences, maintaining objectivity is difficult through no fault of the researchers. If subjects know that they are being observed, they often will feel self-conscious and may alter their behavior, either consciously or unconsciously. This **reactivity** problem exists because social interaction with subjects is often part of the social science research process.

The reactive effect of research on the social phenomena being studied is known as the **Hawthorne effect**, derived from the study of workers assembling telephone relays in the Hawthorne plant of the Western Electric Company in Chicago (Roethlisberger and Dickson, 1939). In studying the impact of varying working conditions on work performance among employees, researchers were surprised to note that productivity increased even when rest periods were eliminated. They later realized that it was a reactive effect. The researchers' presence altered the very behavior (worker productivity) they wished to study. The Hawthorne effect is also common in health studies, especially when interventions are introduced. This is called the **placebo** effect, in which the belief in the presence of a promising treatment (even though it is in fact an inert substance) creates a real result (e.g., recovery from disease).

Fortunately, scientists adopt numerous measures to enhance objectivity. During the research process, scientists use procedures to control for, minimize, or eliminate, as far as possible, sources of bias that may mislead their findings. Research findings are often open to a variety of interpretations. The concept of control involves the use of procedures (either by design or by statistical modeling) to exclude alternative explanations. For example, in medical research, a double-blind procedure is often used to assign patients to experimental or control groups. Patients in the control group use a placebo; neither the patients nor the doctors know which group patients belong to. This procedure is designed to rule out the possibility of doctors' and patients' expectations contributing to the effectiveness of a treatment. The Hawthorne effect may be reduced through an improved design (for example, by using more control groups including those whose subjects are not aware of the research, or by extending the study period since the reactive effect tends to be relatively short-lived). The use of control procedures to reduce biases is a common method for enhancing objectivity.

Peer review is another measure to improve objectivity. When a group of scientists can independently agree on the results of a given observation, validity is enhanced. Replication is another measure that can be used. If it is possible for two or more independent researchers working under the same conditions to agree that they are observing the same event, validity is further enhanced. To meet the requirements of objectivity and openness in scientific inquiry, researchers provide detailed accounts of their study, delineating their methods of observation and analysis. Such a process enables others to assess whether the researchers have maintained objectivity or whether they should repeat the study themselves under similar conditions. These and many other measures to enhance objectivity will be discussed throughout this book.

Ethical Standards

Ethical standards, or the proper conduct of research with full consideration of the subjects' interests, became paramount in the wake of one marker event. The Nuremberg war crimes trials following World War II brought to public view the ways German scientists had used captive human beings as subjects in oftentimes gruesome experiments. These revelations prompted worldwide development and refinement of ethical standards and principles (see Chapter 15 for discussion of ethics in research) that ensure that potential human subjects are protected from being used as "guinea pigs" in scientific research.

When developing research plans, scientists should consider all relevant ethical issues to assure the safety and rights of study participants. An **Institutional Review Board (IRB)**, a panel of persons that reviews research plans with respect to ethical implications, makes sure this is done properly and decides whether additional actions need to be taken. Also, IRBs help protect both the organization and the researcher against potential legal implications of important ethical negligence.

In designing the study, researchers should not put participants in a situation where they might be at risk of harm, whether physical or psychological. No one should be coerced into participating in research. **Voluntary participation** is especially important among "captive audiences" (e.g., those in prisons, universities, and workplaces). All prospective study participants must provide **informed consent.** This means they must be made fully aware of the procedures and risks involved in the research.

During the study, researchers have to respect a person's **right to service.** When an experimental treatment or program may have beneficial effects, persons assigned to the no-treatment control should be provided equal access to the benefits.

Both during and after the study, the privacy of the subjects should be protected through either **anonymity** (which means that the participant will remain anonymous throughout the study, even to the researchers) or **confidentiality** (which means that identifying information will not be made available to anyone not directly involved in the study).

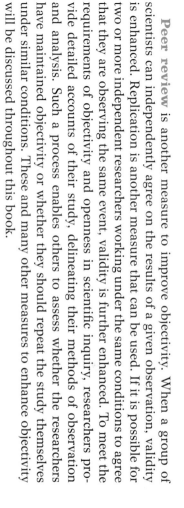

THE PROCESS OF THEORY CONSTRUCTION

Since much of scientific inquiry follows the interactive process of theory verification and/or construction, and there are some important concepts embedded in the process, a detailed discussion (Babbie, 2004; Dubin, 1969) is warranted. The steps involved in theory verification are examined below.

The process of theory construction:

Step 1. Specify the topic

Step 2. Specify the assumptions

Step 3. Specify the range of phenomena

Step 4. Specify the major concepts and variables

Step 5. Specify the propositions, hypotheses, and relationships

Step 6. Specify the theory

Specify the Topic

The first step in theory verification and/or construction is to specify the research topic of interest. Existing theories and literature related to the topic should be identified and used as a guide for determining the nature and scope of the inquiry. Since knowledge is cumulative, the inherited body of information and understanding is the takeoff point for the development of more knowledge. The practice of reviewing the literature in research papers serves the purpose of both identifying relevant theories and findings and discovering whether they are lacking.

Specify the Assumptions

The second step in theory verification and/or construction is to specify the assumptions related to the research focus. **Assumptions** are suppositions that are not yet tested but are considered true. In general, assumptions should make sense to most people. When in doubt, researchers should test their assumptions rather than consider them true. For example, when the telephone interview is used as a data collection method, the assumption is that it can reach a representative sample of the population of interest. If this assumption is not necessarily true, as in studies of Medicaid recipients or indigent patients, then researchers need to conduct a pretest to verify whether the telephone is a proper channel for reaching the study population prior to full-scale data collection.

Specify the Range of Phenomena

The third step in theory verification and/or construction is to specify the range of phenomena that the current research and existing theories address. For example, will the research and theories apply to people of the world or only to Americans, or more specifically, to young Americans? Will the study be relevant to all racial/ethnic groups or to people with different immigration status? Are the findings generalizable only to the insured or would they be applicable to the uninsured as well? Will the study results be generalizable to all hospitals or only to urban community hospitals? Research or theories are more useful the greater the range of phenomena they cover, although broader theories are more difficult to construct. For one thing, data have to be collected from a wider spectrum of the population. Many of the clinical practice guidelines are based on best practices rendered to well-insured patients and are considered inadequate for many of the uninsured, who are often more vulnerable with greater comorbidities and psychological needs.

Specify the Major Concepts and Variables

The fourth step in theory verification and/or construction is to specify the major concepts and variables. **Concepts** are mental images or perceptions (Bailey, 1994). They may be difficult to observe directly, such as *equity* or *ethics*, or they may have referents that are easily observable, such as a *hospital* or a *clinic*. A concept that has only a single, never-changing value is called a **constant**. A concept that has more than one measurable value is called a **variable**. A concept or variable may contain several categories, falling along a recognizable continuum. The variable *old-age*, for example, is a continuum containing many different values or categories, such as ages 65–74, 75–84, or 85 and older. Usually, the values or categories of a variable are designated quantitatively (i.e., signified by numbers, as in the case of age), but some variables have categories designated by word labels rather than by numbers. For example, gender is a variable whose categories are designated by the labels "male" and "female."

Variables may be classified as independent and/or dependent. Generally, a variable capable of effecting change in other variables is called an **independent variable**. A variable whose value is dependent upon one or more other variables, but which cannot itself affect the other variables, is called a **dependent variable**. The dependent variable is the variable we wish to explain, and the independent variable is the hypothesized explanation. In a causal relationship, the cause is an independent variable and the effect a dependent variable. For example, since smoking causes lung cancer, smoking is an independent variable and lung cancer a dependent variable.

Often we can recognize a variable as independent simply because it occurs before the other variable. For example, we may find a relationship between race and level of education. Race clearly comes before schooling and, therefore, must be an independent variable. Education level can in no way influence race, since race has already been determined at birth. When one variable does not clearly precede the other, it may be difficult to designate it as dependent or independent. An example is the relationship between health status and income. If a person has adequate income, he or she may have the financial resources to maintain good health status. Or when a person has good health status, he or she will have the opportunity to earn better income. The question is, which comes first: good health status or adequate income? Perhaps each influences the other. The treatment of these variables will be discussed in the next step when we consider causal relationships.

Specify the Propositions, Hypotheses, and Relationships

The fifth step in theory verification and/or construction is to specify the propositions, hypotheses, and relationships among the variables (Bailey, 1994). A **proposition** is a statement about one or more concepts or variables. Propositions are the building blocks of theories. Depending upon their use in theory building, propositions have been given different names, including hypotheses, empirical generalizations, constructs, axioms, postulates, and theorems.

A proposition that discusses a single variable is called a univariate proposition. An example is: "Forty-five million of the citizens in the United States do not have any type of health insurance." It is a univariate proposition because only one variable, "have any type of health insurance," is contained in the statement.

A bivariate proposition is one that relates two variables. An example is: "The lower the population density in a county, the lower the physician-to-population ratio in that county." It is a bivariate proposition because two variables, "population density" and "physician-to-population ratio," are contained in the statement.

A proposition relating more than two variables is called a multivariate proposition. An example is: "The lower the population density in a county, the lower the physician-to-population ratio and hospital-to-population ratio in that county." It is a multivariate proposition because three variables, "population density," "physician-to-population ratio," and "hospital-to-population ratio," are contained in the statement. A multivariate proposition can be written as two or more bivariate propositions. For example, (1) "the lower the population density in a county, the lower the physician-to-population ratio in that county" and (2) "the lower the population density in a county, the lower the hospital-to-population ratio in that county." This would allow for one portion of the original proposition to be rejected without rejecting the other portion, based on later statistical tests.

When a proposition is stated in a testable form (that we can in principle prove right or wrong through research) and predicts a particular relationship between two or more variables, it is called a **hypothesis**. Normative statements, or those that are opinions and value judgments, are not hypotheses. For example, the statement "Every person should have access to health care" is a normative statement. It is a value judgment that cannot be proved right or wrong.

This definition also excludes statements that are too abstract to be tested. Consider the statement "The poor do not have adequate access to health care." Although this is a valid proposition, we would not call it a testable hypothesis until the concepts of poor, adequacy, and health care are measured or defined on an empirical level. For example, we can define poor as those with income below the poverty line, adequacy as the U.S. average, and health care as number of visits to the doctor. We can then state, "Compared with the U.S. average, those with income below the poverty line experience fewer visits to the doctor." This becomes a testable hypothesis.

Hypotheses may be generated from a number of sources. They may be deduced from a formal theory that summarizes the present state of knowledge about the research problem. This is the standard deductive process. Or they may be inspired by past research, by commonly held beliefs, or by current evidence, as in many HSR studies. Or they may be generated through direct analysis of data. The latter two approaches are used typically when there is an absence of relevant theories related to the topic of research, often common in HSR. Regardless of how hypotheses are expressed, they should indicate at least the form of the relationship between variables. A hypothesis is an expected but yet unconfirmed relationship between two or more variables. An adequate hypothesis statement about two variables indicates which variable predicts or causes the other or how changes in one variable are related to changes in the other.

The properties of the relationship (Bailey, 1994; Miller and Salkind, 2002; Singleton and Straits, 2005) between two variables involve the strength of the relationship and the designation of each variable as either independent or dependent (as in a causal relationship). Other properties include whether the relationship is positive or negative, symmetrical or asymmetrical, linear or curvilinear, and is spurious or involves an intervening or suppressor variable.

Positive versus Negative Relationships

In a **positive**, or **direct**, **relationship**, both variables vary in the same direction, that is, an increase in the value of one variable is accompanied by an increase in the value of the other variable. Similarly, a decrease in one variable is accompanied by a decrease in the other variable. For example, if an increase in one's income level is accompanied by an increase in health insurance coverage, the relationship is positive. In a **negative**, or **inverse**, **relationship**, the variables vary in opposite directions. An increase (decrease) in one variable is accompanied by a decrease (increase) in the other variable. For example, if an increase in educational level is accompanied by a decrease in smoking, the relationship is inverse. A negative relationship does not imply that the variables are less strongly related than those in a positive relationship.

Strength of Relationships

The strength of the relationship reflects how much the variables are related. When two variables are unrelated, knowing the value of one does not tell us the value of the other. The more two variables are related, the more accurately we can predict the value of one variable based on the value of the other. Statistics (see Chapter 14) can be used to measure the strength of a bivariate relationship.

Symmetrical versus Asymmetrical Relationships

In a **symmetrical relationship**, change in either variable is accompanied by change in the other variable. In an **asymmetrical relationship**, change in one variable is accompanied by change in the other, but not vice versa. For example, the relationship between poverty and health status may be considered symmetrical in that a poor person is more likely to have a poor health status, which in turn makes that person even poor. The relationship between smoking and lung cancer would be asymmetrical because smoking could cause lung cancer, but lung cancer could not cause smoking.

Linear versus Nonlinear Relationships

In a **linear** (or straight-line) **relationship**, the two variables vary at the same rate regardless of whether the values of the variables are low, intermediate, or high. In a **nonlinear relationship** (e.g., curvilinear), the rate at which one variable changes in value is different for different values of the other variable. For example, the relationship between packs of cigarettes smoked and chances of getting lung cancer may be considered as linear in that the more cigarettes one smokes the greater is the chance of getting lung cancer. The relationship between education and income may be described as nonlinear. Higher education level leads to higher income, up to a point, when additional education has no marginal impact on income. In other words, going to school forever would not guarantee that one will become a millionaire.

Spurious, Intervening, and Suppressor Relationships

When a correlation between two variables has been caused by a third or extraneous variable, rather than by their interrelationship, the relationship is called spurious. The variable that causes a **spurious relationship** is an antecedent variable, which is causally related to both the independent and dependent variables (see Figure 1.1).

An apparent relationship between two variables may be caused by an **intervening variable** that is between the independent and dependent variables. For example, as Figure 1.1 shows, variables X and Y may be highly correlated, but only because variable X causes a third variable, Z (the intervening variable), which in turn causes variable Y.

A **suppressor variable** suppresses or conceals the relationship between two variables because it is positively associated with one variable and negatively associated with the other. The true relationship between the two variables can be made clear after controlling for the suppressor variable (i.e., by including the suppressor variable in the analysis). For example, we might hypothesize a positive relationship between level of access and health status (the greater the access, the better the health status), conduct a study, but find no existing relationship. The relationship may be suppressed by the variable *age*, which is inversely correlated with health status (the higher the age, the lower the health status) and positively correlated with access (the higher the age, the greater the access level).

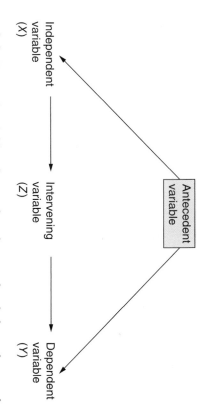

Figure 1.1. Types of variables: Antecedent, intervening, independent, and dependent

In other words, younger age tends to elevate health status but lower access level, whereas older age raises access level but reduces health status. The combined effect is likely to cancel out the relationship between access and health status. If access and health status are studied for each age group separately, the relationship between them will reappear.

Existing theories play a significant role in the identification of independent, dependent, spurious, and intervening variables. Theories also help researchers understand the complex relationships among variables and indicate the process that connects events. Research findings can then be used to validate, modify, or reconstruct existing theories.

Causal Relationships

When we say that two variables are related, we mean simply that they vary together, so that a change in one is accompanied by a change in the other, and vice versa. Such variation is often referred to as concomitant variation, or correlation. The discovery that there is a correlation between two variables does not ensure that the relationship is a causal one, that change in one variable causes change in the other variable.

There are three basic requisites to a **causal relationship**: statistical association, sequence of influence, and nonspuriousness. For one variable to be a cause of the other, the two variables must have a statistically significant relationship, or correlation. However, a perfect association between variables is not required of a causal relationship, because a perfect association may be expected only under the theoretical condition that all other things are held constant. In health services research, a phenomenon is typically caused by multiple factors, not all of which may be identified. Causal relationships may also be affected by relatively imprecise measurements. Commonly, statistics are used to judge whether an association is strong enough to imply a meaningful causal relationship.

The second criterion needed to establish causality is that there should be a clear cause–effect sequence. The causal factor must occur first, before the effect. The temporal sequence is often one major way to determine which factor is the cause and which is the effect. That is, the one that occurs first is the cause and the one that occurs second is the effect. Causal relationship is easily determined for asymmetrical relationships, where the cause precedes the effect in time. Given the complexity of social science research, some definitions allow for the possibility that the cause and effect occur simultaneously. Thus, it is possible to define cause for symmetrical relationships, or mutual causation, in which variable A causes variable B and simultaneously B causes A, so that each factor is both a cause and an effect. The relationship between poverty and disease is one such example.

The third criterion of causality is nonspuriousness; that is, a change in one variable results in a change in another regardless of the actions of other variables. If two variables happen to be related to a common extraneous variable, then a statistical association can exist even if there is no inherent link between the two variables. Therefore, to infer a causal relationship from an observed correlation there should be good reason to believe that there are no spurious factors that could have created an accidental relationship between the variables. When an association or correlation between variables cannot be explained by an extraneous variable, the relationship is said to be nonspurious. To infer nonspuriousness the researcher ideally must show that the relationship is maintained when all related, extraneous variables are held constant. Circumstances seldom allow a researcher to control all variables. Therefore, the researcher tries to include as many relevant variables as possible in the analysis. For example, heavy alcohol consumption is strongly associated with cirrhosis of the liver. The causal link between heavy alcohol consumption and liver cirrhosis is strengthened by the fact that this rate remains the same when other variables, including gender, urban/rural residence, and socioeconomic status are taken into account or controlled for.

Specify the Theory

The final step in theory verification and/or construction is to specify the theory as applied to a particular phenomenon under investigation. The theory may be a corroborated or revised existing theory or a newly constructed one. Theory is the result of hypothesis testing that examines, based on empirical evidence, the anticipated relationships among variables. The formal description of a theory consists of the definitions of related concepts, the assumptions used, and a set of interrelated propositions logically formed to explain the specific topic under investigation (McCain and Segal, 1988).

The theory–research process described is somewhat idealistic. Researchers use this process to guide and measure their research activities, even when, because of the various realities of research, they cannot always live up to the ideal.

The first reality is that theoretical knowledge is not yet well developed in many areas of social science research (Singleton and Straits, 2005). Frequently, unanticipated findings occur that cannot be interpreted meaningfully in light of current theories. The terms *theory* and *hypothesis* are often used interchangeably. *Theory* may have a loose meaning and refer to speculative ideas used to explain phenomena. The course of inquiry may be irregular rather than follow a smooth path from theory to hypothesis to observation and to generalization. Reports of the research process may be merely the result of hindsight.

Sometimes theories are created based on observation rather than on deduction from existing theories. These theories are referred to as **grounded theories.** B. G. Glaser (1992) and Strauss and Corbin (1998) summarized the process of developing grounded theory as: (1) entering the field or proceeding with research without a hypothesis, (2) describing what one observes in the field, and (3) explaining why it happens on the basis of observation. These explanations become the theory, which is generated directly from observation.

The second reality is that it is often very difficult to establish causality in social science research. One reason is the limitations of existing theories, which may not be sufficient to identify the proper causes. Another reason is that the identified causes cannot be properly controlled. Further, since much of the data in social sciences are gathered via the survey and interview method, we often cannot determine the temporal sequence of the factors of interest. Hence, we cannot be certain of the causes and effects and may have to treat the relationship as symmetrical without implying causality.

The third reality is that applied social science research such as HSR has developed from practical needs and problem solving. The imperatives of theory development are often less critical than the need to solve problems that arise in the real world. Where useful, researchers draw from the theoretical perspectives of social science disciplines but do not aim to develop theories. Often they begin with a real-life problem, formulate a hypothesis about a suspected relationship, investigate the relationship, and revise the hypothesis as necessary.

Examples of established health determinants theories are shown below. Based on cumulative empirical studies over time, Aday (2001) proposes a comprehensive framework tracing the pathways that influence community and individual health (Figure 1.2). In her model, Aday accounts explicitly for the connections between individual and community-level risk factors and resources that determine vulnerability for poor physical, psychological, and social health. Policy's influence on health is included as a mediator. This comprehensive framework could also be used to generate testable hypotheses for future research. For example, studies focusing on individual risk factors should also take into account the influence of community-level risk factors, and vice versa. The role of health and health care policy in mediating the adverse effects of risk factors can also be studied, as can the differential effects of risk factors on the different health dimensions, including the physical, mental, and social.

In addition to Aday's theory, numerous other frameworks are postulated regarding health determinants and are summarized below. Shi and Stevens (2005) built on Aday's model in their creation of a general framework to study vulnerable populations (Figure 1.3). In this multilevel model, the authors account

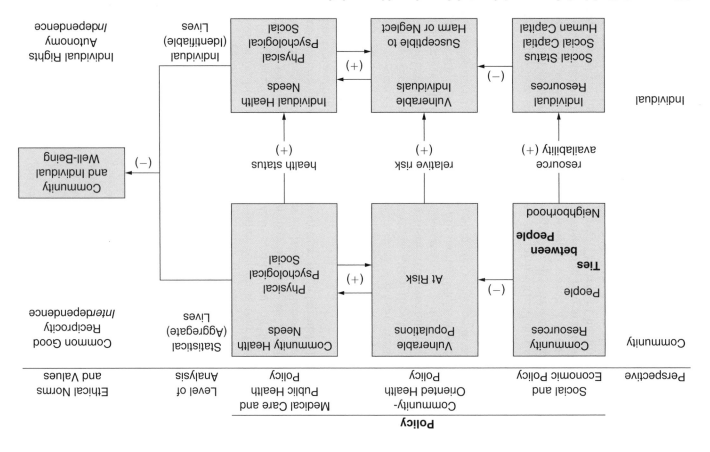

Figure 1.2. Aday's framework for studying vulnerable populations

Note: A plus sign indicates a direct relationship (the likelihood of outcomes increases as the predictor increases). A minus sign indicates an inverse relationship (the likelihood of outcomes decreases as the predictor increases).

Source: Aday (2001), p. 3.

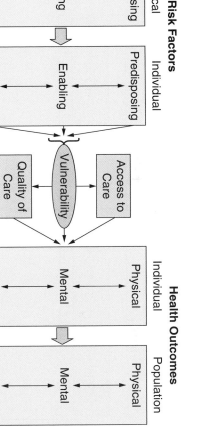

Figure 1.3. A general framework for studying vulnerable populations

Source: Shi and Stevens (2005).

for both individual and ecological/environmental risk factors that influence a person's vulnerability status. This suggests the importance not only of individual behaviors and beliefs, but also of the many environmental influences that are beyond an individual's control. As a growing body of literature attests, for vulnerable populations, access to care and quality of care often are compromised. As Shi and Stevens' model illustrates, these differentials in access and quality affect both individual- and population-level health outcomes.

The theory of the social context of child health was developed by Schor and Menaghan (1995). This theory postulates that child health outcomes are shaped by the family environment, which is influenced by three broad categories of factors: (1) the family characteristics (i.e., individual family member characteristics, sociodemographics, and family structure); (2) the family life cycle (i.e., the developmental status of the family members and transitions or disruptions to the family); and (3) the family community and society, which includes the social network, community characteristics, and social policies (such as health care, education, and housing) that affect the family's life. Child health outcomes are also shaped by the individual child's innate biological and psychological characteristics, by the child's community and society (i.e., his or her peers and school), and by the child's physical, social, and cognitive development. The theory of the social context of child health emphasizes the myriad documented influences on child health, and the need for a holistic approach to improving child health outcomes.

Figure 1.4 displays a framework for studying community and health conceptualized by Patrick and Wickizer (1995). This framework organizes multiple theories concerning community influences on the health of populations. The broad categories of cultural systems, political and policy systems, and economic

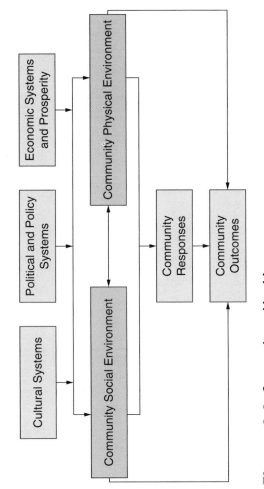

Figure 1.4. Community and health

Source: Adapted from Patrick and Wickizer (1995).

systems and prosperity shape the social and physical environments of communities. Characteristics of the social environment of a community include levels of poverty and social inequality, gender distribution and inequality, social homogeneity and cohesion, and cultural and social norms. Physical traits of a community include pollution, population density, and climate. The physical and social environments of a community shape one another, and also inform community responses to problems and community outcomes, such as social behaviors, health, and quality of life. Not all of the theories behind the community and health framework are proven, as it is difficult to make the causal link between certain factors (e.g., between the political and policy systems and community health and quality of life). However, this framework is a useful illustration of areas of research that need to be strengthened.

Another set of health theories developed in recent years explores the relationship between race and health. King and Williams (1995) suggest the etiological relationship between race and health involves the interaction between several different components of race and multiple intervening variables. Figure 1.5 suggests race may be a proxy for a range of factors (biological, cultural, socioeconomic, social [racism], and political), all of which shape health practices, psychosocial stress, environmental stress, psychosocial resources, and medical care. These intervening factors shape the biological processes that result in health outcomes.

Figure 1.6 illustrates theories involving gender and health developed by Walsh, Sorensen, and Leonard (1995). As has been shown in the previous figures included in this section, the authors postulate that broad social forces shape gender differences in health outcomes. The "gender order" box refers to power differentials between genders, or the degree to which the division of labor and gender stereotypes shape society. These power differentials lead to inequalities in income,

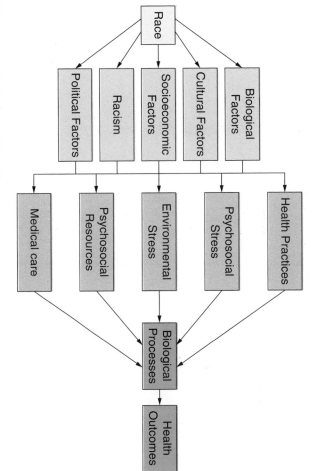

Figure 1.5. Race and health

Source: Adapted from King and Williams (1995).

health, education, occupation, social status, and other factors. Such inequalities produce differential risks and responses to disease, which result in the gender disparities in health, including morbidity, mortality, and quality of life indicators.

HEALTH SERVICES RESEARCH

Health services research examines how people get access to health care, how much care costs, and what happens to patients as a result of this care (Agency for Healthcare Research and Quality [AHRQ], 2002). It produces knowledge about the **resources**, organization, **financing**, provisions, and policies of health services (Frenk, 1993; Institute of Medicine, 1979; White, 1992, pp. xvii–xxiv). As an applied multidisciplinary field, HSR may be defined as studies that address the planning, distribution, organization, provision, quality, effectiveness, efficiency, and outcome of health care services, with the aim of improving the health care of the public through enhanced clinical and organizational practices and health care and public policy.

The development of HSR may be attributed to the following major factors: the expanded role of the federal government, the rapid ascension of managed care, the drive toward quality and outcome, the development of medical education, and the need to demonstrate the value of health care services.

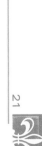

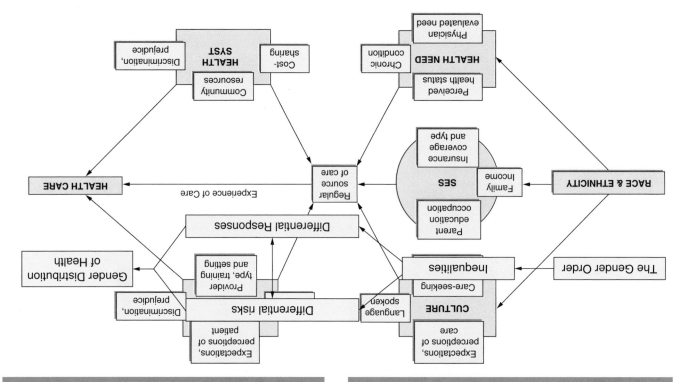

Figure 1.6. Gender and health

Source: Shi and Stevens (2003).

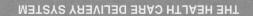

Health services research has been significantly influenced by the expanding role of the federal government as a major financer, provider, regulator, and planner of health services since the 1960s (Choi and Greenberg, 1982; Mechanic, 1973). The increasing involvement of the federal government in health services (e.g., in Medicare and Medicaid) and the rapid rise in health care expenditures contribute to the need for information and research related to the quality, availability, and cost of health services delivery (Gaus and Simpson, 1995). The establishment of the National Center for Health Services Research (NCHSR) in 1968 and the increasing reliance on the request for proposal (RFP) approach to grant-letting, in contrast to the investigator-oriented approach, have ensured that health services research is problem-oriented and focused on desired policy issues. The creation of the Agency for Health Care Policy and Research (AHCPR) in 1989 doubled the funding base for health services research to nearly $100 million and added statutory authority for outcomes research, guideline development, and research dissemination to the work of the NCHSR (Gaus and Simpson, 1995). In December 1999, the AHCPR was reauthorized by Congress and renamed the Agency for Healthcare Research and Quality (AHRQ). The official mission of AHRQ is: "To support research designed to improve the quality, safety, efficiency, and effectiveness of health care for all Americans. The research sponsored, conducted, and disseminated by AHRQ provides information that helps people make better decisions about health care" (AHRQ, 2001). As of July 2005, AHRQ's proposed FY 2006 funding was $324 million, a $5 million increase over FY 2005 (Coalition for Health Services Research, n.d.).

One of the driving forces in the recent U.S. health care system transformation is the shift from traditional fee-for-service (FFS) systems to managed care networks, which run the gamut from tightly structured staff model health maintenance organizations (HMOs) to loosely organized preferred provider organizations (PPOs). Managed care has called upon market forces for cost control, led to regulatory initiatives on cost and quality, and contributed to consumer demands for quality care and greater flexibility in provider choice. Because these changes occurred so rapidly and extensively, little is known about the long-term effects of managed care on access to and quality of care or on cost. If policy makers, purchasers, and consumers are to make thoughtful and reasonable decisions, we need to know what works and how much it costs. Answers to these questions have provided impetus to HSR in recent years.

The drive toward quality and outcome has also provided impetus for HSR to identify best practices, explain practice variations, develop and test practice guidelines, and demonstrate cost-effectiveness. For example, HSR on volume-outcome has garnered a preponderance of evidence supporting the association of higher volume with better outcomes with respect to a variety of conditions and procedures. There is considerable evidence that patients undergoing various types of complex treatments or high-risk surgical procedures have lower mortality rates and otherwise better outcomes if care is provided in hospitals that have a heavy caseload of patients with the same conditions than if care is provided by institutions with lighter caseloads of such patients (Gandjour, Bannenberg, and Lauterbach, 2003; Halm, Lee, and Chassin, 2002; Luft, Bunker, and Enthoven, 1979).

To identify and explain practice variations, HSR, in the example of **small area analysis** (SAA), uses large administrative databases to obtain population-based measures of utilization and resource allocation. Small area analysis is useful for studying the effects of differing practice styles on health care utilization rates. When rates of utilization among neighboring communities are compared, variation not related to demand (and/or errors in the data) can be explained by the way physicians make diagnoses or recommend treatments. With SAA, differing clinical decision making on hospital utilization can be revealed.

Outcomes research seeks to understand the end results of particular health care practices and interventions (Clancy and Eisenberg, 1998). By linking the care people get to the results they experience, outcomes research has become the key to developing better ways to monitor and improve the quality of care. For clinicians and patients, outcomes research provides evidence about benefits, risks, and results of treatment so they can make more informed decisions. For health care managers and purchasers, outcomes research can identify potentially effective strategies they can implement to improve the quality and value of care.

The application of HSR can also benefit the operation of the health delivery systems, including managed care. HSR tools and principles are appropriate to the management of practices and managed care functions, for example, in analyzing disease prevalence and incidence in covered or served populations, assessing quality of care, developing and assessing adherence to clinical guidelines and protocols, evaluating resource utilization and clinical practice patterns, and implementing process improvement activities.

Health services research also fills a critical niche within the medical education, research, and public service functions of a university health program or an academic health center. The educational role is based upon the growing importance of understanding the impact of changes in the health care delivery system on the role and functions of all health care professionals. Topics such as health care policy, health economics, and evidence-based medicine have become essential ingredients of the education of future health care and health management professionals. The training of health care managers requires in-depth knowledge of the health care system and interactions among the various components of the system that HSR is to shed light on. The challenge of academic health centers to increase the number of generalist practitioners requires greater expertise in disciplines related to HSR, such as population-based studies and health systems management. Also, academic-based HSR programs are in a unique position to meet the public service missions of their institutions.

Finally, HSR helps evaluate the impact of medical care services and ascertain their cost-effectiveness. Examples in which HSR has contributed toward this objective include:

- physician manpower planning (including recommendations to increase the number of generalists and reduce the number of specialists in practice)

- alterations in hospital and physician payment systems (such as development of Diagnosis-Related Groups, or DRGs, and resource-based relative value scales, and applications of risk adjustment methods)

- development, implementation, and assessment of finance systems for the poor and the elderly (including State Children's Insurance Program, or SCHIP, and TennCare)

- evaluation of alternative health care delivery systems (including managed care)

- critical assessment of new technologies and drugs

- examination of disparities in health and health care among different racial/ethnic and socioeconomic groups

- assessment and improvement of quality of care (by, for example, implementation of process improvement programs and evidence-based clinical guidelines)

- measurement of the progress toward achieving Health People initiatives and the reduction/elimination of disparities

Chapter 2 further summarizes current foci of HSR. The following describes the four major characteristics of HSR: scientific, interdisciplinary, population-based, and applied.

Scientific

Health services research is scientific inquiry. Practitioners of HSR are primarily social scientists. The philosophical foundations of social science disciplines go beyond the subject matter and provide guidance to health services researchers. The scientific principles of positivism, theory, empiricism, objectivity, and ethical standards apply to health services research as well. Health services researchers believe that there are regularities in the delivery of health services. Scientific theories, many from the social sciences, provide guidance for HSR, which in turn contributes to the development of social scientific theories related to the health phenomena. The major research processes ordinarily associated with empirical research, including problem conceptualization and formulation, measurement and data collection, and analysis and interpretation, are also necessary components of HSR. Maintaining objectivity is crucial for health services researchers, given the complexity and personal nature of health services and the diverse interest groups involved. Ethical standards were refined in the wake of the Nuremberg war crimes trials (described earlier) and the Tuskegee Syphilis Study. In the 1950s and 1960s, the Tuskegee Syphilis Study involved the withholding of known effective treatment for syphilis from African-American participants who were infected.

The application of scientific principles in HSR, as in social science disciplines, is not without constraints. The complexity of problems addressed in health services and their variations in time and place complicate analytic research efforts. Because HSR takes place in particular locations and periods and is focused on different levels of generality, particular studies cannot satisfy the needs and interests of all potential audiences. Findings from a study done in a particular health care institution, city, or state often may not be generalizable to other settings because of circumstances that are peculiar to the site in which the study was done. For the same reasons, data from national studies often do not apply to local situations, and vice versa.

Much of HSR is not theory driven but rather is designed to answer practical questions. This is not because health services researchers do not value theories as other scientists do. Health services research is often constrained by the state of the art of the theories and methods of the disciplines that contribute to it. Since much of HSR is based on the theories and methods of the social sciences, its ability to explain events is limited by the level of development of those sciences. There is still considerable debate about the validity of fundamental social science concepts when applied to HSR. The uncertainty is compounded by the concerns of much of health services research with such elusive and judgmental issues as the general health status of populations, the quality of and access to care, and the economic value of life, to name just a few.

The limitations of available data for research also contribute to the difficulty. Data for HSR are drawn principally from population surveys, records and documents, and direct observation. Each of these methods admits various biases that militate against clear-cut description and analysis. Answers to seemingly straightforward questions may not be found from existing data sources, and special studies conducted to determine these answers are often expensive and time-consuming. For example, the annual series of national health care expenditure estimates produced by the Center for Medicare & Medicaid Services, formerly called the Health Care Financing Administration, provides valuable information on the amount and categories of public and private expenditures for health care (Heffler et al., 2002). Similarly, the series of publications from the National Health Care Survey conducted by the National Center for Health Statistics (2004) yields national estimates of the prevalence of illness and the use of health services. However, those studies are expensive and their publication or electronic dissemination typically falls behind by many years. Furthermore, the protection of privacy afforded individuals and institutions by law, and the economic and political advantages that accrue to some for concealing certain types of information, frequently lead to incomplete data that limit the validity of analyses.

The classic experimental design (where research subjects are randomly assigned to an experimental/intervention group or a control group) remains the ideal foundation on which to conduct scientific research, even though such a design is often deemed impractical in HSR because of practical and ethical concerns and the difficulty of establishing truly experimental situations. Often, ethical concerns prevent investigators from controlling events and circumstances that are extraneous to the principal research problems, introducing bias into the results. Since patients cannot be forced to participate in experimental or control groups, self-selection is often used to recruit study subjects. Differences between participants and nonparticipants could obscure study findings. Ethical behavior also includes not deceiving subjects or putting them in dangerous and uncomfortable positions. Practical problems such as time and resource constraints may also limit the options available to researchers. These difficulties inherent in HSR account to a large extent for the use of quasi-experimental designs, cohort studies, longitudinal analyses, surveys, and multidisciplinary approaches.

Multidisciplinary

Social and biomedical scientists have contributed to the development of health services research through the use of applied social science research in problem solving and public decision making (Bice, 1980). Health services research is **multidisciplinary**. It is a unique speciation of study that makes use of the different branches of socio- and biomedical sciences in the study of health care services. Health services include biological and social factors. Since no **conceptual framework** from a single discipline takes into account all aspects of a health services problem or is inherently superior to the others, a cohesive mixture of various academic disciplines that encompass a great variety of perspectives is often required to carry out health services research successfully. HSR may be considered as the application of biomedical, social, and other scientific disciplines to the study of how to deliver health services to groups of people.

The first required disciplines are those of the biomedical sciences. Input from this area is important for several reasons. First, there is a biological dimension of human populations, which is expressed in the distribution of genetic characteristics, herd immunity, and the interaction of humans with other populations, such as microorganisms (Frenk, 1993, p. 476). To achieve a proper understanding of any health condition in a population (e.g., a particular disease), we must understand the biological processes that underlie the condition. Biological sciences contribute to the understanding of human populations through the study of biological determinants, risk factors, and the consequences of health processes in populations, as well as through the use of methods and techniques derived from the biological sciences to characterize such phenomena (Institute of Medicine, 1979). Examples of such applications include health surveys that require laboratory tests to measure the prevalence or incidence of a given condition, and toxicological analysis of environmental risks. Second, medical sciences also contribute to health services research in important ways. For example, the normative clinical standards of care as accepted by the medical professions have to be taken into account before any assessment of health services can be made. Practice patterns of individual doctors must be known before data can be aggregated coherently.

Social science disciplines contribute significantly to HSR (Bice, 1980; Choi and Greenberg, 1982). First, since human populations are organized in societies, social sciences are indispensable for a full understanding of health services in populations. Second, similar to HSR, social science disciplines are more likely to focus on groups rather than individuals. Third, many health services researchers were trained in social science disciplines, including sociology (e.g., medical sociology), economics (e.g., health economics), law (e.g., health law), psychology (e.g., clinical psychology), and political science (e.g., health policy). Their research is influenced by the conceptual frameworks, theories, and methods espoused by their respective disciplines.

Health services researchers benefit from demography, that is, population studies, in two important ways. First, the facts about population size, composition, growth rates, and so on are needed for proper health planning. Planners need data about current and projected populations to estimate needs for health services and potential use of those services. National health legislation has had a direct impact on demographers' work. Because of increasing emphasis on local and regional health planning, demographers are producing more data with local-level detail and are developing estimation techniques for small populations. Second, health researchers and planners with some training in demography can use techniques generally employed in this discipline to compute rates, map population distribution, and the like. For example, using data on hospital patients and estimates of population size, local health professionals can compute hospital discharge rates for their local geographic or service areas. Thus, demographers provide important descriptive information for health services researchers and planners. Further, this allows them to develop methods that health workers can use to describe populations.

Anthropology also influences HSR, particularly in the conduct of qualitative research. Anthropology is distinguished from other social science disciplines by its emphasis on cultural relativity, in-depth examination of context, cross-cultural comparisons, and intensive case studies based on field research or ethnographies.

Economics is critical to HSR, particularly in the conceptualization and investigation of the cost-benefit and cost-effectiveness ratios of health care interventions and justifications of health resources allocations. Work in the area of health economics evaluates the cost effectiveness of alternative health care interventions. This provides information that facilitates decisions on how to spend the limited resources available for health care, with the aim of maximizing the benefit for society as a whole. The role of economics is so prominent that a distinct branch of economics, called health economics, developed hand in hand with HSR.

In addition to biomedical and social sciences, positive contributions to HSR have also come from the quantitative sciences, including mathematics, statistics, operations research, and computer science. Advances in computerized multivariate analyses, for example, have enhanced modeling capabilities and opened up to research certain types of questions that previously could not be addressed.

Behavioral sciences are crucial to the understanding of health services. Behavioral research draws upon knowledge from epidemiological studies that identify behavioral determinants of illness, such as diet and smoking habits, and examines the social and psychological components of these determinants. The interests of behavioral and health services research come together in studies of effects of lifestyles on the utilization of health services and in research on the influence of health services on individuals' health-related habits.

The influence of the physical sciences should also be considered, particularly in the study of problems that have an environmental component. Research findings pertaining to the environmental causes of health problems are important in HSR because they give insight into the kinds of health problems that prompt people to seek medical care (Institute of Medicine, 1979).

Administrative sciences, which themselves are an amalgam of the social and quantitative sciences, have made significant contributions to the study of health services through the refinement of a body of knowledge related to organization theory, decision theory, information theory, and financial analysis. Educational sciences have had a significant impact as well. Effective educational programs are usually directed toward groups of people, health services institutions, and health professionals.

The fact that many biomedical and social science disciplines are involved in HSR does not mean multidisciplinary research has been achieved. Multidisciplinary research requires the integration of different disciplines in the study of a particular phenomenon. Too often, much HSR is carried out within a single disciplinary boundary by economists, sociologists, psychologists, or administrators. The logical and practical necessities that set the limits of analytic studies encourage investigators, working from different theoretical perspectives, to focus on selected aspects of problems and to disregard others. A conventional belief is that the development of science necessarily implies a growing specialization and fragmentation of the objects of study and the consolidation of independent disciplines (e.g., medical sociology and health economics). For instance, research relating to the impact of prospective payment systems would employ the theories and methods of economics to assess the effects of those systems on hospital cost containment, while ignoring their effects on patients and community, which are typically studied with the perspectives and approaches of sociology or political science. Obviously, health services phenomena are not divided neatly into the same categories as research disciplines but have complex and comprehensive characteristics that pose an essential challenge to scientific knowledge.

The fragmentation of knowledge as a basis for organizing research has a restrictive impact on problem solving and decision making. In applied fields, decision makers face complex problems that do not recognize the arbitrary boundaries imposed by scientific subspecialization or disciplinary fragmentation. The comprehensive information needed to solve complex problems cannot be obtained if studies are narrowly conceived and knowledge is generated in small pieces that are difficult to aggregate. In such studies, research results become less definitive and the implementation of findings more difficult. The challenge for HSR is to break with isolation and disciplinary fragmentation and integrate the theoretical perspectives and methods across scientific disciplines around comprehensive problems, thus achieving significant advances in knowledge.

The conceptual framework of biomedical research has its own limitations when applied to HSR. No explicit attention is given to matters other than therapeutic interventions and disease processes. Indeed, a major assumption of the

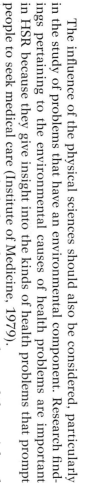

randomized clinical trial is that all factors that may influence an organism and be associated with the intervention under investigation are controlled by randomization. To the extent that this assumption is tenable, the randomized clinical trial can assess the effects (e.g., safety and efficacy) of therapeutic interventions on an individual's disease without the disturbing influence of extraneous matters, such as the characteristics of physicians and hospitals. In practice, however, relatively few such studies are carried out. Consequently, most information about the efficacy of medical procedures is derived from studies done in practice settings where the conditions of the randomized clinical trial cannot be achieved.

Population Based

Health services research focuses on health care services within populations rather than individuals. As Figure 1.7 indicates, its concentration on population is what differentiates HSR from some other health-related research. For example, **clinical research** is primarily about studying the efficacy of the preventive, diagnostic, and therapeutic services applied to the individual patients (Institute of Medicine, 1979). **Biomedical research** is largely concerned with the conditions, processes, and mechanisms of health and illness at the sub-individual level (Frenk, 1993). **Environmental health research** concentrates on services that attempt to promote the health of populations by treating their environments rather than by treating specific individuals.

Like health services research, **epidemiological research** focuses on population level. Unlike HSR, which studies various aspects of health care services, epidemiological research examines the frequency, distribution, and determinants of health and diseases among populations (Donabedian, 1976). The explanatory factors related to health and disease are drawn principally from individuals' physical, biological, and social environments and their lifestyles and behavioral patterns.

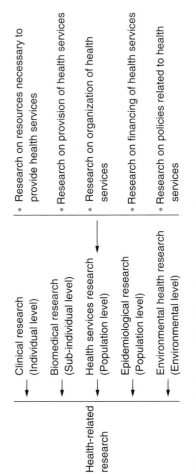

Figure 1.7. Types of health-related research

Epidemiological research may be classified according to the point of departure for analysis. On the one hand, it is possible to start with a set of determinants to study their various consequences; this is the case with environmental, occupational, genetic, and social epidemiology. On the other hand, research may begin by examining some specific health condition (e.g., positive health, infectious diseases, chronic and degenerative ailments, or injury) to investigate its multiple determinants (Frenk, 1993, p. 473).

The results of epidemiological research provide the conceptual foundation for HSR. Studies employing epidemiological methods to assess the impacts of particular health interventions on general health status or other outcomes would be classified as HSR (Institute of Medicine, 1979).

There are, however, other fields, such as bioepidemiology, clinical epidemiology, decision analysis, and technology assessment, that, similar to HSR, deal with connections and interfaces among the major types of health-related research. Indeed, the future development of health-related research will depend on its ability to build bridges across different levels of research. Such integration across research levels, as well as across scientific disciplines as discussed above, will contribute to achieving a full understanding of the broad field of health, rather than provide only a fragmented piece.

Applied

Health services research is an **applied** field. It is almost always defined by its practical, problem-solving orientation and is determined as much by what one wants to do, is paid to do, and can do as by the needs of theory development. Its priorities are established by the health services questions and concerns society raises. Studies in HSR are frequently occasioned by existing problems related to specific populations identified by societal groups and decision makers. "Research in the field of health services has generally stemmed not from curiosity, but from a need to have facts on which to base organization, administration, and legislation and this search for facts has been frankly for public policy purposes, to provide a factual basis for a given policy" (Anderson, 1985, p. 237).

Knowledge generated through HSR can be applied to the study of specific populations, such as children, pregnant women, the poor, the elderly, or migrants; particular problems, such as AIDS, mental illness, or heart disease; and specific programs, such as community, environmental, occupational, or international health. The products of HSR are often assessed primarily in terms of their usefulness to people with decision-making responsibilities, be they clinicians, administrators of health care institutions or government programs, or officials charged with formulating national health care policy. Indeed, the institutionalization of HSR within the nation's major universities and research institutions (e.g., Rand) and the sharp increase in HSR activities over the past two decades have been largely due to increases in federal funding. This increase is a result of the expanded federal roles in health care delivery, financing, planning, and regulation, and the need for relevant research for guidance and evaluation.

Ideally, HSR findings should contribute to more evidence-based health policy decisions. However, policy makers and researchers often have conflicting interests. Bensing, Caris-Verhallen, and Dekker (2003) suggest the results of research do not lend themselves to the pragmatic, feasible types of solutions policy makers can adopt and implement. Researchers who seek to have a policy impact must be attuned to the needs of those dictating the policy for timely, salient, practical advice, and must involve policy makers in the research process to ensure the work is useful and adaptable.

This theory is echoed in the work of Lavis, Ross, and Hurley (2002), which used organizing frameworks from three disciplines (organizational behavior and management research, knowledge utilization, and political science research) to study the role of HSR in public policy making in Canada. They found that sustained interactions between researchers and policy makers make a difference in terms of whether research has an impact on policy. However, they also found that HSR has the potential to inform and shape certain policies more than others. For instance, small-scale, content-driven policies (e.g., HIV prenatal testing and needs-based funding formulas) appeared to be particularly amenable to suggestions from research. By contrast, larger-scale policy decisions (e.g., broad health care financing schemes) seemed less affected by research, perhaps because other political factors, such as stakeholder influence and institutional constraints, are more influential factors in those types of decisions. The authors conclude that we should continue to explore the ways in which research is used in the context of other, competing factors that influence the policy-making process.

The belief that studies in HSR should have direct implications for action and problem solving does not mean that theories and general knowledge should be ignored. Producing research results of direct utility to the client is important but not all-inclusive to HSR. If health services researchers restrict themselves to resolving problems for specific clients but do not concern themselves with accumulating evidence and building theories, then ultimately the problem-solving process will be based on techniques that have to be worked out from scratch. In the long run, HSR will be inefficiently conducted and costly to the clients for lack of established methodology and theories. Without collective norms and standards, it will also be difficult to judge the quality of research and the soundness of analyses and corresponding recommendations or to teach HSR as a coherent endeavor. The challenge to health services researchers is to balance the two competing demands of their efforts: the problem-solving, practical orientation demanded by users and sponsors of research, and the professional standards of theory development set by their scientific disciplines and enforced by their peers. Available theory and methodology provide the framework within which researchers try to model practical problems of health care in ways that will produce insights that can be used to improve the system. The following section describes the distinctions and connections between health services research and health policy research.

Health Services Research and Health Policy Research

As the previous section explored, a major goal of HSR is the applicability of results to policy development, implementation, and evaluation. HSR, therefore, is closely related to health policy research. In fact, the World Health Organization (WHO) describes health policy research as a subset of HSR. The WHO (2005) defines health policy research as a process of scientific investigation that applies methodologies from different health and social sciences to formulate and evaluate health policies. The ultimate goal of health policy research is to improve the population's health status through needs assessment, policy/program development, implementation, and evaluation. Harrison (2001) identifies several aspects of the policy process that policy researchers attempt to explain. These include:

- how issues come to be seen and defined as problems
- how some issues reach policy agendas and others do not
- how policies and decisions are made, and what options are rejected
- the (normative and explanatory) theories espoused by relevant actors
- the effect of implementation attempts on the policy itself
- why policies survive or are abandoned

In addition, policy researchers evaluate existing policies and programs in order to learn what types of interventions work and under what conditions. In the new edition of the classic text *A Practical Guide to Policy Analysis*, Bardach (2005, p. 13) elaborates on the multiple roles and tasks of policy analysts:

Policy analysts help in planning, budgeting, program evaluation, program design, program management, public relations, and other functions. They work alone, in teams, and in loose networks that cut across organizations. They work in the public, nonprofit, and for-profit spheres. Although their work is ideally distinguished by transparency of method and interpretation, the analysts themselves may explicitly bring to their jobs the values and passions of advocacy groups as well as "neutral" civil servants. The professional networks in which they work may contain—in most cases, do contain—professionals drawn from law, engineering, accounting, and so on and in those settings the policy-analytic point of view has to struggle for the right to counter—or better yet, synthesize—the viewpoints of the other professionals. Although policy-analytic work products typically involve written reports, they may also include briefings, slide presentations, magazine articles, and television interviews. The recipients of these products may be broad and diffuse audiences as well as narrowly construed paying clients or employers.

As Bardach describes, the work of policy researchers is closely connected to (and mutually dependent upon) the work of policy makers and professionals in other fields, such as health care service delivery. The products of policy research include not just traditional research products (e.g., papers and presentations), but also materials more relevant for and usable by policy makers, health professionals, and, in some cases, the general public.

The following section summarizes the major components of scientific inquiry as applied in HSR.

THE PROCESS OF HEALTH SERVICES RESEARCH

Scientific knowledge is verifiable. If a study is repeated with a different sample of the population, a second confirmation of the findings, called **replication**, will lend further support to the research finding. To make verification possible, the researcher should design his or her study in acceptable ways and clearly communicate the process of conducting research.

The term **process** refers to a series of activities that bring about an end result or product (Singleton and Straits, 2005). In scientific inquiry, typically the product itself, knowledge, is never finished but constantly refined to fit new evidence. The end of one investigation often marks the beginning of another. The most characteristic feature of the scientific process is its never-ending cyclical nature. We always accept each finding tentatively, knowing that it may be proved wrong in further investigations.

The traditional model of science consists of three major elements: theory, operationalization, and observation (Babbie, 2004; Singleton and Straits, 2005). Researchers begin with an interest in some aspect of the world. They then develop a theoretical understanding of the relevant concepts. The theoretical considerations result in a general hypothesis, or an expectation about the way things ought to be in the world if the theoretical expectations are correct. The notation $Y = f(X)$ indicates that Y (e.g., health status) is a function of and in some way caused by X (e.g., socioeconomic status). At that level, however, X and Y have general rather than specific meanings.

In the **operationalization** process, general concepts are converted to specific indicators or variables, and the procedures for identifying and concretely measuring the variables are delineated. This operationalization process results in the formation of a testable hypothesis. For example, health status may be operationalized as the number of doctor visits and hospitalization days per year, and socioeconomic status as a combination of income, education, and occupation measures.

The final step in the traditional model of science is observation, or the examination of the world, and recording what is seen or heard based on identified measurements. For example, the number of doctor visits and hospitalization days are counted, and data measuring income, education, and occupation, as well as other relevant control variables, are collected and analyzed. The results of the analysis are used to test the research hypothesis.

This deductive approach is often referred to as the traditional model of science. The inductive approach starts with a set of observations. Then, a pattern that best represents or summarizes the observations is sought. A tentative explanation of the pattern of the relationship between the variables of interest is suggested. This tentative suggestion helps generate further expectations about what should be observed in the real world. Thus, the deductive phase starts with theory and conducts observations guided by theory, whereas the inductive phase starts with observations and works toward developing a theory. Both deduction and induction are routes to the construction of scientific theories. The following are the specific stages of HSR, based on the scientific model of theory, operationalization, and observation. Figure 1.8 displays the components of conducting HSR and Table 1.1 shows the critical elements within each component. The section below summarizes these components and the ensuing chapters provide detailed coverage.

Table 1.2 relates each of the stages to specific chapters of the book. Even though the sequencing of the stages is not fixed and practicing health services researchers often skip over one or more, sometimes moving backward as well as forward, each stage is dependent upon the others and some must be conducted before others are initiated. For example, one cannot analyze data before one has collected the data. One cannot formulate an adequate hypothesis without an understanding of the related subject matter. The researcher needs to have adequate knowledge of the earlier stages before he or she can perform the later tasks. A researcher can do irreparable harm to the study by performing one of the early steps inadequately—for example, by writing an untestable hypothesis or by securing an inadequate sample. Research, then, is a system of interdependent related stages.

Conceptualization

The conceptualization stage of the research process requires the researcher to understand the general purpose of the research, determine the specific research topic, identify relevant theories and literature related to the topic, specify the meaning of the concepts and variables to be studied, and formulate general hypotheses or research questions.

Groundwork

The groundwork stage requires the researcher to identify relevant data sources, explore potential funding sources, develop a research plan or proposal (to obtain funding), and prepare organizationally and administratively to carry out the research.

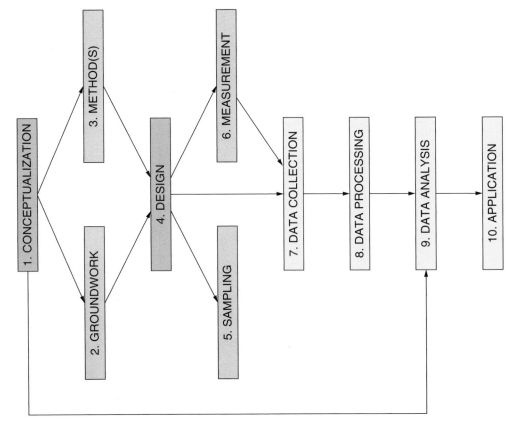

Figure 1.8. A conceptual framework for conducting research

Research Methods

The researcher then needs to choose the appropriate research methods for the particular study. By method we simply mean the general strategy for studying the topic of interest. Many research methods are available for HSR researchers, such as research review (including meta analysis), secondary analysis (including research analysis of administrative records), qualitative research (including case study), experimental, survey (including longitudinal study), and evaluation research. Each of these methods has strengths and weaknesses that determine its suitability for a given problem. Often the best strategy is a combination of different approaches.

Table 1.1. **Content areas of the conceptual framework for conducting research**

1. CONCEPTUALIZATION
- Research Aims and Objectives
- Problem Statement and Significance
- Literature and Theory
- Conceptual Framework
- Research Hypotheses and/or Questions

2. GROUNDWORK
- Data
- Funding
- Proposal
- Infrastructure

3. METHOD(S)
- Research Review
- Secondary Analysis
- Qualitative Research
- Experiment/Quasi-experiment
- Survey
- Evaluation
- Longitudinal Study

4. DESIGN
- Choices of Methods
- Validity Threats
- Designs and Pitfalls

5. SAMPLING
- Random/Probability (Simple, Systematic, Stratified, Cluster)
- Nonrandom (Convenience, Quota, Purposive, Snowball)
- Sample Size

6. MEASUREMENT
- Levels (Nominal, Ordinal, Interval)
- Validity (Construct, Content, Concurrent, Predictive)
- Reliability (Test-retest, Split-half, Inter-rater)
- New Measures and Validation

7. DATA COLLECTION
- Available vs. Empirical
- Published vs. Nonpublished
- Instrument vs. Observation
- Impact on Research Projects
- Impact on Respondents
- Impact on Interviewers
- Impact on Instrument
- Choices among Methods
- Improving Response Rate

8. DATA PROCESSING
- Questionnaire Coding
- Code Book
- Data Entry and Merging
- Data Cleaning
- Data Exploration

9. DATA ANALYSIS
- Univariate Statistics
- Bivariate Statistics
- Multivariate Statistics
- Hypothesis Testing

10. APPLICATION
- Communicating
- Publishing
- Implementing

Research Design

Once the research problem has been clearly formulated, the researcher then develops an overall plan or framework for investigation. Research design addresses the planning of scientific inquiry: anticipating subsequent stages of the research project, including choosing the research method (the previous stage); identifying the unit of analysis and the variables to be measured; establishing procedures for data collection; and devising an analysis strategy. Thinking through and planning for the critical stages of research in advance can prevent important omissions and reduce serious errors. However, not all problems can be foreseen, especially in exploratory and qualitative research, and later changes are often necessary.

Table 1.2. Stages of health services research

Stage of Research	Chapter of Coverage
Conceptualization	Chapter 2
Groundwork	Chapter 3
Research Methods	Chapter 4–9
Research Design	Chapter 10
Sampling	Chapter 11
Measurement	Chapter 12
Data Collection	Chapter 13
Data Processing	Chapter 13
Data Analysis	Chapter 14
Application	Chapter 15

Sampling

In the sampling stage of the research process, the researcher must be clear about the population of interest for a study, which may be defined as the group about which we want to draw conclusions. Since we are almost never able to study all the members of the population that interest us, we must sample subjects for study. In addition to the unit of analysis, the researcher must decide upon the appropriate sample size and sampling procedures.

Measurement

The measurement, or operationalization stage, involves devising measures that link particular concepts to empirically observable events or variables. The validity and reliability of measurement should be ascertained. Since survey research is frequently used, health services researchers should be knowledgeable about the general guidelines and specific techniques for writing survey questionnaire instruments.

Data Collection

Data collection entails the gathering of empirical data. The research method often influences the observation method. The two commonly used direct data collection tools are interview (telephone or face-to-face) and questionnaire survey. The relative advantages and disadvantages of these and other possibilities should be taken into account in selecting the observation method.

Data Processing

Generally, it is difficult to analyze and interpret data in their raw format. Before analyzing the data, the researcher needs to transform or process it into a format suitable for analysis. In the case of a survey, the raw observations are typically in the form of questionnaires with responses checked or answers written in blank spaces. The data-processing phase for a survey typically involves coding or classifying responses and converting the information into a computer-readable format.

Data Analysis

The data analysis stage employs statistical procedures to manipulate the processed data so that conclusions may be drawn that reflect on the hypotheses or research questions. Researchers need to be knowledgeable about commonly used descriptive and analytic statistical procedures. Such knowledge is important to facilitate independent research and improve the design of research and measurements.

Application

The final stage of the research process emphasizes the interpretation and use of the research findings. The researcher may communicate the findings to the sponsor through a specially prepared report or publish the results in a scientific journal. The results may also be communicated through the media, delivered at professional conferences, or prepared as a monograph or book. Contributions to scientific theories and policy formulation are often the greatest enjoyment a researcher obtains from his or her painstaking efforts. Finally, the researcher should provide suggestions for further research on the subject and outline the shortcomings that might be avoided in future studies.

SUMMARY

The aim of scientific inquiry is to produce and enhance knowledge. The assumption is that there is a logical pattern in life that can be studied, and that scientific theory can explain this logical pattern. Scientific inquiry is conducted using empirical evidence to corroborate, modify, or construct scientific theories. Empirical evidence exists independent of researchers, and it is crucial that investigators maintain their objectivity in searching for and explaining such evidence, uninfluenced by their personal beliefs and biases. Ethical standards should be upheld in the conducting of research.

Health services research and scientific inquiry have much in common. Both believe in social regularity and the importance of theories in explaining such regularity. Both are empirically oriented and stress the importance of objectivity in collecting and interpreting empirical evidence. Both uphold ethical standards. The practical orientation of HSR comes from its emphasis on solving problems and producing knowledge useful to users and sponsors of research. Thus, HSR may be considered a social scientific inquiry designed to gain a better understanding of certain aspects of health services resources, provision, organization, finance, and policy. Its process follows that of scientific inquiry and includes conceptualization, preparation or groundwork, design (consisting of choice of research method, sampling, measurement, data collection, processing, and analysis), and the application of research findings.

REVIEW QUESTIONS

1. What are the major characteristics of scientific inquiry?
2. What is the purpose of scientific theory?
3. What is the relation between theory and research?
4. Can research be value-free? Why or why not?
5. Why must scientists uphold ethical standards in research?
6. What is the process of generating scientific theory?
7. Identify the major types of relationships between variables.
8. What conditions are necessary to establish a causal relationship?
9. What is grounded theory?
10. What are the major characteristics of health services research?
11. How are the principles of scientific inquiry reflected in health services research?
12. What is the interdisciplinary nature of health services research?
13. What is the distinction between health services research and other health-related research, such as clinical, biomedical, environmental health, and epidemiological research?
14. Why do we consider health services research as applied research?
15. What is the distinction between inductive and deductive research?
16. How does the process of health services research reflect the characteristics of scientific inquiry?

REFERENCES

Aday, L. A. (2001). *At Risk in America: The Health and Health Care Needs of Vulnerable Populations in the United States* (2nd ed.). San Francisco: Jossey-Bass.

Agency for Healthcare Research and Quality. (2001, March). AHRQ Profile. Retrieved July 13, 2007, from http://www.ahrq.gov/about/profile.htm

Agency for Healthcare Research and Quality. (2002, March). *Helping the Nation with Health Services Research* [Fact sheet]. U.S. Department of Health and Human Services. AHRQ Pub. No. 02-P014.

Anderson, O. W. (1985). *Health Services in the United States*. Ann Arbor, MI: Health Administration Press.

Babbie, E. (2004). *The Practice of Social Research* (10th ed.). Belmont, CA: Thomson/Wadsworth.

Bailey, K. D. (1994). *Methods of Social Research* (4th ed.). New York: Free Press.

Bardach, E. (2005). *A Practical Guide to Policy Analysis* (2nd ed.). Washington, DC: CQ Press.

Bensing, J. M., Caris-Verhallen, W. M., and Dekker, J. (2003). Doing the right thing and doing it right: Toward a framework for assessing the policy relevance of health services research. *International Journal of Technology Assessment in Health Care, 19*(4), 604–612.

Bice, T. (1980). Social science and health services research: Contribution to public policy. *Milbank Memorial Fund Quarterly, 56,* 173–200.

Choi, T., and Greenberg, J. N. (1982). *Social Science Approaches to Health Services Research.* Ann Arbor, MI: Health Administration Press.

Clancy, C. M., and Eisenberg, J. M. (1998). Outcomes research: Measuring the end results of health care. *Science, 282,* 245–246.

Coalition for Health Services Research. (n.d.). Funding Chart. Retrieved July 13, 2007, from http://www.chsr.org/fundingchart

Dilthey, W. (1988). *Introduction to the Human Sciences: An Attempt to Lay a Foundation for the Study of Society and History.* Detroit: Wayne State University Press.

DiRenzo, G. J. (Ed.) (1967). *Concepts, Theory, and Explanation in the Behavioral Sciences.* New York: Random House.

Donabedian, A. (1976). *Aspects of Medical Care Administration: Specifying Requirements for Health Care.* Cambridge, MA: Harvard University Press.

Dubin, R. (1969). *Theory Building: A Practical Guide to the Construction and Testing of Theoretical Models.* New York: Free Press.

Durkheim, É. (1951). *Suicide: A Study in Sociology.* Glencoe, IL: Free Press.

Durkheim, É. (1974). *Sociology and Philosophy.* New York: Free Press.

Frenk, J. (1993). The new public health. *Annual Review of Public Health, 14,* 469–490.

Gandjour, A., Bannenberg, A., and Lauterbach, K. W. (2003). Threshold volumes associated with higher survival in health care: A systematic review. *Medical Care, 41,* 1129–1141.

Gaus, C. R., and Simpson, L. (1995). Reinventing health services research. *Inquiry, 32,* 130–134.

Glaser, B. G. (1992). *Emergence vs. Forcing: Basics of Grounded Theory Analysis.* Mill Valley, CA: Sociology Press.

Glaser, M. (1972). *The Research Adventure: Promise and Problems of Fieldwork.* New York: Random House.

Halm, E. A., Lee, C., and Chassin, M. R. (2002). Is volume related to outcome in healthcare? A systematic review and methodologic critique of the literature. *Annals of Internal Medicine, 137,* 511–520.

Harrison, S. (2001). Policy analysis. In N. Fulop, P. Allen, A. Clarke, and N. Black (Eds.), *Studying the Organization and Delivery of Health Services.* New York: Routledge.

Heffler, S., Smith, S., Won, G., Clemens, M. K., Keehan, S., and Zezza, M. (2002). Health spending projections for 2001–2011: The latest outlook. *Health Affairs (Millwood), 21*(2), 207–218.

Hempel, C. G. (1965). *Aspects of Scientific Explanation and Other Essays in the Philosophy of Science.* New York: Free Press.

Hempel, C. G. (1967). Scientific explanation. In S. Morgenbesser (Ed.), *Philosophy of Science Today.* New York: Basic Books.

Institute of Medicine. (1979). *Health Services Research.* Washington, DC: National Academy of Sciences.

Kaplan, A., and Wolf, C. (1998). *The Conduct of Inquiry: Methodology for Behavioral Science.* Somerset, NJ: Transaction Publishers.

King, G., and Williams, D. R. (1995). Race and health: A multidimensional approach to African-American health. In B. C. Amick III (Ed.), *Society & Health.* New York: Oxford University Press.

Kuhn, T. S. (2000). *The Road Since Structure: Philosophical Essays, 1970–1993, with an Autobiographical Interview.* Chicago and London: University of Chicago Press.

Lavis, J. N., Ross, S. E., and Hurley, J. E. (2002). Examining the role of health services research in public policymaking. *Milbank Memorial Fund Quarterly, 80*(1), 125–153.

Lester, D. (1994). *Émile Durkheim: "Le Suicide" One Hundred Years Later.* Philadelphia: Charles Press.

Luft, H. S., Bunker, J. P., and Enthoven, A. C. (1979). Should operations be regionalized? The empirical relation between surgical volume and mortality. *New England Journal of Medicine, 301,* 1364–1369.

McCain, G., and Segal, E. M. (1988). *The Game of Science* (5th ed.). Pacific Grove, CA: Brooks/Cole.

Mechanic, D. (1973). *Politics, Medicine and Social Science.* New York: Wiley.

Miller, D. C., and Salkind, N. J. (2002). *Handbook of Research Design and Social Measurement* (6th ed.). Thousand Oaks, CA: Sage.

National Center for Health Statistics. (2004). *Health, United States, 2004.* Hyattsville, MD: Public Health Service.

Neurath, O., Carnap, R., and Morris, C. F. W. (Eds.). (1970). *Foundations of the Unity of Science: Toward an International Encyclopedia of Unified Science* (Vol. 2, p. 2). Chicago and London: University of Chicago Press.

Patrick, D. L., and Wickizer, T. M. (1995). Family pathways to child health. In B. C. Amick III (Ed.), *Society & Health.* New York: Oxford University Press.

Patton, M. Q. (2002). *Qualitative Evaluation and Research Methods* (3rd ed.). Thousand Oaks, CA: Sage.

Roethlisberger, F. J., and Dickson, W. J. (1939). *Management and the Worker: An Account of a Research Program Conducted by the Western Electric Co. Hawthorne Works, Chicago.* Cambridge, MA: Harvard University Press.

Salmon, W. C. (1967). *The Foundation of Scientific Inference.* Pittsburgh: University of Pittsburgh Press.

Salmon, W. C. (1973). *Logic* (2nd ed.). Englewood Cliffs, NJ: Prentice-Hall.

Schor, E. L., and Menaghan, E. G. (1995). Community and health. In B. C. Amick III (Ed.), *Society & Health.* New York: Oxford University Press.

Selltiz, C., Wrightsman, L. S., and Cook, S. W. (1976). *Research Methods in Social Relations* (3rd ed.). New York: Holt, Rinehart, and Winston.

Shi, L., and Stevens, G. D. (2005). *Vulnerable Populations in the United States.* San Francisco: Jossey-Bass.

Singleton, R. A., and Straits, B. C. (2005). *Approaches to Social Research* (4th ed.). New York: Oxford University Press.

Sjoberg, G., and Nett, R. (1996). *A Methodology for the Social Researcher: With a New Introductory Essay.* Long Grove, IL: Waveland Press.

Skinner, B. F. (1953). *Science and Human Behavior.* Toronto: Macmillan.

Strauss, A. L., and Corbin, J. M. (1998). *Basics of Qualitative Research: Techniques and Procedures for Developing Grounded Theory* (2nd ed.). Thousand Oaks, CA: Sage.

Walsh, D. C., Sorensen, G., and Leonard, L. (1995). Gender, health, and cigarette smoking. In B. C. Amick III (Ed.), *Society & Health.* New York: Oxford University Press.

Weber, M. (1949). *The Methodology of the Social Sciences*. Glencoe, IL: Free Press.

White, K. L. (1992). *Health Services Research: An Anthology*. Washington, DC: Pan American Health Organization.

World Health Organization. (2005). Health in Sustainable Development website. Retrieved July 15, 2005, from http://209.61.208.100/researchpolicy/hpr_meet19a.htm

Zetterberg, H. L. (1954). *On Theory and Verification in Sociology*. New York: Tressler.

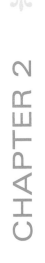

Conceptualizing Health Services Research

KEY TERMS

activities of daily living (ADL)
agency relationship
analytic/causal research
applied research
basic/pure research
behavioral risk factors
burden of illness
Certificate of Need (CON)
conceptualization
descriptive research
diagnosis-related groups (DRGs)
dimension
environment
environmental theory

explanatory research
exploratory research
germ theory
health maintenance organization (HMO)
health services
health status
incidence
instrumental activities of daily living (IADL)
International Classification of Functioning, Disability, and Health (ICF)
lifestyle theory

Medicaid
Medicare
nominal definition
operational definition
policy
prevalence
quality of life
SF-36
social contacts
social resources
social well-being
socioeconomic status (SES)
term
theoretical research

LEARNING OBJECTIVES

- To understand and describe the major steps in the conceptualization stage of health services research.
- To identify the determinants of health.
- To become familiar with the general subject areas of health services research.

Before collecting and analyzing data, the researcher needs to know what data to collect and analyze. Conceptualization is the process used to determine this. The first part of the chapter takes a close look at the major steps in the conceptualization stage. Then, to illustrate conceptualization, the second part of the chapter provides a summary of the major content areas in health services research.

THE CONCEPTUALIZATION STAGE

Conceptualization is the process of specifying and refining abstract concepts into concrete terms. As stated in the previous chapter, in the conceptualization stage, researchers need to understand the general purpose of their investigation, determine the specific research topic, identify relevant theories and literature related to the topic, specify the meaning of the concepts and variables to be studied, and formulate general hypotheses or research questions.

Research Purpose

Like other scientific inquiry, health services research serves many purposes. Three of the general purposes are exploration, description, and explanation (Babbie, 2004; Singleton and Straits, 2005, pp. 16–19). A given study can have more than one of these purposes. **Exploratory research** is usually conducted when relatively little is known about the phenomenon under study; that is, the research topic is itself relatively new and unstudied. The researcher explores the topic in order to become familiar with it and to gain ideas and knowledge about it. Exploratory research often results in generating meaningful hypotheses about the causal relationships among variables or in identifying a more precise research problem for investigation. Thus, exploratory study is not undertaken to test hypotheses or provide satisfactory answers to research questions. Rather, it hints at the answers and gives insights into the research methods that could provide more definitive answers. The reason exploratory study is seldom definitive in itself is its lack of representation. An example of exploratory health services research is the study of the impact of **diagnosis-related groups (DRGs)** on particular interchanges between providers and consumers, such as discussions between doctor and patient about a hospital discharge that may be premature.

Exploratory study may also be undertaken when the researcher is examining a new area of interest. In other words, the topic of interest has been studied by others, but not by the researcher. The investigation is exploratory to the researcher. A third situation in which an exploratory study may be considered is in testing the feasibility of a new methodology. This aspect may have been studied before, but the researcher is interested in applying a new methodology this time. The results of the study will provide guidance for larger-scale, more complex studies. **Descriptive research** is conducted to explain some phenomenon. Descriptive studies summarize the characteristics of particular individuals, groups, organizations, communities, events, or situations as completely, precisely, and accurately as possible, with the ultimate purpose of formulating these descriptions into conceptual categories. The nature of the description, however, differs from exploratory research. A descriptive study is much more structured, carefully conceived, deliberate, systematic, accurate, and precise. It provides detailed numerical descriptions of relatively few dimensions of a well-defined subject. Descriptive research can be an independent research endeavor or, as is more commonly the case, part of a causal research project.

Examples of descriptive health services research include the series on national trends in public health statistics prepared by the National Center for Health Statistics (NCHS, 2006) and published in *Health, United States*. The series covers four major subject areas: health status and its determinants, utilization of health resources, health care resources, and health care expenditures. The NCHS also periodically publishes findings from national health surveys that provide useful national estimates of the prevalence of illness and the utilization of health services. Another example is the series of estimates of national health care expenditures produced by the Centers for Medicare & Medicaid Services, which provides valuable information on the amount and categories of public and private expenditures for health care (Smith, Cowan, Heffler, and Catlin, 2006). Data from these types of descriptive studies identify trends and variations that raise theoretical and policy questions, inviting further analysis to reveal their correlates and causes. This further analysis is the objective of explanatory research.

Explanatory research, also called **analytic** or **causal research**, seeks answers to research hypotheses or problems. It may be conducted to explain factors associated with a particular phenomenon, answer cause–effect questions, or make projections into the future. While exploratory research is concerned with questions of "what" and descriptive research with questions of "how," explanatory research answers questions of "why" or "what will be." Explanatory research differs from descriptive research in the scope of the description. Whereas descriptive research seeks information about isolated variables, explanatory research examines the relationships among these variables and is inherently more in-depth.

An example of explanatory health services research is the study of the relationship among health insurance coverage, utilization of services, and health status. Since these factors influence one another, a descriptive study is unlikely to uncover the true relationship. For example, those with poorer health status may choose more complete health insurance coverage for total expenses or high-cost procedures and may also utilize more services. Those who believe their health is better will choose "shallow" coverage that does not cover high-cost procedures. In this case, greater utilization is associated with poorer health status, and both utilization and health status are associated with greater insurance coverage. An explanatory study conducted to address the complex relationship among insurance coverage, utilization, and health status is the Health Insurance Experiment conducted by a research team at the Rand Corporation (Brook, Ware, and Roger, 1983; Newhouse, Manning, and Morris, 1981; Office of Technology Assessment, 1992). The research used an experimental design in which individual households were randomly assigned to insurance plans with different financial incentives. One purpose of the experiment was to examine the impact of levels of cost sharing among privately insured patients on levels of utilization. The study indicates that for persons with average income and health, health outcomes were neither significantly improved when care was free nor adversely affected by requirements of cost sharing. However, vision, dental, and oral health improved for individuals receiving free care.

The differences in research objectives can lead to differences in research design. For example, exploratory research typically uses qualitative methods, such as case studies, focus groups, or guided interviews. When exploring a topic about which they have little knowledge, researchers often use these methods to help determine the relevant variables and whom to study. Descriptive research frequently employs survey methods. Information is gathered from a set of cases carefully selected to enable the researcher to make estimates of the precision and generalizability of the findings. Explanatory research, on the other hand, is more likely to be associated with experimental research designs that randomly select and assign subjects to different experimental and control groups. However, in health services research, experimental designs tend to be very expensive and are often impossible because of the difficulty in getting subjects to agree to random assignment. Explanatory research relies heavily on multivariate analyses and model-building techniques based on sound theoretical frameworks. Table 2.1 summarizes the major differences among exploratory, descriptive, and explanatory research.

Research Topic

Health services research typically starts with a question or problem that can be answered or solved through empirical investigation. Research ideas are plentiful and may emerge from the researcher's own experience or curiosity, his or her interactions with other researchers, reading the literature, attending workshops or conferences, or any number of other sources. However, formulating a research question or problem is often a difficult process. Experienced and novice researchers alike often spend considerable time narrowing down the topic. The choice of a research topic is influenced by a number of factors. These include whether the researcher is seeking to address a social problem; test or construct a scientific theory; satisfy the researcher's personal interests in accordance with his or her ability and available resources; or whether the researcher is intent on making a contribution to the field and gaining professional recognition.

Health services researchers typically engage in projects of an applied nature. The focus and development of HSR are intimately related to interest in basic social problems related to health services. These problems have been a major source of research topics. Indeed, many people today are attracted to HSR because of its perceived relevance to social problems, its problem-solving focus, and its likely impact on policy. **Policy** entails decision making at various levels, ranging from health services facilities (e.g., whether to use nurse practitioners and physician

Table 2.1. Differences among exploratory, descriptive, and explanatory research

	Exploratory Research	Descriptive Research	Explanatory Research
Purpose	Gain familiarity, insight, ideas; conduct new area of research; test new method	Describe characteristics of units under study	Test hypothesis, answer cause–effect research questions; make projections
Questions to answer	"What"	"How"	"Why," "What will be"
Sequence	Initial	Follow-up	Last
Rigor in study design	Little	Enhanced	Great
Theoretical guidance	Little	Some	Required
Knowledge about subject matter	Little	Somewhat	A lot
Research methods	Qualitative (case study, field observation, focus group)	Survey research	Experiment or other case-control designs; longitudinal research
Sample size	Small	Large	Medium or large
Number of variables examined simultaneously	Univariate	Univariate, bivariate	Multivariate
Statistical analysis	Little	Descriptive statistics	Multivariate statistics
Expenses	Inexpensive	Reasonable to expensive	Expensive
Representativeness of findings	No	Yes	Yes

assistants as substitutes for physicians) to state legislation (e.g., **Certificate of Need [CON]** regulation) to congressional action (e.g., **Medicare and Medicaid** reimbursement). The results of policy-relevant research may be valuable to decision makers in planning future courses of action.

Although not as frequent, HSR may be conducted to test or construct scientific theories. Many health services researchers are trained in social science disciplines that have the goal of advancing knowledge. Their disciplinary framework provides direction in topic selection, research focus, and study design. They draw upon HSR social science theories and, in the process, modify existing theories or develop new ones.

Researchers' personal interests and experience can play a significant role in the selection of topic. The completion of a research project usually entails overcoming numerous obstacles, both anticipated and unanticipated. A genuine commitment is critical to the success of a research project. Researchers are more likely to be committed to a project in which they have a personal interest.

Researchers' ability and the resources available to them are also important determinants of topic selection. Their research skill affects all important phases of the research process, including study conceptualization. Ideally, the research focus should reflect the background and training of those involved. The level of available resources impacts practical considerations. For example, an important concern for any research project is funding. Do researchers have sufficient funding for the study? The availability of relevant data also dictates whether a topic can be studied adequately. Many researchers select their topic based on available data. Research using secondary data avoids many of the problems associated with data collection and greatly speeds up the process. The drawback is that the research is confined by the variables already studied. Other important resources include time, computers, and support personnel. The availability of these resources plays a significant role in topic selection.

The desire for professional recognition also influences the choice of a research topic. Researchers may pursue topics regarded as "hot" or prestigious in their disciplines. The goal may be to publish in premier scholarly journals or to advance their careers in terms of tenure or promotion. In this climate, where securing funding is almost more important than conducting research, researchers may have to follow the directions of funders, whether they are federal agencies or private foundations.

The selection of a research topic is typically influenced by several of the above-mentioned factors. In other words, those factors are not mutually exclusive. A research project may have problem solving as its primary objective while simultaneously addressing a theoretical question. The same research may be influenced by the availability of funding and other resource constraints. It may also coincide with the researcher's personal interests and values, as well as personal and professional rewards.

Theories and Literature

Having identified or formed a general idea of the research topic, researchers proceed to conduct a thorough review of the current literature related to that topic. Chapter 4 delineates the process of conducting literature review. Literature review is necessary because a researcher's personal experiences, however extensive, are limited compared with the cumulative scientific knowledge. Research conducted after extensive review of the literature is more likely to be built on previous studies and contribute toward the further development of scientific knowledge. Appendix 1 summarizes many journals, arranged in alphabetical order, that publish health services research papers.

Literature review serves a number of purposes. First of all, it helps narrow the topic. Research often begins with a question or problem that is so vague or broad in scope that it provides little direction for specific study. Literature review informs researchers about the state of the art and the extent of study on the topic as well as the current limitations. Efforts can then be directed to areas yet to be explored or those with conflicting results.

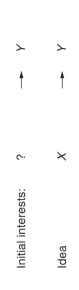

Initial interests: ? $\longrightarrow$ Y

Idea X $\longrightarrow$ Y

Literature review: X_1, X_2, X_3, Z_s $\longrightarrow$ Y_s

Figure 2.1. Identify relevant variables via literature review

Besides helping narrow and refine the topic, literature review may help identify theories related to the topic of interest. Theories provide guidance in the formulation of hypotheses to be tested. The ensuing research results will then have theoretical significance. In searching for relevant theories, researchers need not confine themselves to the thinking of their paradigms. When proponents of different paradigms insist that only their view is correct, researchers cannot communicate effectively with each other. Taking alternative paradigms and theories into account stimulates research and generates more thorough findings. Researchers should be open to different perspectives on their topic of choice.

Literature review helps identify relevant as well as control variables to be included in the analysis. Figure 2.1 illustrates this process. The initial topic of interest is represented by the variable Y. We are interested in finding out what causes Y. We identify the variable X as a potential cause based on our experience or the evidence we observe. But since our experience is limited, it is very likely we have not considered all the potential causes of Y. A literature review will help identify not only the potential causes (variable Xs), but also the factors (variable Zs) that need to be accounted for. Further, literature review suggests different dimensions of our topic (variable Ys). Thus, reviewing the literature enables us to operationalize our abstract concepts, a prerequisite for empirical research.

Literature review also suggests pertinent research design, procedures, and analysis by indicating how other researchers have addressed the topic. Researchers may use a previous investigator's method or even replicate an earlier study. Or they can revise the research design. Just as researchers need to have an open mind for alternative theories, they need to be open to different methods. The development of health services research and the pursuit of knowledge will suffer if investigators only recognize the paradigms of their own disciplines. The tendency to promote one method at the expense of others can prevent researchers from seeing the essential complementarity of various methods.

Concepts and Variables

Having reviewed the relevant literature, researchers will have identified the concepts of interest and gained a better understanding of the research topic. Since a concept is a mental image (conception), it needs to be specified using an understandable term. A **term** is a name representing a collection of apparently related phenomena and serves the purposes of filing and communication (Babbie, 2004). Terms are specified to communicate what is meant by a particular concept. Since each concept is typically derived from many observations and experiences, one concept usually consists of several dimensions or layers of meanings. A **dimension** is a specifiable aspect of a concept. Each dimension contains only one aspect of a concept. Conceptualization is the process through which we specify the meanings of particular terms to represent the various dimensions of a concept. All terms must be defined in detail based on the current literature and the unique situation of the research project. A typology may be developed where terms are carefully organized in a meaningful way as guided by theories and literature. Identifying the different dimensions of a concept and specifying the terms associated with these dimensions enable researchers to gain a more thorough and focused understanding of the research topic.

Concepts are defined on two levels: nominal and operational. A **nominal definition** serves as the working definition for the project and captures the major dimensions as agreed upon by the scientific community and reflected in the literature. Sometimes, however, there might be disagreement or lack of consensus as to the dimensions a particular concept should include. In these situations, the researchers' nominal definition serves to rule out other possible dimensions of the concept. Nominal definition is not specific as to how a concept is to be observed. Different researchers may observe a concept differently based on the nominal definition.

To be specific as to how a concept should actually be observed, researchers assign an operational definition. This is the second level of concept specification. An **operational definition** specifies a unique method of observation. It indicates what specific variables are to be observed, how they are to be observed, and how these observations are to be interpreted. A variable must have two or more different values. Each dimension of a concept may be represented by several variables. An operational definition lays out all the *operations* or steps to be undertaken to measure a concept. Also, the operational definition follows the nominal definition and makes each of the specified dimensions more concrete and observable. Assigning an operational definition to a concept is often the product of the operationalization stage of the research process, discussed in Chapter 12 (Babbie, 2004). Like the nominal definition, the operational definition is a working definition of the concept as used in the research project. Researchers may disagree about the proper nominal and operational definitions to be used, but they can still interpret research findings based on these definitions.

Let us use the concept of socioeconomic status (SES) to illustrate these two levels of specification. Suppose we are interested in examining the relationship between socioeconomic status and health status. To reach a nominal definition, we may represent SES with three major dimensions or indicators: income, occupation, and educational attainment. This definition does not include many other possible dimensions of SES: savings, investment, property, inheritance, lifestyle, reputation, neighborhood, dependents, and so on. The nominal definition points out the direction for observation but the operational definition is necessary to indicate how to make the observation. In this example, we may decide to ask the research subjects two questions about income (What was your total family income, including salary, pension, bonus, and interest, during the past twelve months? and What was your personal income during the past twelve months?),

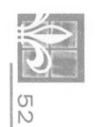

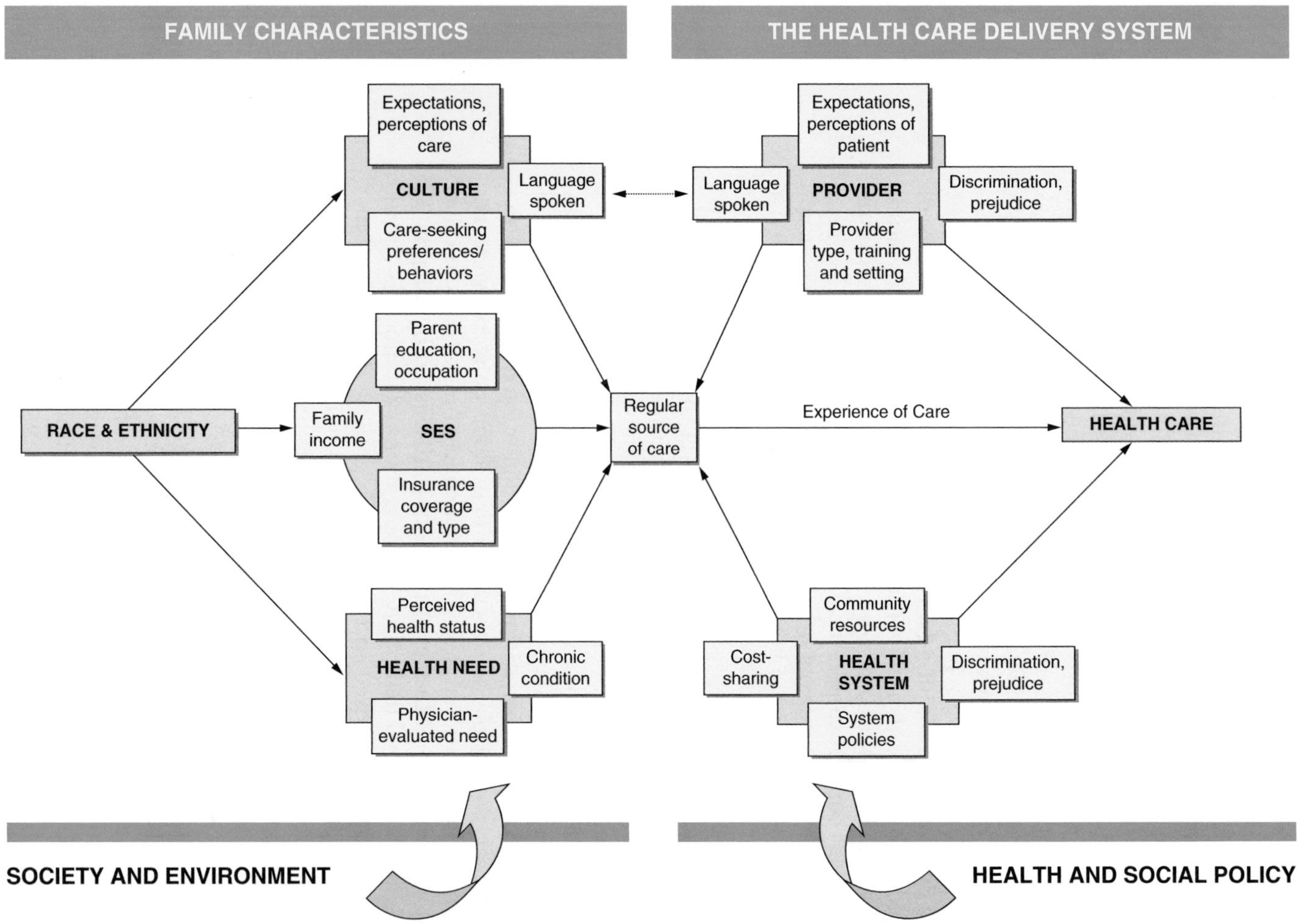

FAMILY CHARACTERISTICS

THE HEALTH CARE DELIVERY SYSTEM

Expectations, perceptions of care

CULTURE

Language spoken

Care-seeking preferences/ behaviors

Parent education, occupation

RACE & ETHNICITY

Family income

SES

Insurance coverage and type

Regular source of care

Experience of Care

HEALTH CARE

Expectations, perceptions of patient

Language spoken

PROVIDER

Discrimination, prejudice

Provider type, training and setting

Perceived health status

HEALTH NEED

Chronic condition

Physician-evaluated need

Community resources

Cost-sharing

HEALTH SYSTEM

Discrimination, prejudice

System policies

SOCIETY AND ENVIRONMENT

HEALTH AND SOCIAL POLICY

Figure 2.2. **Conceptual model linking race and ethnicity with health care experiences**

Source: Shi and Stevens (2004) Reprinted with permission courtesy of John Wiley & Sons, Inc.

one question about occupation (What is your current occupation?), and two questions about education (What is your highest level of education? and How many years of formal education have you completed?). These five questions represent a working definition of SES. Others might disagree with the conceptualization (in terms of the nominal dimensions specified) and operationalization (in terms of the variables included) but can interpret the research results unambiguously, based on the definition of the concept SES.

Development of a Conceptual Framework

A key step in the development of a research study is the creation of a conceptual framework. Wolfson (1994, p. 309) described the importance of a conceptual framework when he asserted, "Data and facts are not like pebbles on a beach, waiting to be picked up and collected. They can only be perceived and measured through an underlying theoretical and conceptual framework, which defines relevant facts, and distinguishes them from background noise." As Wolfson's quote describes, the conceptual framework is a preliminary model of the problem under study, and is reflective of relationships among critical variables of interest. Figure 2.2 is an example of a conceptual framework linking race and ethnicity with health care experiences. As the figure illustrates, a conceptual framework is based on the literature and existing theories, and it is inclusive of definitions, assumptions, values, and presumed causes of the problem. The purpose of a conceptual framework is to synthesize and guide the course of research, as well as to guide analysis of research and interventions.

A critical function of a conceptual framework is its depiction of relationships between variables and concepts of interest. Often, a conceptual framework distinguishes between positive and negative relationships and depicts the strength of various relationships. A conceptual framework may also distinguish between different types of relationships between variables. For instance, the model may show whether relationships are symmetrical or asymmetrical, linear or nonlinear. The model may also indicate whether a particular relationship is spurious, or whether there is a causal path from one variable in the model to another.

The development of a conceptual framework is an iterative, dynamic process. While the researcher may begin developing a framework very early in the process of topic development, the framework will evolve as the researcher learns more. At the completion of a research project, the conceptual framework continues to be a powerful tool for conveying information. Presented as part of an article or lecture, the conceptual framework allows the audience to quickly understand the overarching theories and particular relationships involved in the topic at hand.

Research Hypotheses or Questions

The final step in the conceptualization stage is the formulation of research hypotheses or questions that describe the variables and the units to be studied. The major difference between research hypotheses and questions is that hypotheses specify the relationships among variables whereas questions do not. Hypotheses are usually related to a body of theory. Thus, **theoretical research** (sometimes called **basic** or **pure research**) generally involves testing hypotheses developed from theories that are intellectually interesting to the researcher. The findings might also have application to social problems, although this is not required. Research questions are typically associated with today's social problems. **Applied research** that focuses on current social problems generally specifies its purpose through research questions. Applied research may also use hypotheses statements. The choice is made based on current knowledge about the relationships among the variables of interest. Hypotheses may be formulated if current knowledge (from theories and evidence) indicates anticipated directions of the relationships among the variables of interest. When the relationships are unknown, research questions are posed in lieu of hypotheses.

The hypothesized relationships among the variables of interest determine how they are labeled. In a causal relationship, the variable presumed to cause changes is labeled the independent variable. The variable presumed to change as a result of the intervention is labeled the dependent variable. Other variables on which research subjects may differ and that might also affect the dependent variable are treated as control variables in the analysis. As a way of clarifying the hypothesis, researchers can draw a diagram of the presumed relationships among the variables (Grady and Wallston, 1988).

Research hypotheses or questions share several common characteristics (Goode and Hatt, 1962). First of all, research hypotheses or questions must be conceptually clear. The concepts should be clearly defined and the nominal definition should be commonly accepted in the scientific world. Before achieving a definition, a researcher may want to share his or her definition, based on the literature review, with other researchers in the field. It is possible to neglect a portion of the literature that explores another important dimension of the concept. Peer consultation helps reduce such omissions.

Second, research hypotheses or questions must be statements of fact susceptible to empirical investigation—that is, statements that can be proven right or wrong through research. This requirement means researchers should exclude concepts that express attitudes, feelings, or values.

Third, research hypotheses or questions must be specific and narrowly defined to allow actual testing. A nominal definition alone is not sufficient. Operational specification of the relevant variables is also needed. Although the formulation of research hypotheses or questions is primarily part of the conceptualization process, it also relies on operationalization. Research hypotheses or questions that only rely on the nominal definition are general hypotheses or questions. Only those based on both the nominal and operational definitions can be actually observed and tested. To make the hypotheses or questions sufficiently specific, researchers often break a general hypothesis or question (measuring a concept) into sub-hypotheses or sub-questions (different dimensions of a concept).

Fourth, research hypotheses or questions must be practical. Many things we want to know about are not feasible. We cannot randomly assign people to a health status or illness. Many conditions and diseases are relatively rare and not enough patients exist to generate sufficient sample size. In addition to patients, researchers also need full support from institutions and providers to conduct any investigation.

Fifth, research hypotheses or questions must be suited to available techniques and research methods. Researchers ignorant of the available techniques including research design and analysis are in a disadvantaged position to formulate usable hypotheses or questions. To make sure that hypotheses or questions can be tested with available techniques, researchers need to be aware of those techniques (or have consultants available to them). Literature review helps identify the techniques used along with their strengths and limitations. Often, a topic can be approached with various methods and data analyzed in different ways. A competent researcher needs to know the most commonly used methods and techniques.

Finally, hypotheses are probabilistic in nature and may not be confirmed with certainty. We use the terms *tends to* or *more likely* to indicate this probabilistic nature. The reason is that the measures used to test hypotheses are usually not perfectly accurate and not all relevant variables can be identified or controlled.

The following statements, adapted from the excellent summary of research hypotheses by Singleton and Straits (2005, pp. 66–67), represent the most common forms of hypotheses.

Conditional Statements

Conditional statements (e.g., if–then statements) indicate that if one condition or situation is true, then another will also be true. An example would be: "If a person has a high level of income, then she will have a high level of health insurance." In a conditional statement, the condition following *if* is the cause, and the condition following *then* is the effect.

Continuous Statements

Continuous statements (e.g., the more X, the more Y) indicate that increases in one variable (X) are associated with increases (or decreases) in another variable (Y). Although continuous statements generally imply X causes Y, this also can mean Y causes X or that X and Y cause each other. Researchers should explicitly state the causal relationship in their discussion of the hypothesis. An example of a continuous statement is: "As income increases, health insurance coverage increases"; or, expressed in a slightly different form: "The higher the level of income, the greater the insurance coverage."

Difference Statements

Difference statements indicate that one variable differs in terms of the categories of another variable. For example, when infant mortality is one variable and race is another (with African American and white as its two categories), we can use the difference statement to state the hypothesis: "Infant mortality rate is higher among African Americans than it is among whites." Whether continuous or difference statements are used to express a hypothesis will depend on whether the variables in the hypothesis are quantitative or dichotomous. If both variables could be quantified (such as income and extent of insurance coverage), then the relationship could be stated in the continuous form. If neither variable could be quantified (such as race), then the relationship would need to be stated in the difference form. Like continuous statements, difference statements are ambiguous about the causal connection between variables. Although the dichotomous variable is typically the cause, researchers still need to make explicit the causal connection between variables.

Mathematical Statements

Mathematical statements have the form $Y = f(X)$, which means "Y is a function of X" (McGuigan, 1978, p. 53). Here, Y is the dependent variable and X the independent variable that is hypothesized to cause Y. An example of using a mathematical formula is: $Y = f(X_1, X_2, X_3)$, where Y is medical care utilization, X_1 is insurance coverage, X_2 is age, and X_3 is a measure of health status. Relatively few hypotheses are stated in mathematical terms because researchers often consider their measurement to be less precise than the mathematical formula implies.

THE FIELD OF HEALTH SERVICES

Health services may be defined as the total societal effort, whether private or public, to provide, organize, and finance services that promote the health status of individuals and the community. Health status is important because a state of good health is a basic prerequisite for performing the tasks and duties associated with the roles that individuals assume at different phases of their lives. Even though it is health we are concerned with, many of the health-related theories tend to focus on disease. The three general theories of disease causality are germ theory, lifestyle theory, and environmental theory.

Germ theory was widely accepted in the 19th century with the rise of bacteriology (Metchnikoff, 1939). The doctrine of the theory states that for every disease there is a specific cause for which we can look. Knowing that specific cause will help us identify the solution to that problem. Microorganisms are the causal agent in germ theory, and are thought to be generally environment free, presumably because Pasteur and others could induce the disease in laboratory animals 100 percent of the time. In reality, the disease does not necessarily occur every time microorganisms are present. For example, not everyone exposed to tuberculosis ends up getting it. Germ theory is very reductionistic. The source of a disease is predominantly at the individual level and the disease may be communicated from one person to another (a phenomenon referred to as contagion). Strategies to address disease focus on identification of those people with problems and on follow-up medical treatment. A common approach is to look at two groups of people, those with a disease and those without it, and to try to reduce disease causality to a fundamental difference between the two groups. Much of biomedical research is based on germ theory. The traditional epidemiological triangle (i.e., agent, host, and environment) was also developed based on the single-cause, single-effect framework of germ theory (Dever, 2006).

Lifestyle theory is perceived differently today from the way it was in the 1800s. Lifestyle was seen as a religious, moral issue. People were thought to get diseases as retribution for the way they lived. (Does this sound familiar to the contemporary health problem of AIDS?) Today we think about lifestyle in relation to chronic diseases versus infectious diseases. Lifestyle theory tends to be reductionistic because it tries to isolate specific behaviors (e.g., diet, exercise, smoking, or drinking) as causes of the problem, and defines solutions in terms of changing those behaviors. Thus, problems are defined as related to individuals, and solutions are based on individual interventions. It is environment sensitive, not environment free as in germ theory, or environment dependent as in environmental theory. For example, cigarette smoking is considered to be related to, although not caused by, advertising.

Environmental theory has a much more general approach. The focus is not so much on infectious diseases as on general health and well-being. It is not reductionistic. Rather, it states that health must be understood by looking at the larger context of the community. Traditional environmental approaches focused on poor sanitary conditions, which were connected to disease but not in a one-to-one relationship. Recent environmental approaches examine the impact of production and consumption, considered to be the source of many contemporary health problems. Since the 19th century, there has been increasing industrialization. With societies becoming increasingly oriented toward goods, production, and consumption, overcrowded cities and filth are common by-products. Environmental theory sees health as a social issue, and solutions tend to be at the policy and regulatory levels. Systems interventions rather than medical interventions are emphasized.

Comprehensive theories of health determinants incorporate the major elements of the three general theories—namely, germ, lifestyle (including nutrition), and environmental theories—along with medical care services, in assessing the determinants of health status of the population. As early as 1973, Barbara Starfield suggested that the study of health status should recognize four major determinants in patients: genetic makeup, behavior, medical practice, and environment. Figure 2.3 is a Venn diagram depicting the interrelations among these determinants. Health status is related to outcome and is determined by the interactions of individuals' genetic constitutions, their behavior, the social and physical environment, and medical practices.

In 1974, Henric Blum (1981) proposed an "environment of health" model, later titled the "Force Field and Well-being Paradigms of Health." Blum advocated that the four major inputs contributing to health status are environment, lifestyles, heredity, and medical care, and emphasized that these inputs have to be considered simultaneously when addressing the health status of a population.

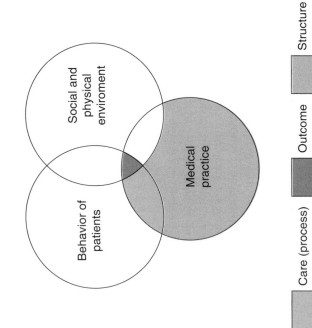

Figure 2.3. Determinants of health status
Source: Adapted from Starfield (1973).

Figure 2.4 diagrams Blum's model. The health or well-being of individuals, situated in the center, is determined by the interaction of three components: the psychic or mental component, the somatic or physical component, and the social component. For example, the loss of a job may affect a person's social health through reduced social functioning, that person's mental health through greater level of stress, and that person's physical health through such ailments as a stomachache. The diagram shows four major wedges, or force fields, that affect health: environment, heredity, medical care services, and lifestyles. The width of the wedges reflects their relative significance.

The prominent force field in Blum's model is environment, followed by life-style, heredity, and finally medical care. The Centers for Disease Control and Prevention (CDC) (1979) identified the same four factors contributing to health. Like Blum, the CDC identified medical care as the least important factor. In fact, the CDC estimated 50 percent of premature deaths in the U.S. population were directly related to individual lifestyle and behaviors, 20 percent to individual inherited genetic profiles, and 20 percent to social and environmental factors. Only 10 percent could be ascribed to inadequate access to medical care. This underscores the point that even though major efforts and expenditures in the United States have been directed toward the delivery of medical care, medical care services have relatively little impact on health status, compared to health behaviors, genetics, and the social, cultural, and physical environment in which people live.

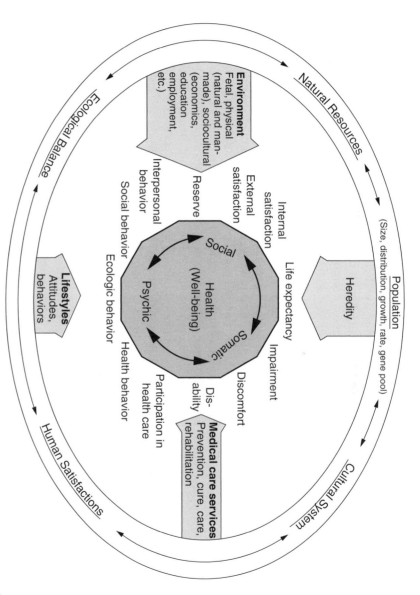

Figure 2.4. **The force field and well-being paradigms of health**

Source: Adapted from Blum (1981).

Since the major purpose of health services is to improve the health status of the population, the measurement of health status will be examined along physical, mental, and social dimensions. The content areas of health services will then be delineated along with other determinants of health, namely, environment, lifestyles, and heredity.

Health Status

Health status measures reflect the needs and outcomes of health services for individuals and populations. As early as 1948, the World Health Organization (WHO) defined health as not merely the absence of disease or infirmity but a state of complete physical, mental, and social well-being (Hanlon and Pickett, 1990). This definition recognizes that health is a crossroads where biological and social factors, individuals and community, and social and economic policies all converge (Frenk, 1993). In addition to its intrinsic value, health is a means for personal and collective advancement. It is not only an indicator of an individual's well-being, but a sign of success achieved by a society and its institutions of government in promoting well-being and human development.

While good or positive health is a major component of broad conceptual definitions of health, the most commonly used indicators are actually measures of poor health (Bergner, 1985; Daly, Duncan, McDonough, and D. R. Williams, 2002; Dever, 2006; Feinstein, 1993; McGinnis and Foege, 2004; U.S. Department of Health and Human Services, 2000; Wilson, 1984; Winkleby, Jatulis, Frank, and Fortmann, 1992). The major reason for this is that, historically, measurements of health status have been conceptually framed in terms of health problems such as disease, disability, and death. Granted, health problems are many and varied, but they all usually affect the length and/or quality of life. The length of life, or longevity, can be expressed in terms of average life expectancy, mortality rates, deaths due to specific causes, and other such indicators. **Quality of life** encompasses such life factors as independent functioning, family circumstances, finances, housing, and job satisfaction. The economic consequences of ill health are reflected in the term **burden of illness**, which refers to both direct and indirect economic costs associated with the use of health care resources and functional restrictions imposed by illness.

The development and widespread use of the **SF-36**, a multipurpose short-form health survey, reflect a shifting focus in the field of health services research from measuring physical illness only to measuring physical, mental, and social well-being (Turner-Bowker, Bartley, and Ware, 2002). The following sections describe commonly used measures (both in the SF-36 and in other instruments) related to these three major dimensions of health: physical health, mental health, and social well-being. A summary of these measures can be found in Table 2.2.

Physical Health Measures

Symptoms

Measures of symptoms reflect acute and chronic problems involving one or more of the body's functional systems. Examples of physical symptoms include toothache, sore throat with fever, and swollen ankles upon waking.

Table 2.2. Common health status indicators

Dimensions	Physical Health	Mental Health	Social Health
Measures	Symptoms Mortality Morbidity Disability Use of health services	Symptoms Psychological state Health perceptions	Symptoms Social well-being

Mortality

Mortality-based measures are among the most often used indirect indicators of health. They include crude death rate, condition-specific death rates, infant mortality, and maternal mortality. Life expectancy at birth and the remaining years of life at various ages are also commonly used measures.

Morbidity

Measures of morbidity include those measuring the incidence or prevalence of specific diseases. **Incidence** refers to the number of new cases of a disease in a defined population within a specified period of time. **Prevalence** refers to the number of instances of a given disease in a given population at a designated time (Gordis, 2004).

Most studies of health status make some attempt to measure morbidity or illness by determining whether or how many times the respondents were sick within a given period and by asking about the occurrence of certain diseases. Researchers are also interested in the conditions of illness. The estimates of acute conditions from ongoing surveys conducted by the U.S. government are based on reported conditions that had their onset within the two weeks prior to the interview (with the exception of certain conditions that are defined as chronic regardless of onset) and resulted in either medical intervention or a day or more of restricted activity. Chronic conditions are generally those that have been present during the past year and have had a duration of at least three months.

Disability

Disability related to illness and injury consists of event-type and person-type indicators. Examples of event-type indicators are restricted activity days, or "cut-down" days, which are used to measure the impact of both acute and chronic illness, including bed days, work-loss days, and school-loss days. Person-type indicators are usually used to reflect the long-term impact of chronic conditions, including measures of limitation of mobility and functional activity. Examples of mobility limitation include confinement to bed, confinement to the house, and the need for help to get around inside or outside the house.

Measuring health and disability has long been a challenge for health services researchers. In 2001, working over the course of seven years, the World Health Assembly of the WHO approved the **International Classification of Functioning, Disability, and Health (ICF)**, which provides a comprehensive, holistic framework for classifying health and disability. The ICF focuses on functionality, measured through body functions and structure; on a person's ability to participate in activities; and on additional information regarding severity of illness/disability and environmental factors (WHO, 2001). Using the ICF framework, WHO estimates that as many as 500 million healthy life years are lost each year due to disability associated with health conditions (WHO, 2001).

Activities of daily living (ADL) is often used to measure functional activity limitations of the elderly and the chronically ill. Measures of ADL focus on the ability of a person to function independently or with assistance in activities such as bathing, dressing, toileting, transferring into and out of a bed or chair, continence, and eating (Travis and McAuley, 1990). A set of measures somewhat related to ADL indicators are measures of functional capacity, including items such as the ability to walk a quarter mile ascend or descend a flight of stairs, stand or sit for long periods, use fingers to grasp or handle, and lift or carry a moderately heavy or heavy object. These are called **instrumental activities of daily living (IADL)**, which require a finer level of motor coordination than is necessary for the relatively gross activities covered in ADL scales (McDowell and Newell, 1987). The IADL scales are used to measure less severe functional impairments and to distinguish between more subtle levels of functioning. The content of IADL scales stresses an individual's functioning within her or his particular environment. When people are unable to perform numerous IADL activities (usually more than five) for an extended period of time, and they are not acutely ill, they are designated as handicapped.

Use of Health Services

While measures of health status have frequently been used to indicate the need for medical care, measures of the use of health services are often used as proxies for health, with implications for health status going in both directions; that is, high utilization as an indicator of poor health and lack of utilization as a presumption of poor health, or at least a poor health practice. Specific indicators in this category include: (1) number of doctor visits per person per year, (2) percentage of persons who have not seen a doctor within the past year, (3) interval between doctor visits, (4) short-stay hospital admission and discharge rate, and (5) short-stay hospital average length of stay.

Mental Health Measures

Symptoms

Mental health symptoms include psychophysiologic symptoms and psychological symptoms. Examples of psychophysiologic symptoms include low energy, headaches, and upset stomach. Examples of psychological symptoms include feeling nervous, depressed, and anxious. The major distinction between physical and psychophysiologic symptoms is that the latter are more likely to reflect an underlying psychological problem.

Self-Assessed Psychological State

Whereas physical functioning is reflected in behavioral performance, mental health involves feelings that cannot be observed. Thus, the assessment of general mental health requires measures of psychological state; that is, self-reports of the frequency and intensity of psychological distress, anxiety, depression, and psychological well-being.

General Health Perceptions

Self-ratings of health in general are among the most commonly used measures of health and well-being. Many studies have asked respondents about self-assessed health status, for example, "Would you say that your health in general is excellent, very good, good, fair, or poor compared to people your age?" Measures of general health perceptions are sometimes criticized as subjective and unreliable. However, the subjectivity of the measure reflects an important aspect of health: personal feelings. It is a good predictor of patient-initiated doctor visits, including both general medical and mental health visits. It is also highly correlated with many objective measures of health status.

Social Health Measures

The concept of social well-being extends beyond the individual to include the quantity and quality of social contacts and resources across distinct areas of life, including family, work, and community. Social health measures are often indicators of quality of life.

Symptoms

Symptoms of social health may be linked to health-related limitations in the performance of the usual social role activities, including employment, schoolwork, and housework.

Social Well-Being

Social well-being includes two distinct categories of concepts, social contacts and social resources. **Social contacts** refer to the frequency of social activities a person undertakes within a specified time period. Examples include visits with family members, friends, and relatives, and participation in social events such as membership activities, professional conferences, and workshops. **Social resources** refers to the adequacy of interpersonal relationships and the extent that social contacts can be relied upon for support. Social contacts can be observed and, thus, represent the more objective of the two measures. However, one criticism of the social contact measure is its focus on events and activities without considering how they are qualitatively experienced. Unlike social contacts, social resources cannot be directly observed. They are best measured by asking the individuals directly. Questions include whether they can rely on their social contacts (i.e., friends, relatives) to provide needed support and company and whether they feel sufficiently cared for and loved.

Environment

Environment is defined as events external to the individual over which one has little or no control. It provides the context of health services provision, which consists of physical and social (including political, economic, cultural, psychological, and demographic) dimensions. These environmental conditions create risks that are a far greater threat to health than any present inadequacy of the medical care system.

Physical Dimension

In a physical environment, certain hazards show a close relationship with the use of energy (such as oil) by an expanding population. Per capita energy consumption is increasing concomitantly with the population and the standard of living.

Thus, health hazards stemming from air, noise, and water pollution almost assuredly will also increase steadily. The resulting diseases and problems include hearing loss, infectious diseases, gastroenteritis, cancer, emphysema, and bronchitis. In limited cases, ionizing and ultraviolet radiation have serious health implications in terms of skin cancer and genetic mutation. These health problems will be reduced only by adopting strict environmental regulations, implementing standards and controls on the responsible agencies and industries, and educating the public about the risks involved.

Collective action using government power can serve to greatly improve public health even as energy consumption increases. For example, in the United States the removal of lead from gasoline and paint has resulted in dramatic declines in mental and physical illnesses and disabilities in children as a result of lead exposure. However, it is important to note the continued threat of lead poisoning among children who live in older homes that still contain lead in the paint on windowsills and walls. Continued public health and governmental vigilance is required to protect children from the threat of lead poisoning (Bellinger and Bellinger, 2006).

Social Dimension

A nation's political, economic, and cultural preferences exert significant influence on the health of its population. For example, a market-dominated country such as the United States is likely to favor a health care system that is pro-competition and antigovernment. The U.S. cultural preference for individualism contributes to a health care system that is individualistic and disjointed rather than collective and organized.

At the individual level, **socioeconomic status (SES)** is an important social measure and a strong and consistent predictor of health status. The major components of SES include income, education, and occupational status. Individuals lower in SES suffer disproportionately from almost all diseases and show higher rates of mortality than those with higher SES. Countries that have universal health insurance (such as England) show the same SES–health gradient as that found in the United States (where such insurance is not provided), indicating that SES is an independent predictor of health status, after controlling for access to medical care. The potential pathways by which SES may influence health are through differential exposure to physical and social contexts; different knowledge of health conditions; adverse environmental conditions, such as exposure to pathogens and carcinogens at home and at work; and social conditions such as crime. Current U.S. medical policy may be moving toward the provision of health insurance to provide universal access to medical care. However, even if this goal is achieved, SES inequalities in health will persist.

The social dimension of environmental health also encompasses major factors involving behavior modification, psychological stress, perceptional problems, and interpersonal relationships. For example, crowding, isolation, accelerated rates of change, and social interchange may contribute to homicide, suicide, decisional stress, and environmental overstimulation.

Demographics also pose significant challenges to health care delivery. The increase of the elderly as a proportion of the total population and the aging of the elderly population is referred to as the "graying of America." Since the elderly, particularly the oldest elderly (those age 85 and older), use a disproportionate share of health care resources, their increase in numbers means greater pressure will be brought to bear on the health care system.

Lifestyles

The shift of the leading causes of death from infectious to chronic diseases such as heart disease and cancer indicates that **behavioral risk factors**, including cigarette smoking, alcohol abuse, lack of exercise, unsafe driving, and poor dietary habits are increasingly predictive of higher risk for certain diseases and mortality. Behavioral risk factors are related to socioeconomic status. For example, the prevalence of smoking is greater for those with less education than for those with more education.

Lifestyles, or behavioral risk factors, can be divided into three categories: leisure activity risks, consumption risks, and employment participation and occupational risks (Dever, 2006). This division involves the aggregation of decisions by individuals affecting their health over which they have more or less control. Individuals have least control over employment and occupational factors, more control over consumption, and greatest control over leisure activity. Thus, the federal government has created regulatory agencies (e.g., OSHA) that force employers to maintain safe workplaces and practices. Leisure and consumption activities, in contrast, are relatively unregulated with the exception of efforts to control the use of illegal drugs and the purchase of tobacco and alcohol products by underage youth.

Leisure Activity Risks

Some destructive behaviors are the result of leisure activity risks. Sexual promiscuity and unprotected sex can result in sexually transmitted diseases, including AIDS, syphilis, and gonorrhea. Lack of exercise is strongly associated with hypertension and coronary heart disease. It aggravates coronary heart disease, leads to obesity, and results in a lack of physical fitness.

Consumption Risks

Another kind of behavioral risk involves consumption patterns. These include (1) overeating (obesity); (2) cholesterol intake (heart disease); (3) alcohol consumption (motor vehicle accidents); (4) alcohol addiction (cirrhosis of the liver); (5) cigarette smoking (chronic obstructive pulmonary disease: chronic bronchitis and emphysema, lung cancer, and aggravating heart disease); (6) drug dependency (suicide, homicide, malnutrition, accidents, social withdrawal, and acute anxiety attacks); and (7) excessive glucose (sugar) intake (dental caries, obesity, and hyperglycemia).

Employment/Occupational Risks

Destructive lifestyles related to employment and occupational risks are usually difficult for individuals to control. Examples include dangerous occupations, unsafe workplaces, and stressful jobs. Work-related stress, anxiety, and tension can cause peptic ulcers and hypertension.

Heredity

The impact of heredity or human biology on health status is concerned with the basic biologic and organic makeup of individuals. For example, a person's genetic inheritance can lead to genetic disorders, congenital malformations, and mental retardation. The maturation and aging process is a contributing factor in arthritis, diabetes, atherosclerosis, and cancer. Obvious disorders of the skeletal, muscular, cardiovascular, endocrine, and digestive systems are subcomponents of complex internal systems.

Medical Care Services

Medical care services differ from other commodities in a number of important ways. First, the demand for medical care services stems from the demand for a more fundamental commodity, namely, health itself; the demand for medical care is therefore a derived demand.

The second difference is the so-called **agency relationship** (Sorkin, 1992). Because patients generally lack the technical knowledge to make the necessary decisions, they delegate this authority to their physicians with the hope that physicians will act for them as they would for themselves if they had the appropriate expertise. If physicians act solely in the interests of patients, the agency relationship would be virtually indistinguishable from normal consumer behavior. However, physicians' decisions will typically reflect not only the preferences of their patients, but also their own self-interests, including the pressures from professional colleagues and institutions, a sense of medical ethics, and a desire to make good use of available resources.

One implication is that health care utilization may well depend on the organizational environment. For example, in an organizational setting where patients are prepaid, such as in a **health maintenance organization (HMO)**, physicians may have the incentive to restrict the number of hospital admissions to fewer than they would if they were acting as "perfect" agents. Likewise, in hospitals where reimbursement is prospectively based, physicians may be pressured to restrict duration of stay. Organizational setting may therefore be one of the key variables in explaining medical care utilization.

The third difference concerns the nature of the price paid for health care. In most medical services, the money paid out-of-pocket at the point of usage is often significantly lower than the total eventual payment, largely due to insurance coverage. It is generally believed that the combination of comprehensive insurance for patients and fee-for-service payment for providers is what has driven the health care system to be the way it is at present—a voracious black hole for economic resources. Thus, the use of medical care services is related to how the services are financed.

Finally, medical care services are influenced by the environment in which services are provided, namely, in the social, economic, demographic, technological, political, and cultural contexts surrounding the provision of health services. For example, among the major forces shaping the health care industry, the social reality of the growing number of uninsured is one of the major factors spearheading the current debate about health care reform. The economic picture of the country and the large federal deficit necessitate greater cost containment and fiscal accountability in addition to clinical accountability. Globalization of the economy results in the increasing prominence of big business, which is getting more involved in both the financing and delivery of medical services. Changing population composition—the growing proportion of the elderly—predicts a greater need for professional labor. Technological growth and innovation contribute to medical care quality and expenditures at the same time.

The distinctive American political culture tends to distrust power, particularly government power, and prefers voluntarism and self-rule in small, homogeneous groups with limited purposes. This implicit American assumption that self-rule in small groups maximizes freedom may explain why there is no national health care system and why there are so many subsystems in the United States. However, many Americans do believe that health is a basic human right and access to medical care should be guaranteed. This belief in the social nature of health may explain the larger role of the government in health care relative to other sectors of the economy.

Indeed, the conflicts between market and social justice can account for many of the problems and contradictions surrounding the provision, organization, and financing of health services. The principles of market and social justice are summarized in Table 2.3. Table 2.4 presents the major content areas of health services, including organizations, providers, service types, government's role, financing, and critical issues in health services. Appendix 2 provides a list of the major health services–related professional associations. For a detailed discussion of these

Table 2.3. Principles of market and social justice

Market Justice	Social Justice
Individual responsibility for health	Shared responsibility for health
Self-determination of health	Social determination of health
Benefits related to individual efforts	Certain benefits are guaranteed to all
Limited obligation to the collective	Strong obligation to the collective
Rugged individualism	Community well-being supersedes that of individual
Emphasis on individual behavior	Emphasis on social conditions
Limited government intervention	Active government involvement

Table 2.4. Classification of major health service content areas

1. Health Services Organizations

- System: system for the employed, insured; system for the unemployed, uninsured, and poor; system for active duty military personnel; system for retired, disabled veterans
- Hospitals: community (proprietary, nonprofit, multihospital system), government
- Hospital integration: vertical versus horizontal
- Nursing homes
- Mental health facilities
- Managed care approaches: HMO, PPO, IPA, EPA
- Ambulatory care facilities (clinics, outpatients, surgical centers, physician group practices, community and migrant health centers)
- Community-based programs: local and state health departments, home health agency, hospice programs
- Supportive organizations: government, business, regulatory organizations; insurance companies; educational institutions; professional associations; pharmaceutical and medical equipment suppliers
- Public health departments

2. Providers of Health Services

- Physicians (generalists, specialists, doctors of osteopathy)
- Dentists, nurses, pharmacists, therapists
- Nonphysician primary care providers: nurse practitioners, physician assistants, certified nurse midwives

3. Types of Health Services

- Preventive services: health promotion, disease prevention, health protection
- Primary care and community-oriented primary care
- Long-term care (home, community, institution)
- Mental health (inpatient facilities, residential treatment facilities, outpatient facilities, community-based services)
- Home care
- Hospice
- Dental care, vision care, foot care, drug dispensing
- Special segments: school health, prison health, Native American health, migrant health, AIDS patients

4. Role of Government

- Medicare
- Medicaid
- Certificate of Need programs
- Veterans Affairs services
- State-, county-, and city-owned or operated general and special hospitals
- County and city health departments ambulatory care and public health services
- Health promotion/enhancement services (e.g., WIC)

Table 2.4. Classification of major health service content areas (continued)

5. Financing of Health Services

- Financing sources: private health insurance, out-of-pocket payment, government
- Financing objects: hospital care, physician services, nursing home care
- Methods of physician reimbursement: fee-for-service, capitation, salary, RBRVS
- Retrospective (cost-based versus prospective payment [DRGs])
- Public health financing: block grant versus categorical grant
- Health insurance terms: risk, moral hazard, adverse selection, deductible, copayment, experience-rated, community-rated
- Health insurance types: voluntary (Blue Cross and Blue Shield, private, HMDs), social (Medicare, Workers' Compensation, CHAMPUS), welfare (Medicaid)
- Cost-containment approaches: cost sharing, utilization review, case management, selective contracting
- Financing reform: one-payer system, "laissez-faire" free-market approach, employer-based approach ("play or pay")

6. Critical Issues in Health Services

- Access to care
- Rural health, urban health
- Minority health
- Quality of care (structure, process, outcome, patient satisfaction)
- Ethics in health care

topics, please refer to the numerous books and articles on U.S. health care systems (e.g., Andersen, 1995; Barnato, McClellan, Kagay, and Garber, 2004; Berkman and Kawachi, 2000; Berwick, 2005; Blum, 1981; Blumenthal, 2006; Boden-heimer, 2006; Cohen and Steinecke, 2006; Crutchfield, 2006; Donabedian, 1985; Enthoven, Schauffler, and McMenamin, 2001; Gillies, Chenok, Shortell, Pawlson, and Winbush, 2006; Goldman and Grob, 2006; Iglehart, 2005; Institute of Medicine, 2000, 2001, 2003; McDowell and Newell, 1987; Mor, Zinn, Angelelli, Teno, and Miller, 2004; NCHS, 2006; Rabinowitz, Diamond, Markham, and Paynter, 2001; Shi, 2004; Shi and Singh, 2004; Sorkin, 1992; Spillman and Lubitz, 2000; Tang, Eisenberg, and Meyer, 2004; U.S. Department of Health and Human Services, 2000; U.S. General Accountability Office, 2006; U.S. Preventive Services Task Force, 2005; Weiner, 2004; Williams and Torrens, 2002).

SUMMARY

Conceptualization is the first stage of health services research. It requires the researcher to understand the general purposes of research (i.e., exploration, description, and explanation), determine the specific research topic (based on factors such as whether the research aims to address a social problem; test or construct a scientific theory; satisfy the researcher's personal interests, ability, and available resources; or achieve professional recognition), identify relevant theories and issues (through extensive review of the relevant scientific literature), specify the meaning of the concepts and variables to be studied (i.e., identify dimensions and define terms both nominally and operationally), and formulate general hypotheses (which specify the relationships among the variables to be studied or research questions. Health, the major purpose of health services, may be conceptualized along three major dimensions: physical health, mental health, and social well-being. Its major determinants include factors related to the environment, lifestyles, and heredity, in addition to medical care services.

REVIEW QUESTIONS

1. What are the major steps in the conceptualization stage of health services research?
2. Draw the distinctions among exploratory, descriptive, and explanatory (or analytic or causal) research. What conditions are most appropriate for each of the three major research purposes?
3. How do investigators identify research topics?
4. Why is literature review an integral part of research?
5. Draw the distinction between the nominal and operational definitions of a concept under study. What are their respective roles in research?
6. What are the major characteristics of a research hypothesis? Identify some common ways of specifying research hypotheses.
7. What are the common indicators of health status?
8. Identify the determinants of health and explain how they affect health status.
9. Draw the distinctions between the following pairs of terms: incidence and prevalence; mobility limitation and functional limitation; ADL and IADL; social contact and social resources.
10. What are the behavioral risk factors that may contribute to diseases or poor health status?
11. What are the unique characteristics of medical care services compared with other market products or services?

REFERENCES

Andersen, R. M. (1995). Revisiting the behavioral model and access to medical care: Does it matter? *Journal of Health and Social Behavior, 36*(1), 1–10.

Babbie, E. (2004). *The Practice of Social Research* (10th ed.). Belmont, CA: Thomson/Wadsworth.

Barnato, A. E., McClellan, M. B., Kagay, C. R., and Garber, A. M. (2004). Trends in inpatient treatment intensity among Medicare beneficiaries at the end of life. *Health Services Research, 39*(2), 363–375.

Bellinger, D. C., and Bellinger, A. M. (2006). Childhood lead poisoning: The torturous path from science to policy. *Journal of Clinical Investigation, 116*(4): 853–857.

Bergner, M. (1985). Measurement of health status. *Medical Care, 23*, 696–704.

Berkman, L. F., and Kawachi, I. (2000). *Social Epidemiology.* New York: Oxford University Press.

Berwick, D. M. (2005). The John Eisenberg lecture: Health services research as a citizen in improvement. *Health Services Research, 40*(2), 317–336.

Blum, H. L. (1981). *Planning for Health* (2nd ed.). New York: Human Sciences Press.

Blumenthal, D. (2006). Employer-sponsored insurance—riding the health care tiger. *New England Journal of Medicine, 355*(2), 195–202.

Bodenheimer, T. (2006). Primary care—will it survive? *New England Journal of Medicine, 355*(9), 861–864.

Brook, R. H., Ware, J. E., and Roger, W. H. (1983). Does free care improve adults' health? Results from a randomized controlled trial. *New England Journal of Medicine, 309*, 1426–1434.

Centers for Disease Control and Prevention. (1979). *Healthy People: The Surgeon General's Report on Health Promotion and Disease Prevention.* Washington, DC: U.S. Department of Health and Human Services.

Cohen, J. J., and Steinecke, A. (2006). Building a diverse physician workforce. *Journal of the American Medical Association, 296*(9), 1135–1137.

Crutchfield, D. (2006). Impact of Medicare Part D on long-term care. *Managed Care, 15*(Suppl. 3), 28–30.

Daly, M. C., Duncan, G. J., McDonough, P., and Williams, D. R. (2002). Optimal indicators of socioeconomic status for health research. *American Journal of Public Health, 92*(7), 1151–1157.

Dever, G. E. A. (2006). *Managerial Epidemiology: Practice, Methods, and Concepts.* Sudbury, MA: Jones and Bartlett.

Donabedian, A. (1985). Twenty years of research on the quality of medical care. *Evaluation and the Health Professions, 8*, 243–265.

Enthoven, A. C., Schauffler, H. H., and McMenamin, S. (2001). Consumer choice and the managed care backlash. *American Journal of Law and Medicine, 27*(1), 1–15.

Feinstein, J. S. (1993). The relationship between socioeconomic status and health: A review of the literature. *The Milbank Memorial Fund Quarterly, 71*, 279–322.

Frenk, J. (1993). The new public health. *Annual Review of Public Health, 14*, 469–490.

Gillies, R. R., Chenok, K. E., Shortell, S. M., Pawlson, G., and Wimbush, J. J. (2006). The impact of health plan delivery system organization on clinical quality and patient satisfaction. *Health Services Research, 41*(4, Pt. 1), 1181–1199.

Goldman, H. H., and Grob, G. N. (2006). Defining "mental illness" in mental health policy. *Health Affairs (Millwood), 25*(3), 737–749.

Goode, W. J., and Hatt, P. K. (1962). *Methods in Social Research.* New York: McGraw-Hill.

Gordis, L. (2004). *Epidemiology* (3rd ed.). Philadelphia: Elsevier Saunders.

Grady, K. E., and Wallston, B. S. (1988). *Research in Health Care Settings.* Newbury Park, CA: Sage.

Hanlon, J. J., and Pickett, G. E. (1990). *Public Health: Administration and Practice.* St. Louis: Times Mirror/Mosby College Publishing.

Iglehart, J. K. (2005). Pursuing health IT: The delicate dance of government and the market. *Health Affairs (Millwood), 24*(5), 1100–1101.

Institute of Medicine. (2000). *To Err Is Human: Building a Safer Health System.* Washington, DC: National Academies Press.

Institute of Medicine. (2001). *Crossing the Quality Chasm: A New Health System for the 21st Century.* Washington, DC: National Academies Press.

Institute of Medicine (2003). *Unequal Treatment: Confronting Racial and Ethnic Disparities in Healthcare.* Washington, DC: National Academies Press.

McDowell, I., and Newell, C. (1987). *Measuring Health: A Guide to Rating Scales and Questionnaires.* New York: Oxford University Press.

McGinnis, J. M., and Foege, W. H. (2004). The immediate vs. the important. *Journal of the American Medical Association, 291*(10), 1238–1245.

McGuigan, F. J. (1978). *Experimental Psychology: A Methodological Approach* (3rd ed.). Englewood Cliffs, NJ: Prentice-Hall.

Metchnikoff, E. (1939). *The Founders of Modern Medicine: Pasteur, Kosh, Lister.* New York: Walden Publications.

Mor, V., Zinn, J., Angelelli, J., Teno, J. M., and Miller, S. C. (2004). Driven to tiers: Socioeconomic and racial disparities in the quality of nursing home care. *Millbank Quarterly, 82*(2), 227–256.

National Center for Health Statistics. (2006). *Health, United States, 2006.* Hyattsville, MD: U.S. Department of Health and Human Services.

Newhouse, J. P., Manning, W. G., and Morris, C. N. (1981). Some interim results from a controlled trial of cost sharing in health insurance. *New England Journal of Medicine, 305,* 1501–1507.

Office of Technology Assessment. (1992). *Does Health Insurance Make a Difference?* (OTA-BP-H-99) [Background paper]. Washington, DC: U.S. Government Printing Office.

Rabinowitz, H. K., Diamond, J. J., Markham, F. W., and Paynter, N. P. (2001). Critical factors for designing programs to increase the supply and retention of rural primary care physicians. *Journal of the American Medical Association, 286*(9), 1041–1048.

Shi, L. (2004). *Essentials of the U.S. Health Care System.* Sudbury, MA: Jones and Bartlett.

Shi, L., and Singh, D. A. (2004). *Delivering Health Care in America: A Systems Approach.* Sudbury, MA: Jones and Bartlett.

Shi, L., and Stevens, G. D. (2005). *Vulnerable Populations in the United States.* San Francisco: Jossey-Bass.

Singleton, R. A., and Straits, B. C. (2005). *Approaches to Social Research* (4th ed.). New York: Oxford University Press.

Smith, C., Cowan, C., Heffler, S., and Catlin, A. (2006). National health spending in 2004: Recent slowdown led by prescription drug spending. *Health Affairs (Millwood), 25*(1), 186–196.

Sorkin, A. L. (1992) *An Introduction to Health Economics.* New York: Lexington Books.

Spillman, B. C., and Lubitz, J. (2000). The effect of longevity on spending for acute and long-term care. *New England Journal of Medicine, 342*(19), 1409–1415.

Starfield, B. (1973). Health services research: A working model. *New England Journal of Medicine, 289,* 132–136.

Tang, N., Eisenberg, J. M., and Meyer, G. S. (2004). The roles of government in improving health care quality and safety. *Joint Commission Journal on Quality and Safety, 30*(1), 47–55.

Travis, S. S., and McAuley, W. J. (1990). Simple counts of the number of basic ADL dependencies for long-term care research and practice. *Health Services Research, 24*, 349–360.

Turner-Bowker, D. M., Bartley, P. J., and Ware, J. E., Jr. (2002). *SF-36® Health Survey & "SF" Bibliography (1988–2000)* (3rd ed.). Lincoln, RI: QualityMetric.

U.S. Department of Health and Human Services. (2000). *Healthy People 2010: Understanding and Improving Health*. Washington, DC: U.S. Government Printing Office.

U.S. General Accountability Office. (2006). *Consumer Directed Health Plans: Early Enrollee Experiences with Health Savings Accounts and Eligible Health Plans*. Washington, DC: U.S. Government Printing Office.

U.S. Preventive Services Task Force. (2005). *Guide to Clinical Preventive Services, 2005*. Rockville, MD: Agency for Healthcare Research and Quality.

Weiner, J. P. (2004, February 4). Prepaid group practice staffing and U.S. physician supply: Lessons for workforce policy [Web exclusive]. *Health Affairs (Millwood), W4*, 43–59. Retrieved July 14, 2007, from http://content.healthaffairs.org/cgi/reprint/hlthaff.w4.43v1?maxtoshow=&HITS=10&hits=10&RESULTFORMAT=&author1=Weiner&fulltext=Prepaid+group&andorexactfulltext=and&searchid=1&FIRSTINDEX=0&resourcetype=HWCIT

Weiner, J. P., and Lissovoy, G. (1993). A taxonomy for managed care and health insurance plans. *Journal of Health Politics, Policy and Law, 18*, 75–103.

Williams, S. J., and Torrens, P. R. (Eds.). (2002). *Introduction to Health Services* (6th ed.). Albany, NY: Delmar Thomson Learning.

Wilson, R. W. (1984). Interpreting trends in illness and disability: Health statistics and health status. *Annual Review of Public Health, 5*, 83–106.

Winkleby, M. A., Jatulis, D. E., Frank, E., and Fortmann, S. P. (1992). Socioeconomic status and health: How education, income, and occupation contribute to risk factors for cardiovascular disease. *American Journal of Public Health, 82*, 816–820.

Wolfson, M. (1994). Social proprioception: Measurement, data and information from a population health perspective. In R. G. Evans, M. L. Barer, and T. Marmor (Eds.), *Why Are Some People Healthy and Others Not?* New York: Aldine de Gruyter.

World Health Organization. (1948). *Constitution of the World Health Organization*. In *Basic Documents*. Geneva, Switzerland: World Health Organization.

World Health Organization. (2001, November 15). WHO publishes new guidelines to measure health [Press release]. Retrieved July 1, 2007, from http://www.who.int/inf-pr-2001/en/pr2001-48.html

CHAPTER 3

Groundwork in Health Services Research

KEY TERMS

Area Resource File
Behavioral Risk Factor
  Surveillance System
  (BRFSS)
cross-sectional data
Health and Retirement Study
  (HRS)
Medical Expenditure Panel
  Survey (MEPS)
Medicare Current Beneficiary
  Survey (MCBS)
Medicare Enrollment and
  Claims Data (MECD)

National Ambulatory Medical
  Care Survey (NAMCS)
National Center for Health
  Statistics (NCHS)
National Health and Nutrition
  Examination Survey
  (NHANES)
National Health Interview
  Survey
National Hospital Discharge
  Survey (NHDS)
National Nursing Home
  Survey (NNHS)

National Vital Statistics
  System (NVSS)
panel data
primary data source
research proposal
secondary data source
Survey of Mental Health
  Organizations (SMHO)
time-series data
unit of observation

LEARNING OBJECTIVES

- To get acquainted with the major national-
  level secondary data sources currently available for health services research.
- To identify the major funding sources for
  health services research.

- To understand the major components of a
  research proposal and the general approach
  of proposal review.
- To become familiar with the general organizational and administrative issues related to
  the preparation and conduct of research.

74

As Chapter 1 points out, the groundwork stage of the research process requires the researcher to identify relevant data sources, explore potential funding sources, develop a research plan or proposal (to obtain funding), and prepare organizationally and administratively to carry out the research. This chapter introduces the major national-level data and funding sources available for health services research, describes the major components of a research proposal as well as the process of reviewing research proposals, and discusses the general organizational and administrative issues related to the preparation and conduct of health services research.

DATA SOURCES

A prerequisite of any research is the availability of data. Data may be collected either through primary or secondary sources. **Primary data source** refers to the collection of data by researchers themselves. **Secondary data source** refers to the use of data collected by others. While primary data are generally more relevant, familiar, and timely than secondary data, they are also more expensive, time consuming, and difficult to collect. Given that both funding sources and amounts available for research are declining, investigators may become increasingly dependent on secondary or existing data for research.

Data may be classified as cross-sectional, time-series, or panel. **Cross-sectional data** are collected at one point in time. The principal advantage of this type of data is its relative inexpensiveness when a large sample size is used. Its transitory nature, which makes causal association difficult, is its main disadvantage. **Time-series data** follow the same **unit of observation** over time. The primary advantage here is the ability to capture historical trends and changes. The principal drawbacks are limited observations and the relative expensiveness when a large sample size is used. **Panel data** combine cross-sectional and time-series data, surveying the same groups over time. Its ability to capture trends and causal associations is its main advantage. Its primary disadvantages are attrition rates and relative expensiveness.

This section introduces the National Center for Health Statistics, the major federal agency mandated to collect health statistics. It then summarizes the major national-level electronic databases commonly used for health services research. These include: the National Center for Health Statistics data sets, the Area Resource File, the Behavioral Risk Factor Surveillance System, the Medicare Current Beneficiary Survey (also, the Medicare Enrollment and Claims Data), the Survey of Mental Health Organizations, the National Ambulatory Medical Care Survey, the National Health Interview Survey, the National Health and Nutrition Examination Survey, the National Hospital Discharge Survey, the Medical Expenditure Panel Survey, the National Nursing Home Survey, the Health and Retirement Study, and the National Vital Statistics System (see Table 3.1 for details).

Table 3.1. **Major national and international level data sources for health services research**

Area Resource File	Bureau of Health Professions, HRSA	Demographics, health professions, health facilities, health status	County, state	1986	http://www.arfsys.com
Behavioral Risk Factor Surveillance System	Centers for Disease Control	Behavioral or lifestyle risk factors, demographics	Noninstitutionalized adult	Early 1980s	http://www.cdc.gov/brfss
Medicare Current Beneficiary Survey	Centers for Medicare & Medicaid Services	Health status, access to care, costs and use of care	Cohort of Medicare beneficiaries	1991	http://www.cms.hhs.gov/ MCBS/01_Overview.asp# TopOfPage
Survey of Mental Health Organizations	Center for Mental Health Services, SAMHSA	Characteristics of mental health organizations, patients, and services	Mental health organizations	1969	http://mentalhealth.samhsa.gov/ cmhs/MentalHealthStatistics
National Ambulatory Medical Care Survey	National Center for Health Statistics, CDC	Provision and utilization of office-based ambulatory services	Patient visit	1973	http://www.cdc.gov/nchs/about/ major/ahcd/ahcd1.htm
National Health Interview Survey	National Center for Health Statistics, CDC	Health conditions, doctor visits, hospital stays, household characteristics, personal characteristics	Household, individual members of the household	1957	http://www.cdc.gov/nchs/ nhis.htm

National Health and Nutrition Examination Survey	National Center for Health Statistics, CDC	Physical, physiological, psychological diseases; nutritional status	Individual	1959	http://www.cdc.gov/nchs/ nhanes.htm
National Hospital Discharge Survey	National Center for Health Statistics, CDC	Patient, treatment, hospital characteristics	Patient record, hospital	1970	http://www.cdc.gov/nchs/about/ major/hdasd/nhdsdes.htm
Medical Expenditure Panel Survey	Agency for Health Care Research and Quality	Health expenditures, use of health services, insurance coverage	Individual	1977	http://www.meps.ahrq.gov/ mepsweb
National Nursing Home Survey	National Center for Health Statistics, CDC	Types of nursing homes, residents, discharged residents, follow-up	Resident, staff	1973	http://www.cdc.gov/nchs/ products/elec_prods/subject/ nnhs.htm
National Vital Statistics System	National Center for Health Statistics, CDC	Mortality, cause of death, fetal death	Individual	1968	http://www.cdc.gov/nchs/ nvss.htm
Health and Retirement Study	National Institute of Aging, University of Michigan	Demographics, health status, measures of social and economic well-being	Individual	1992	http://hrsonline.isr.umich.edu

All these data sets are available for public purchase and use. Indeed, the availability of national data has given impetus to the fast development of health services research.

The National Center for Health Statistics

The federal health statistics system is primarily located within the Department of Health and Human Services (HHS), although other agencies, such as the Department of Defense, the Veterans Administration, the Environmental Protection Agency, and the Bureau of Labor Statistics, also collect health statistics in carrying out their functions. Within HHS, the **National Center for Health Statistics (NCHS)** undertakes the majority of health statistical activities. The NCHS was established in 1960 within HHS as the principal federal agency to collect, analyze, and disseminate health statistics. Section 306 of the Public Health Service Act, amended to the National Health Survey Act (1956), specifies that the NCHS shall collect statistics on:

- the extent and nature of illness and disability of the population of the United States (or of any groupings of the people included in the population), including life expectancy, the incidence of various acute and chronic illnesses, and infant and maternal morbidity and mortality

- the impact of illness and disability of the population on the economy of the United States and on other aspects of the well-being of its population (or such groupings)

- environmental, social, and other health hazards

- determinants of health

- health resources, including physicians, dentists, nurses, and other health professionals by specialty and type of practice, and the supply of services by hospitals, extended care facilities, home health agencies

- utilization of health care, including (1) ambulatory health services by specialties and types of practice of the health professionals providing such services and (2) services of hospitals, extended care facilities, home health agencies, and other institutions

- health care costs and financing, including the trends in health care prices and costs, the sources of payments for health care services, and federal, state, and local governmental expenditures for health care services

- family formation, growth, and dissolution

Recently, recognizing that existing national health data systems needed to be more responsive to the changes occurring in the health care system, the NCHS revised, expanded, and coordinated its data collection activities on health care utilization that previously were carried out in separate, uncoordinated surveys. The integrated system, called the National Health Care Survey (NHCS), collects data to monitor the nation's health, illness, and disability; the use and costs of care by incident and episode; and the outcomes and cost-effectiveness of the services provided. The NHCS now includes the following components: National Ambulatory Medical Care Survey (NAMCS), National Employer Health Insurance Survey (NEHIS), National Health Provider Inventory (NHPI), National Home and Hospice Care Survey (NHHCS), National Hospital Ambulatory Medical Care Survey (NHAMCS), National Hospital Discharge Survey (NHDS), National Nursing Home Survey (NNHS), and National Survey of Ambulatory Surgery (NSAS). More information on these data sets is available at NCHS (http://www.cdc.gov/nchs/nhcs.htm), and several are described in more detail later in this chapter.

Area Resource File

The **Area Resource File** is prepared by the Bureau of Health Professions, Health Resources and Services Administration, Public Health Service, HHS. It pools data from various sources to facilitate health analysis both cross-sectionally and longitudinally.

Each data series is available at the levels of county, state, and aggregate United States. The major unit of observation is the county, with more than 6,000 counties represented. There are four major types of variables: demographics (e.g., age distribution, income, and education), health professions (e.g., physicians by specialty), health facilities (e.g., hospitals and nursing homes), and health status (e.g., morbidity, natality, and mortality data by cause, sex, race, and age).

The Area Resource File is an excellent data source at the aggregate county and state levels. National averages can also be easily computed from the county data. It is useful in research concerning health status and the relationship between health status and other factors, particularly for smaller geographic areas and specific population subgroups. The Area Resource File is updated annually. More frequent updates can sometimes be obtained on an ad hoc basis. The original file was created in 1986.

Behavioral Risk Factor Surveillance System

The **Behavioral Risk Factor Surveillance System (BRFSS)** is maintained by the Centers for Disease Control (CDC), a federal agency within the Public Health Service responsible for leadership in the prevention and control of diseases. The BRFSS provides state health agencies with the funding, training, and consultation necessary to collect behavioral risk factor data. Each participating state conducts surveys of their noninstitutionalized adult population using telephone interviews. The sample size varies between 600 and 3,000 for all states. The CDC also provides competitive grants to Prevention Centers around the nation for BRFSS-related activities, including development and use of research methods, data dissemination, and training.

The unit of observation is the noninstitutionalized adult population. The BRFSS includes such data elements as weight control, hypertension, physical activity, obesity, mammography, alcohol consumption, seat belt use, tobacco use, HIV/AIDS, preventive health practices, and demographic information (e.g., age, sex, race, and education). In addition, states may add modules of questions to meet their special needs.

This data system provides valuable information for states to monitor, develop, and evaluate health promotion and disease prevention programs aimed at reducing behavioral risk factors. The BRFSS can also be used to conduct trend analysis and track progress in risk reduction over time. The surveillance system was first created in the early 1980s.

Medicare Current Beneficiary Survey

The **Medicare Current Beneficiary Survey (MCBS)** is conducted by the Office of Strategic Planning of the Centers for Medicare & Medicaid Services (CMS). The MCBS targets a representative, national sample of the Medicare population. The survey collects data on expenditures and sources of payment for health care services used by Medicare beneficiaries; on the types of insurance held by Medicare beneficiaries; on the changes over time in beneficiaries' health status, satisfaction with care, and usual source of care; and on the impact of Medicare program changes (such as shifts to managed care) on beneficiaries. Data for the MCBS are released in two different files, Access to Care (which has been released annually since 1991), and Cost and Use (which has been released annually since 1992).

The unit of analysis is the individual beneficiary, who is enrolled in Medicare Part A (hospital insurance) or Part B (medical insurance) or both. Beneficiaries who live in the community, as well as those who live in long-term care facilities, are included in the MCBS sample. A stratified, multistage area probability design is used to select survey participants, who are followed over four years to assess long-term changes in health status, use of services, and satisfaction with care. The survey participants are interviewed three times over the course of the four years, using computer-assisted personal survey technology.

The MCBS provides unique, longitudinal information to researchers interested in the health of aged and disabled populations, as well as in the utilization and costs of health care services associated with these populations. The MCBS was instituted in 1991.

In addition to the MCBS, another population-based administrative data set collected through CMS is called the **Medicare Enrollment and Claims Data (MECD)**, which provides Medicare utilization and enrollment data that are linked to NCHS survey data. The advantages of Medicare claims data are that they are population-based, not subject to recall bias, and can be linked to NCHS population health surveys to expand their analytic potential to health services researchers. The MECD consists of the following data files: the Denominator File, which provides data on all Medicare beneficiaries entitled to Medicare benefits in a given year; the Medicare Provider Analysis and Review (MedPAR) Hospital Stay File, which contains inpatient hospitalization records; the Medicare

Provider Analysis and Review (MedPAR) Skilled Nursing Facility (SNF) File, which contains skilled nursing facility stays; the Outpatient File, which contains Medicare Part B final action claims from institutional outpatient providers for each calendar year; the Home Health Agency (HHA) File, which contains final action claims for home health services; the Hospice File, which contains final action claims data submitted by hospice providers; the Carrier File (formerly the Physician/Supplier Part B File), which contains final action claims data submitted by noninstitutional providers; the Durable Medical Equipment (DMERC) File, which contains final action claims data submitted by Durable Medical Equipment (DME) regional carriers; and the Public-use Linkage Summary File, which includes a limited set of variables for researchers to use in determining the feasibility and sample sizes of their proposed research projects. More detailed information on these data sets may be obtained through the websites of the following organizations: CMS (http://www.cms.hhs.gov), Research Data Assistance Center (ResDAC) (http://www.resdac.umn.edu), and National Cancer Institute SEER-Medicare Linked Database (http://healthservices.cancer .gov/seermedicare).

Survey of Mental Health Organizations

The **Survey of Mental Health Organizations (SMHO)** was introduced in 1998 as a replacement for earlier mental health inventories conducted by the Center for Mental Health Services, which is part of the Substance Abuse and Mental Health Services Administration, HHS. Surveys are mailed every other year to mental health organizations in the United States, including psychiatric hospitals, psychiatric services in nonfederal general hospitals, VA psychiatric services, residential treatment centers for emotionally disturbed children, freestanding outpatient psychiatric clinics, and partial-care organizations.

The unit of observation is the mental health organization. The SMHO contains information on types of mental health services provided; number of inpatient beds; number of inpatient, outpatient, and partial-care additions; average daily census; patient characteristics; staffing characteristics; expenditures; and revenue by sources.

The SMHO provides valuable information on the sociodemographic, clinical, and treatment characteristics of patients served by mental health facilities. The SMHO's predecessors, called the Mental Health Inventories, were initiated in 1969.

National Ambulatory Medical Care Survey

The **National Ambulatory Medical Care Survey (NAMCS)** is conducted by the National Center for Health Statistics, Centers for Disease Control, Public Health Service, HHS. Data are obtained through a national sample of office-based physicians and a systematic random sample of physician office visits during a seven-day period. Physicians or their staff fill out an encounter form for each sampled visit. Physicians in nonoffice settings, government service, anesthesiology, pathology, and radiology are excluded.

The unit of observation is the patient visit as recorded in the patient record. Each record provides a complete description of the office visit and is weighted statistically to reflect annual utilization of private office-based practice in the United States. The number of records per survey ranges from between 29,143 and 71,594. These national estimates describe the provision and utilization of ambulatory medical care services in the United States and provide information on demographic characteristics of the patient, clinical aspects of the visit, and physician specialty and practice type. The survey offers an indirect measure of health status via diagnostic information. It was initially conducted in 1973.

National Health Interview Survey

The **National Health Interview Survey** is conducted by the National Center for Health Statistics, Centers for Disease Control, Public Health Service, HHS. Each week a probability sample of households is interviewed for information on all living members of the sampled households over the previous two weeks. The annual sample size is between 36,000 and 47,000 households, including 92,000 to 125,000 persons. The 31 major metropolitan areas have self-representing samples, allowing derivation of local measures of health status and use of health services by individuals with varying sociodemographic characteristics. The survey is a continuing nationwide household survey of the U.S. noninstitutionalized population.

The units of observation are the household and the individual members of the household. The major categories of information include region of residence, files on health conditions, doctor visits, hospital stays (in the prior 12 months), household characteristics, and personal characteristics. Specific health conditions include acute and chronic conditions, restricted activity days, bed days, work- and school-loss days, doctor visits, hospital stays, and long-term limitation of activity. These core questions are supplemented by additional questions on varying health topics each year. The supplemental questions are used to produce separate files on current health topics.

The survey is the principal source of information on the general health status of the civilian, noninstitutionalized population of the United States. It provides the most sophisticated measure of national health, illness, and disability. The Current Health Topics databases are valuable for policy studies on specific topics. The survey has been conducted annually since 1957 with approximately a two-year lag between survey year and availability of data.

National Health and Nutrition Examination Survey

The **National Health and Nutrition Examination Survey (NHANES)** is conducted by the National Center for Health Statistics, Centers for Disease Control, Public Health Service, HHS. Since 1959, the National Health Examination Survey (NHES) has been conducted in three cycles. In 1970, nutritional status was added as an additional assessment category and the survey was renamed NHANES. This expanded survey has been conducted twice to facilitate comparison. An NHANES I Epidemiologic Follow-up Study (NHEFS) was conducted in two waves to obtain longitudinal information on participants in NHANES I. The NHES and NHANES were conducted through physical examinations at mobile exam sites throughout the United States. The sample sizes ranged from 6,672 persons in NHES I to more than 20,000 persons in each NHANES. The NHEFS was conducted via personal interviews, interviews with proxy respondents, and review of hospital and nursing home records and death certificates.

In 1999, NHANES became a continuous survey with a changing focus on various health and nutrition measurements. Each year, a nationally representative sample of about 5,000 people in 15 counties are surveyed. The unit of observation is the individual person. The surveys provide measures of prevalence of a variety of physical, physiological, and psychological diseases in the U.S. general population and, since 1970, nutritional status. The objective is to collect data that can be best obtained through direct physical examination, clinical and laboratory tests, and related measurement procedures. Examples include blood pressure, visual acuity, and serum cholesterol level.

The surveys are an excellent data source on health and nutrition status. The NHANES I, II, and III allow assessment of changes in the health status of the general population over time on a number of detailed health indicators. NHES Cycle I was conducted from 1959 to 1962, NHES Cycle II from 1963 to 1965, NHES III from 1966 to 1970, NHANES I from 1971 to 1975, NHANES II from 1976 to 1980, and NHEFS from 1982 to 1984 and in 1986. As previously stated, since 1999, the NHANES has been conducted annually.

National Hospital Discharge Survey

The **National Hospital Discharge Survey (NHDS)** is conducted by the National Center for Health Statistics, Centers for Disease Control, Public Health Service, HHS. Data are abstracted from a multistage cluster random sample of medical records of inpatients discharged from nonfederal short-stay hospitals (approximately 200,000 records per year). The survey is a continuous nationwide survey of inpatient utilization of short-stay hospitals and allows sampling at the census division level.

The unit of observation is the patient's medical records. Data elements include patient characteristics (i.e., date of birth, sex, race, ethnicity, and marital status), expected payment sources, admission and discharge dates, discharge status and disposition, length of stay, hospital characteristics (i.e., region, bed size, and ownership type), patient diagnoses, surgical and nonsurgical procedures, dates of procedures, and residence zip code. Hospital may also be used as a unit of analysis.

The survey provides measures of illness status through hospital diagnosis information and thus far enables analysis of trends over a 35-year period. Interregional comparisons can also be made. The survey has been conducted annually since 1970. There is approximately a two-year lag between survey year and data-base availability.

Medical Expenditure Panel Survey

The **Medical Expenditure Panel Survey (MEPS)** is conducted by the Agency for Healthcare Research and Quality (AHRQ) and the National Center for Health Statistics (NCHS). The MEPS is the third iteration of a series of surveys conducted by AHRQ on the financing and use of medical services in the United States. Previous surveys include the National Medical Care Expenditure Survey (NMCES), last conducted in 1977, and the National Medical Expenditure Survey (NMES), last conducted in 1987.

The MEPS conducts three related surveys: (1) the Household Component Survey, which collects medical expenditure data at the person and household levels from a nationally representative survey of the U.S. civilian noninstitutionalized population; (2) the Medical Provider Component Survey, which surveys medical providers and pharmacies identified by household respondents to verify and supplement information; and (3) the Insurance Component Survey, which collects data on health insurance plans obtained through private- and public-sector employers.

The Medical Expenditure Panel Survey provides information on expenditures for health care, use of health services, payment sources or insurance coverage, and individual health status. Results of the survey may be used to provide fairly detailed population-group estimates of health status and access to care and national estimates of long-term care services and expenditures. The survey was initially started in 1977 by the National Center for Health Services Research and Health Care Technology Assessment.

National Nursing Home Survey

The **National Nursing Home Survey (NNHS)** is conducted by the National Center for Health Statistics, Centers for Disease Control, Public Health Service, HHS. The data are collected using a two-stage, stratified probability design. In the first stage, nursing home facilities are selected. In the second stage, the residents, discharges, or staff of the sampled facilities are selected. Data are collected using a combination of personal interviews and self-administered questionnaires.

The major units of observation are nursing home residents and staff of nursing home facilities. Data are collected on four major areas: (1) nursing homes (size, ownership, license and Medicare and Medicaid certification status, number of beds, services offered, staffing patterns and characteristics, and costs); (2) residents (demographics, activities of daily living, status and living arrangements prior to admission, condition at admission and at interview, receipt of services, cognitive and emotional services, charges, sources of payment, history of nursing home utilization, and hospitalization during stay); (3) discharged residents (demographics, history of nursing home utilization, hospitalization during stay, status at discharge, condition at admission and discharge, and sources of payment); (4) follow-up with the next of kin of the current or discharged residents (living arrangements, health, and functional status prior to admission; history of previous nursing home use; activities of daily living; and Medicaid spend-downs).

The survey provides a series of national samples of nursing homes, their residents, and their staff. It facilitates research on the general health status of the nursing home population and the characteristics of nursing home facilities. The first NNHS was conducted in 1973, with subsequent surveys in 1977, 1985, 1995, 1997, and 1999.

Health and Retirement Study

Another useful source of longitudinal data on the elderly population is the **Health and Retirement Study (HRS)**, maintained by the University of Michigan and supported by the National Institute on Aging. The HRS and its companion study, Assets and Health Dynamics for the Oldest Old (AHEAD), were merged in 1998. The HRS currently surveys more than 22,000 Americans over the age of 50 every two years. Information collected by the HRS includes: respondent demographics, health status, housing, family structure, employment of respondent, work history and current employment, disability, retirement plans, net worth, income, and health and life insurance. The HRS is also linked to information from employers and administrative data (such as Social Security earnings and benefits information, Medicare claims, and pension information).

The unit of analysis is the individual. Several different cohorts of individuals are tracked and interviewed every two years from the time they enter the survey until death. The overall 1998 HRS cohort included the War Baby cohort (born between 1942 and 1947), the Children of the Depression, or CODA, cohort (born between 1924 and 1930), the original HRS cohort (born between 1931 and 1941), and the original AHEAD cohort (born between 1890 and 1923). Every six years, the HRS adds the six-year birth cohort that is between 51 and 56 years old that year. Therefore, in 2004 the Early Boomers (born between 1948 and 1953) were added to the HRS. The Baby Boomers (born between 1954 and 1959) will enter the study in 2010.

Data collection for the original HRS occurred in 1992, 1994, and 1996. Data collection for the original AHEAD occurred in 1993 and 1995. Since 1998, when the HRS and AHEAD were merged, the survey has been conducted every two years. The most recent HRS data currently available are from 2004.

National Vital Statistics System

The **National Vital Statistics System (NVSS)** is developed by the National Center for Health Statistics, Centers for Disease Control, Public Health Service, HHS. Data are obtained from birth and death certificates provided by states.

A number of "follow-back" surveys have also been performed to obtain more detailed information from informants identified on the vital records.

The unit of observation is the individual person. The NVSS is a national registration system for vital statistics, including natality, fetal death, mortality, and their contributing causes. The most relevant health status databases are the following mortality types: Mortality: Detail; Mortality: Local Area Summary; and Mortality: Cause of Death Summary. All databases include data on age, race, sex, and residence.

The system provides the most detailed picture of vital statistics information. Vital statistics databases are annual, starting in 1968. There is approximately a two-year lag from date of vital statistics registration to public availability of vital statistics databases.

In addition to the national databases described above and summarized in Table 3.1, there are numerous other important data sources potentially useful for health services research. These include the Medicaid Statistical Information System; the National HIV/AIDS Surveillance System; the National Immunization Survey; the National Notifiable Diseases Surveillance System; the National Survey of Family Growth; the National Survey on Drug Use and Health; Surveillance, Epidemiology, and End Results; and the Survey of Occupational Injuries and Illnesses. Some of these sources are available as public-use databases while others disseminate data only through published reports. While these sources are less appropriate for a broad overview of U.S. health status and services, their data should be considered for more specialized policy work as needed. Excellent sources of international health data include the Organization for Economic Cooperation and Development (which collects health data for 24 Western industrialized countries) and the World Health Organization (the health agency of the United Nations).

FUNDING SOURCES

There are essentially four types of funding for a research project: self-funding, consultation, contracts, and grants. Self-funding involves carrying out a study using existing resources provided by the individual researcher or the researcher's institution, which usually include data processing services, library services, and other support services as well as time and a budget for research and development work. Consulting services, while usually addressing the client's specific needs, may be integrated with research and contribute to scientific knowledge. Research combined with consulting work is common in private, nonprofit research institutions, such as Rand.

Grants and contracts represent explicit research funding and may be provided by both public and private sources. The major distinction between research contracts and grants has to do with who has the final responsibility for the project and control of funding. In the case of research grants, the researcher has sole responsibility for the design of the study, for any modification to it, and for the implementation of the project. In research contracts, there is a joint responsibility for carrying out the project, and the funder may have final control in that the contract can be stopped if the contractor fails or refuses to proceed with the research protocol as jointly agreed upon or amended. The key distinction, then, is whether the organization providing the money also has an active role in the study.

There are many public and private funding sources for health services research (Annual Register of Grant Support, 2007). Public sources include the various entities under the National Institutes of Health (NIH) of the U.S. Department of Health and Human Services (Parklawn Bldg., 5600 Fishers Lane, Rockville, MD 20857; or NIH Bldg., 9000 Rockville Pike, Bethesda, MD 20892). These organizations include NCI (cancer), NHLBI (heart, lung, and blood), NIA (aging), NIAAA (alcohol abuse), NIDA (drug, alcohol), NIMH (mental health), and NINR (nursing research). Other governmental organizations that serve as sources for funding are the National Science Foundation (2101 Constitution Avenue, Washington, DC 20418), the Agency for Health Care Research and Quality (AHRQ), the Centers for Medicare and Medicaid Services (CMS), the Department of Veterans Affairs (VA), and the Office of Rural Health Policy (ORHP).

The Federal Information Exchange (FEDIX: http://www.fie.com) has designed an electronic service to notify researchers by e-mail of grant opportunities available from twelve federal agencies, including the National Institutes of Health. Researchers can register their e-mail addresses and select key words from a thesaurus to develop a profile of research interests. Announcements of research opportunities are sent via e-mail based on the matching of research interest and funding opportunity.

The Office of Extramural Research (OER) is the entity that administers NIH grants. The OER website (http://grants1.nih.gov/grants/oer.htm) outlines the types of grants awarded by NIH for health services research. Among these are research training grants (called NRSA awards) for researchers-in-training, career development grants (called K awards) for researchers who have recently earned their doctorates, and research project grants (called R01 awards), which are typically sought after by more experienced researchers. The OER's CRISP database (http://crisp.cit.nih.gov) contains information on all projects funded by the National Institutes of Health, Substance Abuse and Mental Health Services, the Health Resources and Services Administration, the Food and Drug Administration, the Centers for Disease Control and Prevention, the Agency for Health Care Research and Quality, and the Office of the Assistant Secretary of Health. This is a good source for new and experienced health service researchers to explore projects recently funded by these agencies. The CRISP interface allows users to search by scientific concepts, emerging trends and techniques, or by the names of specific projects and/or investigators.

Private sources of funding include major foundations such as the Ford Foundation, the Pew Charitable Trusts, the Robert Wood Johnson Foundation, the Lilly Endowment, the Carnegie Corporation of New York, the W. K. Kellogg Foundation, the Henry J. Kaiser Family Foundation, the Baxter Foundation, the Commonwealth Fund, the John A. Hartford Foundation, the Rockefeller Foundation, the Sloan Foundation, the Russell Sage Foundation, and the Social Science Research Council. Additional funding information resources are listed in Appendix 3.

THE RESEARCH PROPOSAL

A **research proposal** describes what specific study a researcher intends to accomplish and how. The primary purpose is to obtain the funding necessary to carry out the study. In the proposal, the researcher tries to convince a prospective sponsor that he or she is well acquainted with the state of the art and the accomplishments in the field, has demonstrated competency in study design and analysis, is qualified to perform the described activities, and has the necessary personnel and facilities to carry out the activities related to the project. Moreover, the researcher must show that the proposed activities either aim at solving an immediate problem or at advancing existing knowledge in the field and eventually aiding in the solution of an identified problem. The research purpose should be within the scope of the established program objectives of the funding agency, and the importance of the anticipated results should sufficiently justify the expenditure of the proposed time and money.

Preliminary Work

The prelude to writing a good proposal is adequate preliminary work. This involves reviewing the funding literature and examining information regarding the funder's areas of interest and funding priorities, guidelines for proposal submission, possible restrictions, size of the grants, cost-share requirements, and review procedures. The researcher should be aware of the dates and terms of proposal submission, required forms, the contact person or office, and the correct name and address of the potential funding source. Once this information is obtained, the researcher then decides whether the proposed idea is consistent with the funding priorities; whether the proposed costs are within the given range; whether funding is short term or long term and whether renewal is possible; whether matching funds are required and, if so, what kind; and whether there is a funding cycle and, if so, what deadlines are to be met for proposal submission.

After a funding source has been identified, the investigator should contact the source prior to writing or submitting a formal proposal. Some funding agencies have specific guidelines regarding preapplication contact. These guidelines should be understood prior to initiating contact. The preliminary contact can be made through a telephone call, written communication, and/or personal visit. A phone call can be placed to determine the compatibility of the proposed project with the priorities of the funder, and to find out the appropriate contact person. Phone calls can also be used to follow up on any written communication and to make appointments for personal visits.

Written communication includes letters of intent, abstracts, and preliminary proposals. A letter of intent, required by some funders, generally contains a brief description of the proposed project in terms of its objectives and design, an estimated budget, and some information about the researchers. An abstract of the proposed research project is usually accompanied by a letter of transmittal containing information about the applicant, his or her institution, and the budgetary requirements. A preliminary proposal, also referred to as a concept paper, may be required by some funders. It is an outline of the proposed project or activity and consists of such elements as the project title, the name of the submitting organization, a need statement or a statement of the problem, and a statement of the objectives of the proposed project. The outline also includes a description of the anticipated methodology; a listing of available resources and personnel, including their roles; the benefits of the proposed project; the qualifications of the researchers and site; the support expected to be obtained; the estimated duration of the project; and a budget with an outline of estimated costs.

Personal visits should be preceded by adequate preparation as to their purpose and objectives. In addition to determining the potential match between the proposed project and the funding agency's target, the investigator may want to obtain the following additional pieces of information during the visit: (1) the amount of funding available for new projects (as opposed to those committed to continuing ones), (2) suggestions about what other agencies might be interested if the project proves to be inappropriate for the agency in question, and (3) other topics of interest to the funder.

Format

Most funding sources require the same basic information for a research proposal, although the details and required forms may vary. For examples, see Center for Scientific Review (2006), Coley and Scheinberg (2000), and Reif-Lehrer (2004). Appendix 4 provides a copy of the application forms for Public Health Service Grant PHS 398, which is the application mechanism for many NIH grants. Examples of private foundations that provide grants for health-related research include the Robert Wood Johnson Foundation and the Commonwealth Fund (see appropriate agency websites for grant application materials and online submission instructions). Whether an application form is provided or only sketchy instructions are given, the components of a well-written research proposal generally include the following elements: a title page, a table of contents, an abstract, a detailed project description, references, a detailed budget, a human subjects review, and appendices (see Table 3.2). If a grant research officer is available in the researcher's organization, that person's help and counsel should be sought before putting together a research proposal.

Table 3.2. Components of a research proposal

A. Title Page
B. Table of Contents
C. Abstract
D. Project Description
  1. Introduction
  2. Problem statement and significance
  3. Goals and objectives
  4. Methods and procedures
  5. Evaluation
  6. Dissemination
E. References
F. Budget and Justification
G. Human Subjects
H. Appendices

Title Page

The title page identifies the proposal and provides the endorsement of appropriate organizational (e.g., university) officials. Some funding agencies, for example, the National Science Foundation and the National Institutes of Health, have designed their own title pages. Whether or not an application form is provided, generally similar information is required, including: (1) the title of the project, (2) the name of the designated agency (i.e., funding source) to which the proposal is to be submitted, (3) the name, address, telephone number, and signature of the project director of the institution submitting the proposal, (4) the date of proposal submission, (5) the beginning and ending dates of the proposed funding period, (6) the total amount of funds requested (specify first-year request for multiyear project), (7) the total indirect cost, and (8) the name, address, and signature of the individual accepting responsibility for managing the funds and the designated endorsement of the institution.

Table of Contents

A table of contents may be available in the proposal application package. A brief proposal does not necessarily need a table of contents. A longer or more complex proposal generally requires one to assist reviewers in finding their way through the proposal. When included, the table of contents generally lists all major parts and divisions of the proposal.

Abstract

An abstract is a concise summary of the material presented in the proposal. Though it appears at the front of the proposal, it is written last. It should be clearly written, emphasizing the need for the project, its specific objectives, study design, evaluation methods, and significance. These materials are condensed to a page or less (often 200 to 300 words in length), although specific lengths are sometimes given in the proposal guidelines.

The abstract is important to the review process in several ways: (1) it offers the reviewer a quick introduction to the study and its expected significance; (2) it makes it easy for the reviewer to reference the nature of the study when the project comes up for discussion; and (3) it is sometimes the only part of the proposal that is read by those reviewing a panel's recommendation or the field readers' consensus (Miller and Salkind, 2002). Given how critical the abstract is, it is important that it be prepared with great care and that objectives and procedures are paraphrased using general but precise statements. Key concepts presented in the body of the proposal are highlighted in the abstract to alert the reviewer to them. Many funding decision makers may read only the review comments and the abstract.

Project Description

The project description, or the narrative section, is the main body of the proposal. the section on which the decision to accept or reject is typically based. In this section, the purpose is stated and defined, the conceptual framework and underlying premise are laid out, the methods for conducting the research are described, the procedures of evaluation are explained, and the schedule of dissemination is summarized. In writing the project description, the researcher should let the language of the proposal reflect his or her knowledge of the field, and make it understandable to the least knowledgeable of the anticipated reviewers. The major components of a project description will be discussed in greater detail later.

Reference

The reference section should include the literature cited in the proposal narrative. The number of references should not exceed the page limit, if any. Unless specified by the funding agency, any acceptable bibliographic methods may generally be used.

Research Budget

The research budget reflects, in financial terms, the activities developed in the proposal, specifying how the money will be spent. It documents the actual costs of achieving the objectives stated in the proposal. The total amount requested in the budget is determined by the needs of the project and the limitations set by the granting organization. Many major funding agencies have budget formats on computer templates. The funding agency should be contacted before developing the budget. A more detailed discussion of the budget section will follow later in this chapter. Even for a modest project, it is a good idea to spend some time anticipating the expenses involved: office supplies, photocopying, computer disks, telephone calls, transportation, and so on.

Human Subjects

In the preparation of a proposal, investigators must follow both the sponsor's and their own organization's requirements regarding human research subjects. The human subject review and approval procedures are mandated by federal statute/regulations and university policy. Violations can lead to loss of federal and perhaps nonfederal support. Specifically, all research involving human subjects must be approved by the organization's institutional human subjects review committee. This committee is established in accordance with federal law. Most funding agencies require evidence of institutional human subjects approval prior to making a grant award for a project involving human subjects. Appropriate forms and procedures for obtaining review/approval may be obtained from the committee.

The following is an example of questions included in a typical human subjects application form.

1. Who are your subjects?
   (Briefly outline your criteria for subject selection, including information regarding the number of subjects and their anticipated ages. If your study involves the use of abnormal subjects, explain any psychological or physical characteristics they will possess.)

2. How will your subjects be recruited?
   (Describe your procedures for finding subjects and obtaining informed consent.)

3. Is there a cost involved?
   (Does consenting to be a subject lead to additional costs in tests, medical care, for example, for the subject? If so, who is responsible for the costs?)

4. What are your procedures?
   (Outline what you will do to, or require of, your subjects. Who will be your data collectors, and what training will they have or require?)

5. What are the potential risks to the subjects?
   (In your estimation, do the explained procedures involve any potential risk to the subjects—physically, psychologically, socially, or legally? Could the type of data you are collecting from each subject possibly be construed as an invasion of privacy? If any of your procedures create potential risks for any of the subjects, describe other methods, if any, that were considered and why they will not be used, and present the precautions you plan to take to reduce the possibility of such risks.)

6. What deception may be used in your study?
   (If your research involves deceiving your subjects, explain how it will be handled.)

7. Who will benefit from this study?
   (What is the significance in this investigation of potential benefits to be gained by the subjects, persons similarly situated, the scientific community, and humankind in general.)

8. How will subjects' privacy be protected? (Establish procedures to safeguard each subject's rights with respect to the following: safety and security of the individual, as described in question 5; privacy and confidentiality, including protection and anonymity of data; embarrassment, discomfort, or harassment—would there be any stigma or repercussions from having participated in this study?)

The following provides instructions for specifying informed consent as part of the human subjects application form:

1. Provide a heading at the top of the page that indicates it is an informed consent form.

2. Explain the duration of the project, the procedures to be followed, and their purposes, including identification of any procedures that are experimental.

3. Provide evidence that the subject will be able to exercise free power of choice and that no element of coercion or constraint will be used in the obtaining of consent to participate. Also indicate that the subject is free to withdraw his or her consent and to discontinue participation in the project at any time without prejudice to the subject.

4. Describe any attendant discomforts and risks reasonably to be expected for each aspect of the study.

5. Describe the benefits that may reasonably be expected from participation in this study.

6. Include a statement of security of data (maintaining confidentiality), especially as it relates to specific individuals.

7. Include a statement on availability of compensation in the event of physical injury and how to obtain more information about this.

8. Offer to answer any inquiries concerning the procedures, and include a telephone number and address for the contact person.

9. Provide a place for the subject to sign and date the form.

10. Disclose any appropriate alternative procedures that might be advantageous for the subject.

11. Prominently located on the consent form must be a statement to the effect that the subject must be provided a copy of the consent form.

12. The informed consent form must be worded at the level of understanding of the subject.

13. No statements may be made to waive or appear to waive any of a subject's legal rights, including any release of the institution or its agents from liability for negligence.

Although not common in health services research, projects involving vertebrate animals or hazardous materials must also obtain special approval before the proposal is funded. An animal-use questionnaire should be completed concerning the use, procurement, and care of animals. Research involving potential hazards associated with the use of toxic materials, infectious organisms, or genetic recombination must be reviewed and approved by a committee on biosafety and hazardous waste.

Appendices

Appendices contain information that will strengthen the basic concepts developed in the narrative section of the proposal. They may be items that could have been put in the main body of the proposal but in the interest of conciseness are appended. Examples include expanded vitae, letters of support, lists of supportive data, publications, and so on.

Project Description

The project description, or the narrative portion of the proposal, is the most essential component of a research proposal. It consists of the following major elements: introduction, problem statement and significance, goals and objectives, methods and procedures, evaluation, and dissemination.

Introduction

An introduction section includes a brief summary of the problem of interest and the related subject. It should be clear to the layperson and give enough background to enable the reader to place the proposal in a context of common knowledge. What have other researchers concluded about this topic? What theories can be used to shed light on it and what are their major components? What relevant empirical research has been done previously? Are there consistent findings, or do past studies disagree? Are there limitations and gaps in the body of existing research that the proposed study can resolve? The introduction generally contains information showing what has been accomplished in the field, that the investigator is well acquainted with the past and current work and with the literature in the field, and that the proposed project will advance or add to the present store of knowledge in this field or be important to the solution of the problem.

Problem Statement and Significance

The problem statement and significance section describes the overall purpose of the project and its significance in meeting the funder's goals and objectives. Why is the topic worth studying? What is the practical significance of the proposed research? Does it contribute to improved understanding of health services delivery, problem solving, or the refinement of existing theories?

Goals and Objectives

In the goals and objectives section, the proposal presents a detailed description of the work to be undertaken. What exactly will be studied? Goals are general statements specifying the desired outcomes of the proposed project. Objectives are specific statements summarizing the proposed activities and including a detailed description of the outcomes and their assessment in measurable terms.

Methods and Procedures

The methods and procedures section is perhaps the most important part of the narrative portion of the proposal. In this section, the proposal describes in detail the general research plan, including research design, relevant theory and data sources, instruments to generate data and their validity, and analytical techniques or methods to be used.

If subjects are to be selected for study, the researcher, in order to collect data, needs to address who will be studied. The subjects should be identified both in general, theoretical terms and in specific, more concrete terms. The researcher should indicate who among the subjects is available for study and how they will be reached. Will it be appropriate to select a sample? If so, how will the researcher select the sample? If there is any possibility that the research will have an impact on those under study, how will the researcher ensure that they will not be harmed by the research?

In terms of measurement, what are the key variables in the study? How are they defined and measured? Are these definitions and measurement methods consistent with or different from those of previous research on this topic? It is usually appropriate to include a copy of the questionnaire (either self-developed or available in the literature) as an appendix to the proposal.

In terms of data collection methods, procedures used to collect the data for the study need to be described. Will an experiment or a survey be conducted? Will field research be undertaken, or will available data already collected by others be reanalyzed?

In terms of data analysis, the kind of analysis to be conducted should be described (e.g., multiple regression or factor analysis), and the variables to be included in each model should be specified. The purpose and logic of the analysis should be spelled out. The analysis should address research hypotheses or questions.

The researcher is often required to provide a schedule for the various stages of research, which includes time estimates for major activities to be conducted. For grant reviewers, a schedule or timeline of activities serves as a measure of the completeness and timeliness of research activities. For the investigator, it is a chronological checklist of the progress of research. Without a timeline, the researcher might not be aware when a project runs behind schedule.

Evaluation

The evaluation section describes the plan for assessing the ongoing progress toward achieving the research objectives. The plan specifies how each project activity is to be measured in terms of completion, the timeline for its completion, and the conditions and mechanisms for revising program activities. A good evaluation plan enables both the investigators and the funder to monitor project progress and provide timely feedback for project modifications or adjustments.

Dissemination

Some funding sources require a dissemination plan to be included in a proposal. The dissemination section indicates research findings will be made available to others, particularly those interested in the study outcomes. Dissemination provides research results to regional, national, or international audiences.

Researchers must recognize that grants and contracts have two different sets of rules with respect to publication. The grant usually carries the right of publication by investigators. Grantees generally encourage publication and distribution of the results of research. Under contract research, investigators may be restricted in terms of publishing their contracted research. The funding agency may be only interested in receiving reports that fit the specifications of its internal needs. Investigators should negotiate with the funding agency on publication rights prior to submitting papers for professional publication.

Budget

Typically, a proposal budget reflects direct and indirect costs. Direct costs incurred by grant activities fall within the following categories: personnel, supplies, equipment, travel, communications, publications, subcontracts, consultants, and other costs (those not included in previous categories such as computer time, service contracts, and so on). Figure 3.1 shows a sample budget for a research proposal.

Personnel

Personnel costs include salaries and wages of all investigators, research assistants, and staff who will be working full time or part time on the project. All key personnel (e.g., investigators) who will participate in the proposed project should be identified by name, title, and the expected amount of time to be devoted to the project. The names of supporting personnel (e.g., graduate assistants) generally are not necessary. Unfilled positions may be marked "vacant" or "to be selected." If the individuals involved have exceptional qualifications that would merit consideration in the evaluation of the proposal, this information should be included in budget justification. Federal grants and contracts will not allow salaried personnel to be paid for overtime (i.e., extra compensation beyond the monthly rate) unless this is specifically stated in the proposal and awarded in the grant. The fringe benefit rate associated with various types of employment can be found out from the benefits office or sponsored program office of the employing agency. These percentages may change frequently.

Expendable Supplies

Expendable or consumable supplies include office supplies, computer supplies, chemicals, and educational materials. Supplies and their costs may be listed

DETAILED BUDGET FOR INITIAL BUDGET PERIOD
DIRECT COSTS ONLY

				FROM 95/10/01	THROUGH 96/09/30		
					DOLLAR AMOUNT REQUESTED (omit cents)		
NAME	ROLE ON PROJECT	TYPE APPT. (months)	% EFFORT ON PROJ.	INST. BASE SALARY	SALARY REQUESTED	FRINGE BENEFITS	TOTALS
PERSONNEL (Applicant Organization Only)							
Scientist 1	Principal Investigator	12	20	$60,955	$12,191	$2,213	$14,404
Scientist 2	Co-investigator	12	25	$38,000	$9,500	$2,174	$11,674
Scientist 3	Co-investigator	12	25	$40,000	$10,000	$2,265	$12,265
Scientist 4	Investigator	12	15	$32,000	$4,800	$871	$5,671
GA 1		12	100	$15,000	$15,000	$90	$15,090
GA 2		12	100	$15,000	$15,000	$4,500	$19,500
				SUBTOTALS	$66,491	$12,113	$78,604
CONSULTANT COSTS							
Scientist 5				$5,000			$5,000
EQUIPMENT (Itemize)							
Computer 1				$2,000			
Computer 2				$3,500			$5,500
SUPPLIES (Itemize by category)							
Postage				$500			$500
TRAVEL				$2,000			$2,000
PATIENT CARE COSTS	INPATIENT						$0
	OUTPATIENT						$0
ALTERATIONS AND RENOVATIONS (Itemize by category)							$0
OTHER EXPENSES (Itemize by category)							
Photocopying				$1,000			
Subcontracting	$21,000 (3 × $7,000)						$22,000
SUBTOTAL DIRECT COSTS FOR INITIAL BUDGET PERIOD							**$113,604**
CONSORTIUM/CONTRACTUAL COSTS							
	DIRECT COSTS			$0			
	INDIRECT COSTS			$0		TOTAL	$0
TOTAL DIRECT COSTS FOR INITIAL BUDGET PERIOD (Item 7a, Face Page)							**$113,604**

PHS 398 (Rev 9/91)   (Form Page 4) Page _____   DD

Number pages consecutively at the bottom throughout the application. Do not use suffixes such as 3a, 3b.

Figure 3.1. Example of a research proposal budget

under one general heading or by category. In the budget justification section, the investigator may explain why these supplies are needed for the project.

Equipment

Both the unit and total costs of equipment should be specified. Equipment is usually defined as a property with an acquisition cost of $500 or more and an expected service life of two or more years. Some funding agencies have restrictions on equipment purchases. Check the proposal guidelines for specific rules and definitions for equipment. When developing the budget for the acquisition of expensive equipment, investigators should remember to add their state's sales tax to the vendor's quoted purchase price.

Travel

The total cost of project-related travel is summarized in the budget. The detailed breakdown of travel and its justification is provided in the budget justification section. A travel description includes mode, frequency, and cost of travel. Justification includes the travel purpose and its relation to project objectives. Many funding sources do not allow foreign travel. The investigator should contact the potential funding source to determine its travel regulations.

Communications

This category usually includes postage, telephone, telegram, messenger, and fax charges associated with a project. If funding sources do not have a category for communications, such charges could be properly placed in the "other direct costs" category.

Publications

The costs incurred for preparing and publishing the results of the research are specified. Examples include technical reports, reprints, manuscripts, and illustrations such as artwork, graphics, photography, slides, and overheads.

Subcontract Costs

The guidelines of the potential funding agency should be checked carefully for information related to subcontracting. Usually, a subcontract proposal endorsed by the submitting agency along with a complete budget should be included in the primary proposal.

Consultant Services

The budget identifies each consultant, his or her primary organizational affiliation, compensation rate, and number of days or percent of time expected to serve. The justification section emphasizes each consultant's expertise and expected role in the project.

Other Direct Costs

Other direct costs consist of all items that do not fit into any other direct cost category, including payment to human subjects, copying fees, service charges, repair and maintenance contracts on major equipment, and computer time. These categories may be itemized by unit and total cost.

Indirect costs, or overhead, are those costs incurred in the support and management of the proposed activities that cannot be readily determined by direct measurement. Examples include: (1) general administrative costs such as accounting, personnel, and administrative functions at both central and unit levels, (2) operation and maintenance including utilities and janitorial services, and (3) depreciation and use allowance. Many research institutions (such as universities) have negotiated indirect cost rates with the federal government or private foundations. These rates apply unless an agency or program specifically stipulates another. Indirect cost rates change from time to time. It is advisable to check with the grants management office before calculating indirect costs.

In addition to direct and indirect costs, some funding agencies require that grantee institutions commit to share the overall costs of a sponsored program and display the institution's share of the project in the proposal budget. Check the announcement for cost-share requirements and methods.

Justification

The budget is followed by a justification section in which any unusual costs associated with the proposed project are justified. If the proposal narrative is well developed, explaining in detail the activities and anticipated objectives, the justification can be easily related to these activities. In addition, items such as annual salary increases, equipment costs, unusually high supply or travel costs, and stipend costs should be included. The researcher needs to secure the going wage rates for many budget items, such as interviewers, cost of transportation, mainframe computer usage, and so on. A checklist for common budget items follows:

Personnel

- salaries and wages for academic personnel during the academic year and during the summer
- research associates
- research assistants
- technicians
- secretarial staff
- hourly help
- fringe benefits
- consultants
- fees

- domestic travel
- foreign travel

Equipment

- installation and freight
- equipment rental

Communications

- telephone and telegraph
- photocopying
- postage

Supplies

- chemicals and glassware
- animals and animal supplies
- office supplies
- alterations and renovation

Other Costs

- subcontracts
- training
- publication of reports
- data processing

A common practical mistake in research proposals is to grossly underestimate the budget, both in time and money. Most underestimates can be attributed to inexperience. However, the less promising funding climate for research also contributes to inadequate budget requests. Unfortunately, a project with an inadequate budget is unlikely to be completed successfully.

Appendices

The appendices section includes important documentation that enhances the competitiveness of the research proposal. Examples include letters of support or endorsement, vitae, descriptions of relevant institutional resources, and a list of references.

Letters of support or endorsement are solicited from elected officials and other organizations and individuals either required by a funding source or on the basis that their support would be essential or helpful to a funding decision. In general, letters should be addressed to the investigator's organization and sent to the investigator for submission along with the proposal. Letters should not be sent under separate cover to the funding source because they may not get there in time or may not be filed appropriately with the investigator's proposal. Some funding sources may not accept documents submitted separately. To speed up the process of securing a letter of support and to ensure inclusion of key information, the investigator may prepare a draft letter and fax it to the potential signee. Telephone discussions that summarize project ideas often do not get heard exactly as investigators think they have transmitted them.

Most sponsoring agencies require a curriculum vita and list of publications for each member of the project. Curriculum vitae may also be placed in the appendices. Vitae should be updated and current. If possible, the same format should be used. A two-page summary should be prepared highlighting important experience and publication information in the vitae.

Relevant institutional resources may be included in the appendices. Available facilities and major items of equipment especially adapted to the proposed project should be described. These facilities could include libraries, computer centers, other recognized centers, and any special but relevant equipment.

A list of references is desirable when the proposal contains 10 or more references. Otherwise, unless specifically required, references may be inserted in the text as footnotes.

Proposal Review Process

Understanding the review process helps the researcher write a more fundable grant application. Researchers need to be aware of the review process and time lapses of funding agencies. This information may be obtained in the visit if not already included in the application package. Since much of health services research is funded by the National Institutes of Health (NIH), we summarize the major components of the NIH review process here (Reif-Lehrer, 2004). Researchers should be aware the information provided below may not be entirely relevant in their situations.

A grant proposal to the NIH is prepared by a principal investigator (PI) and submitted by his or her sponsoring institution to the NIH. The proposal is received at the NIH by the Division of Research Grants (DRG), which is the advisory group to the NIH and sets up study sections (both standing and, when necessary, ad hoc) to review research grant proposals (RO1), Research Career Development Awards (RCDA), first awards, and fellowship applications (NRSA). Knowledgeable investigators can suggest an initial review group they think would be appropriate for their applications. The final decision is made by the DRG.

At the institute, the application is assigned to a health scientist-administrator (HSA), who acts as the primary institute contact for the applicant before, during, and after the review process. That person is also responsible for grant administration if the application is funded. The NIH has a dual peer review system. The first level of review is by an initial review group (IRG), often referred to as a study section. The second level of review is by an advisory council. The decision to award a proposal is based on both scientific merit (judged by the study section) and program considerations (judged by the advisory council).

In the first level of review, the study section is composed of scientists who represent different geographical areas and a wide range of expertise. The study section provides initial scientific review of grant applications, assigns a priority score based on scientific merit, and makes budget recommendations. The role of the study section is only advisory. It does not make funding decisions, which are the prerogative of each institute under the NIH.

The primary and secondary reviewers come to the study section review meeting with written critiques of the assigned grant proposals. The critiques focus on the proposal's scientific and technical merit, originality, and methodology or research design; examine the qualifications and experience (or potential, in the case of a new applicant) of the investigators; and assess the availability of resources, the appropriateness of the budget and timeline, and ethical issues (e.g., human subjects). The following lists some commonly used proposal review questions:

- Are research aims logical?
- Is the background or literature review adequate?
- Is there preliminary work or prior relevant experience?
- Are the hypotheses appropriate, relevant to aims and procedures, and testable?
- Are the data adequate?
- Is the instrument reliable and valid (having been previously tested)?
- Is the sample sufficiently large and representative to allow inference to be drawn for the entire population?
- Are the analysis methods adequate to the data elements?
- Are potential contributions feasible, creative, and significant?
- Are the budget and time adequate and justified?
- Are the limitations pointed out and their improvement discussed?

At the study section meeting, the primary and secondary reviewers present the critiques of their assigned proposals. A general discussion among all study section members follows, including asking further questions about, or reanalyzing certain portions of, the proposals. After the discussion, a recommendation is made by majority vote for (1) approval, (2) disapproval, or (3) deferral for additional information. The budget is then discussed in terms of appropriateness. For each approved proposal, all study section members then vote through secret ballot using a numerical score based on a scale of 0.1 increments from 1.0 (the best score) to 5.0 (the worst score). A recommendation for a site visit may be made by the primary reviewer or the executive secretary of the study section who recognizes the need for additional information that cannot be obtained by mail or telephone.

After the study section meeting, the scores assigned by individual members for each approved proposal are averaged and multiplied by 100 to provide a three-digit rating known as a priority score. The executive secretary prepares a summary statement (often called "the pink sheets") based on the primary and secondary reviewers' reports and the discussion at the study section meeting.

The summary statement is later sent to the principal investigator. The grant application is then forwarded to the advisory council for further review.

The second level of review is conducted by a national advisory council within each individual institute. The council reviews the summary statements of all approved applications from each study section, together with the proposals, and adds its own review based on judgments of both scientific merit and relevance to the program goals of the assigned institute. The executive secretary of a study section attends the council meeting when an application reviewed in his or her section is discussed. The council then makes recommendations on funding to the institute staff. It may concur with or modify study section action on grant applications or defer for further review.

ORGANIZATIONAL AND ADMINISTRATIVE ISSUES

Another important preparation for research has to do with organizational and administrative issues related to the conduct of research. Before research can be started, researchers need to determine the organization and management of research work. In general, larger projects will have more formal arrangements than smaller studies. There are three main options for the organization of a research team. The first option is the hierarchically organized research team, in which the status of lead researchers is clearly stated and the (sometimes narrow) roles for research assistants and other members of the team are well defined. The second option is the research team of formal equals, which is often used for multidisciplinary studies. Here there is a need to draw on the different and complementary expertise of a number of people. The third option is the collaborative research team, which draws together members from different institutions who will often have somewhat different interests in the project and different contributions to make.

Regardless of how a research team is formed, it should include people with substantive, methodological, and analytical knowledge and experience related to the research topic. Substantive knowledge ensures study validity, for example, as to whether the most relevant measures of outcome are being collected. Methodological knowledge ensures that the study design is adequate for the topic and that the results can be used to generalize to the population of interest. The wording and ordering of questions may also be better arranged to improve data quality. Analytical knowledge ensures appropriate use of statistical methods to address research questions or hypotheses. The response format and coding scheme should be designed to allow maximum and flexible data analysis. A collaborative research team that combines the knowledge and experience of all those involved can turn out a better research product.

However, members of a research team can bring both problem-solving and problem-generating capacities (Grady and Wallston, 1988). Problems can arise because people have different research styles and work habits, in addition to differences in thinking. To reduce possible confusion, conflicts, and disputes during project implementation, the roles of members of the research team should be clearly specified. Team members should know what their roles are and how they fit into the overall research project.

In funded research, one person is designated as the principal investigator (PI) and is responsible for both the scientific and financial aspects of the research. Coinvestigators or investigators are those who participate in specific aspects of the project. Research associates or assistants are assigned to investigators to assist in carrying out research activities. Prior to the conduct of research, investigators should reach an agreement, in writing, on individual responsibilities, time frame to complete specific tasks, publication credit and authorship, ways to deal with unexpected events or resolve disputes, and other issues of mutual interest.

The important aspect to note is to work out all foreseeable sources of conflict in advance. A research team that carries out its activities based on individual assumptions rather than specified and agreed-upon roles will likely run into problems, adversely affecting both the research project and the interrelations among investigators.

Researchers must also think through any problems that might arise concerning access to key informants, organizations, or information. If funding needs to be sought, questions of access need to be resolved before a proposal is presented to a funding body. If the research design depends crucially on having access to key informants, organizations, sources of information, sampling frames, official statistics, and the like, it is premature to develop a research proposal for funding without obtaining the consent or active support of potential collaborators or checking the feasibility in relation to such access issues.

Obtaining access often depends on the presentation of a study design that is meaningful and interesting to those concerned. It is usually necessary to provide a separate, shorter outline of the study for this purpose, quite different from the main proposal, focusing on the issues and questions addressed and their relevancy to the collaborators rather than on the methods and data collection techniques to be used. Researchers should actively seek input from potential collaborators who may be able to make suggestions about the study design, its conduct, and practical difficulties that could not have been foreseen.

Other practical details to be attended to prior to carrying out research include: negotiating with the funding agency to work out a protocol; getting familiar with the research site; determining the level of staff support and services needed; reallocating the budget to fit with the actual situation of project implementation (including preparing a research budget that may contain subcontracts for needed services such as sampling, interviewing, or data processing); finalizing the research plan with collaborators: recruiting personnel; identifying supplies and logistics; revising or updating the timetable or schedule of research activities; training staff for data collection, processing, and analysis; conducting a human subjects review; revising the data collection instrument; and pilot-testing the instrument. Careful preparation of these activities will facilitate the smooth progress of the research process.

SUMMARY

During the groundwork stage of HSR, researchers identify relevant data and funding sources, develop research proposals, and prepare organizationally and administratively to carry out the research. A rich body of data collected periodically by federal agencies, principally the National Center for Health Statistics, is available for secondary health services research. Notable examples are the National Health Interview Survey, the National Ambulatory Medical Care Survey, the National Hospital Discharge Survey, and the Medical Expenditure Panel Survey. The various institutes under the National Institutes of Health and major private foundations are the principal funders of health services research. An important step toward seeking funding for research is a well-written proposal that matches the funding purpose and level of the funder. Knowledge about preliminary research and preparation and about how grant proposals are reviewed will help the researcher compose the right proposal and improve the chances of getting funded.

REVIEW QUESTIONS

1. What are the major national-level data sources suitable for health services research? Describe the major features of these data sources.
2. Become familiar with the funding sources most likely to support the research topics of your interest. What are their requirements and restrictions?
3. Identify the major steps in a research proposal. As an exercise, write a research proposal on a topic of interest to you.
4. What is the research review process of the National Institutes of Health?
5. What are the organizational and administrative issues related to research?

REFERENCES

Annual Register of Grant Support: A Dictionary of Funding Sources (40th ed.). (2007). Medford, NJ: Information Today.

Center for Scientific Review: National Institutes of Health. (2006, April). Public Health Service Grant PHS 398: OMB No. 0925-0001. Bethesda, MD: U.S. Department of Health and Human Services.

Coley, S. M., and Scheinberg, C. A. (2000). Proposal Writing. Thousand Oaks, CA: Sage.

Grady, K. E., and Wallston, B. S. (1988). Research in Health Care Settings. Newbury Park, CA: Sage.

Miller, D. C., and Salkind, N. J. (2002). Handbook of Research Design and Social Measurement (6th ed.). Thousand Oaks, CA: Sage.

National Health Survey Act. (1956). U.S. Public Law 652. 84th Congress, 2d session, S 3076.

Reif-Lehrer, L. (2004). Grant Application Writer's Handbook (4th ed.). Boston, MA: Jones and Bartlett.

CHAPTER 4

Research Review

KEY TERMS

effect size
integrative review
MEDLINE

meta-analysis
methodological review
policy-oriented review

research review
theoretical review

LEARNING OBJECTIVES

- To understand the types of research review and their purposes.
- To describe the process of research review.
- To identify the general categories of information likely to be focused on in research review.

- To become familiar with commonly used computer-based abstracting and indexing services.
- To comprehend the purpose of meta-analysis and its commonly used procedures.

As described in Chapter 1, scientific inquiry is a cumulative process, with each study built on previous, related investigations. By reviewing what previous studies have accomplished and what mistakes have been made, researchers gain a comprehensive, integrated picture of the topic under investigation. Such accomplishment is particularly important today because of the huge amount of HSR already conducted. Indeed, systematic and objective research reviews may become an independent research project yielding substantial information in its own right. This is especially the case as HSR becomes more specialized, and time constraints make it nearly impossible for most researchers to keep abreast of the state of the art of all HSR topics.

This chapter introduces the method of research review with particular emphasis on its process. In addition, its strengths and weaknesses will be summarized.

DEFINITION

Research review provides a synthesis of existing knowledge on a specific question, based on an assessment of all relevant empirical research that can be found. Good research reviews are multidisciplinary in that relevant studies from all related social science disciplines are covered, although research focuses differ across disciplines.

There are at least three uses of research review. Literature review is commonly part of the ground-clearing and preparatory work undertaken in the initial stages of empirical research. It guides the formulation of research questions or hypotheses, the design of the study, and the analysis used.

Literature review is also the initial part of the research product, appearing as the introduction in a report on empirical research (Harper, Weins, and Matarazzo, 1978). When used in this capacity, literature review has a narrow scope, typically restricted to those studies pertinent to the specific issue addressed by the primary research.

Literature review may also appear as an independent research product serving different purposes (Cooper, 1989a, 1989b). For example, reviews can focus on research methods, theories, outcomes, or prior accomplishments; criticize previous works; build bridges between related areas; or identify central issues in a field.

Four independent research reviews may be identified: the integrative research review, theoretical review, methodological review, and policy-oriented review. The **integrative review**, by far the most frequently used, summarizes past research by drawing conclusions from many separate studies addressing similar or related hypotheses or research questions (Cooper, 1982). The reviewer aims to accomplish such objectives as presenting the state of knowledge on the topic under review, highlighting issues previous researchers have left unresolved or unstudied, and directing future research so that it is built on cumulative inquiry.

Theoretical review summarizes all the existing relevant theories used to explain a particular topic and examines them in terms of major content areas, similarities, differences, and accuracy in prediction. Theoretical review provides a detailed summary of the theories and findings based on which theories were developed or tested, assesses which theories are more powerful and consistent with known findings, and refines theories by reformulating or integrating concepts from existing theories.

Methodological review summarizes the different research designs used to study a particular topic and compares studies using the range of designs with regard to their findings. The purpose is to identify the strengths and weaknesses of the existing designs for a particular topic and explain to what extent differences in findings are the results of differences in design.

Policy-oriented review summarizes current knowledge of a topic so as to draw out the policy implications of study findings. Such review requires knowledge of the major policy issues and debates, as well as common research expertise.

It is possible that a comprehensive review will address several issues. For example, integrative review may cover policy impact, designs, and relevant theories, in addition to major findings. Theoretical review may also contain some integrative review components.

PROCESS

Research review is a familiar process to most health services researchers. The common practice of literature review has been idiosyncratic, relying on the intuitive, subjective, and narrative styles of the researcher, leaving room for partial or selective coverage. Different researchers studying the same topic may review entirely different sets of studies without describing the selection procedures or identifying the studies that are excluded. Subjectivity in selecting, analyzing, and interpreting studies has led to skepticism about the conclusions of many reviews. Because of the great amounts of HSR conducted by diverse organizations in numerous locations, the comprehensiveness and validity of literature reviews cannot be taken for granted. Indeed, differences in review approaches create variations in review conclusions and present a threat to the review's validity.

This section presents an alternative research review process that is more systematic and objective. Specifically, it details an integrated five-step process: identifying the topic, preparing a coding sheet, searching for research publications, synthesizing research publications, and reporting previous research on the selected topic. Adopting these procedures will make research review systematic and thus replicable, satisfying an important principle of scientific inquiry.

Identifying the Topic

Similar to empirical research, research review starts with topic identification. The choice of a topic for review is influenced by the interests of the researcher and the research community. In addition, the topic should have appeared in the literature for some time. A topic is probably not suitable for independent review unless there is sufficient research activity surrounding it. Similar to empirical research, the identification of a topic is also influenced by the literature review process. Researchers may encounter additional relevant elements of a topic that they had not initially identified.

To assist topic identification, researchers may conduct a preliminary review of a dozen or so representative works on the topic. Such a process enables them to ascertain the scope of research related to the topic, identify all needed information for the review, and further refine the topic. Generally, researchers should adopt a broader rather than narrower definition of their topic so that worthy studies are not overlooked. If a topic has a long history within a discipline, it is likely that relevant reviews of the topic have already been conducted. These past reviews should be previewed early in the process since doing so serves a number of purposes. Past reviews enable investigators to identify relevant bibliographies. Studying previous reviews is also consistent with the cumulative nature of scientific inquiry. Researchers will gain a better sense of the scope of previous research from past reviews rather than from individual studies. Past reviews also establish the necessity of new ones. If the topic has been recently reexamined and the approach of review was appropriate, there may be little value in undertaking another one. On the other hand, if previous reviews were conducted many years ago and many recent studies were not included, or the methodology employed was problematic, researchers will have added incentive to conduct a more current and improved review. Past reviews, thus, become the stepping stones for the new review.

Preparing a Coding Sheet

Once the topic is identified and refined, the next step is to construct a coding sheet for collecting relevant information from articles to be reviewed. The preparation of a coding sheet is all the more necessary if there are a vast number of studies to be reviewed. A coding sheet enables the researcher to collect all needed information during the first reading so that the time-consuming practice of rereading is avoided. The preparation of a coding sheet is also useful even for a relatively small number of studies because the information collected will assist the investigator in analyzing and reporting those studies.

The information to be collected in the coding sheet should be determined based on the preliminary review and the strategy to be adopted in analyzing and synthesizing studies (refer to the "Synthesizing Research Publications" section in this chapter for details). Generally, any information to be analyzed and used in the review should be collected. It is better to collect too much than too little information, because the time spent in collecting additional information during the first reading is significantly less than if the researcher were to go back later to retrieve new information.

Figure 4.1 shows the general categories of information related to empirical research in which an investigator is likely to be interested. The categories include a study's background, design, measurement, and outcome characteristics. In the background category, source indicates the media or information channel from which a study is retrieved. In the design category, it is possible that the general

1. Background Information
Source _____
Author(s) _____
Title _____
Journal _____ Volume _____ Pages _____
Year _____

2. Design Information
Primary/Secondary study _____
Random/Nonrandom _____
Control/No control _____
Matching/Statistical control _____
Pretest/No pretest _____
Type(s) of intervention _____
Population _____
Sample size _____
Response rate _____
Sample characteristics _____
Sample representativeness _____
Sampling biases _____
Other _____

3. Measurement Information
Research question or hypothesis _____
Dependent variable(s) _____
Independent variable(s) _____
Validity of measures _____
Reliability of measures _____
Statistical measures _____
Model specifications _____

4. Outcome Information
Hypothesis supported or refuted _____
Significant independent variable(s) _____
Insignificant independent varible(s) _____
R^2 _____

Figure 4.1. Research review coding sheet for items of general interest

categorization as presented will not be sufficient. Researchers may then include additional design characteristics (for example, whether there were any restrictions on the types of individuals sampled in the original study, when and where the study was conducted, and whether time-series or longitudinal designs were used). In the measurement category, investigators may document the use of particular scales, available instruments, and specific features of the analytic models (e.g., number of variables used, types of measures implemented for the same construct, and tests of interaction terms and nonlinearity). In the outcome category, if more quantitative analysis is envisioned, more precise statistical information related to study results may be recorded. Examples are means, standard deviations, sample sizes for each comparison group (to be used for effect size calculation), association between variables (e.g., correlation coefficient), values of inferential test statistics (e.g., c^2, t ratio, F ratio), and the strength of a model (e.g., regression R^2).

It bears reemphasizing that the construction of a coding sheet is the result of, rather than a prelude to, preliminary review. The development of a coding sheet forces researchers to think ahead about the review and analysis strategy and to be precise in their thinking. The first draft of the coding sheet can then be used to pilot-test some additional reports. If coders other than the researcher are involved, they need to be trained to comprehend and retrieve the relevant information. In the pilot test, different coders may be asked to code the same reports. Their differences in coding may identify ambiguities in the wording. The revised coding sheet may be sent for further comment to experts or colleagues knowledgeable about the topic. Researchers need not be alarmed if the completed coding sheets contain many blank spaces. This is an indication that the studies may not report everything researchers intend to find out.

Searching for Research Publications

Similar to empirical research, research reviews need to specify the target population from which studies are selected. The typical target population for research reviews is all previous investigations conducted on the topic. However, not all previous studies may be accessible because some research reports either are hard to locate or would be too costly and time consuming to retrieve. Researchers may re-specify the target once the search is complete. At a minimum, sources from which studies are retrieved should be delineated, as should the scope of the search.

In general, there are four major sources of literature for reviewers to retrieve: (1) books; (2) journals, including professional journals, published newsletters, magazines, and newspapers; (3) theses, including doctoral, master's, and bachelor's theses; and (4) unpublished work, including monographs, technical reports, grant proposals, conference papers, personal manuscripts, and other unpublished materials (Rosenthal, 1991).

The ability to gain access to HSR studies has improved in the past decade. In particular, retrieval of past research work has been facilitated by prominent national databases and computerized literature search. Among the many ways to search for reports of previously conducted studies, the most efficient method is perhaps the use of computer-based abstracting and indexing services. A brief description of some of the most frequently used abstracting and indexing services in HSR follows.

The most common online abstracting service is called MEDLARS (Medical Literature Analysis and Retrieval System), compiled by the National Library of Medicine (NLM) (2006b) for more than 100 years. The abstracting service became computerized in the early 1960s and has since served as a major source of bibliographic searches for health professionals. Within MEDLARS, users have access to a host of specialized databases in the fields of biomedicine, health administration, cancer, population studies, medical ethics, and more. Over the years, MEDLARS has come to represent a family of databases of which **MEDLINE** is the most well known. MEDLINE is the world's leading bibliographic database of medical information, covering more than 4,800 journals since 1966 and containing information found in the publications *Index Medicus, International Nursing Index,* and *Index to Dental Literature.* MEDLINE is the largest component of PubMed, which also includes OLDMEDLINE (for pre-1966 citations) and some life science journals. PubMed also includes citations from journals related to HSR. Other National Library of Medicine websites containing HSR-relevant materials include LocatorPlus (http://locatorplus.gov), which contains citations for books, book chapters, technical reports, and conference papers; and the NLM Gateway (http://gateway.nlm.nih.gov), which includes meeting abstracts from AcademyHealth, Health Technology Assessment International, and the Cochrane Colloquium annual conferences. MEDLINE contains abstracts of articles published by the most common U.S. and international journals on medicine and health services.

Searching for literature using MEDLINE requires a familiarity with the use of MeSH terms. MeSH stands for "Medical Subject Headings," and is the NLM's self-described "vocabulary thesaurus" (National Library of Medicine, 2006a). Each article in MEDLINE is associated with a set of MeSH terms that describes the content of the article. MeSH terms range from very broad levels (e.g., "anatomy") to very specific levels (e.g., "ankle"). Searching MEDLINE using the most appropriate MeSH terms for your topic considerably simplifies and streamlines the literature review process. The MeSH website (http://www.nlm.nih.gov/mesh) provides advice and strategies for using MeSH to its full advantage. Table 4.1 displays examples of commonly used MeSH terms related to HSR.

The *Hospital Literature Index*, published until 2000 by the American Hospital Association, provided the primary guide to literature on hospital and other health care facility administration, including multi-institutional systems, nursing homes and skilled nursing facilities, health maintenance organizations and other group practice facilities, freestanding facilities (e.g., surgicenters and emergicenters), health care centers of all types (e.g., academic, community, and mental health), rehabilitation centers, hospices, mobile health units, homes for the aged, and university student inpatient facilities (American Hospital Association Resource Center, 1994). The *Index* covered the organization and administration, economics, laws and regulations, policy, and planning aspects of health care delivery. It was published quarterly, in print form, between 1945 and 2000. Currently, the literature formerly included in the *Index* is cataloged by the National Library of Medicine and contained within PubMed.

Public Health, Social Medicine and Epidemiology contains such topics as biostatistics and biometrics, health care (health education and promotion, professional education, and medical practice), epidemiology, screening and prevention, populations at risk (maternal and child health, aging and old age, and occupational health), food and nutrition, lifestyles (alcohol, smoking, drugs,

Table 4.1. Selected MeSH terms used in health services research

Health	Health behavior	Health benefits plan, employee
Health care costs	Health care rationing	Health care reform
Health education	Health expenditures	Health facilities
Health facilities, proprietary	Health facilities	Health facility closure
Health facility environment	Health facility administrators	Health facility moving
Health facility planning	Health facility merger	Health fairs
Health maintenance organizations	Health facility size	Health occupations
Health personnel	Health manpower	Health planning
Health planning guidelines	Health plan implementation	Health planning support
Health planning technical assistance	Health planning organizations	Health priorities
Health promotion	Health policy	Health resources
Health services	Health resorts	Health services for the aged
Health services, indigenous	Health services accessibility	Health services, needs and demands
Health services research	Health services, misuse	Health status indicators
Health surveys	Health status	Health systems plans
Hospital administration	Health systems agencies	Hospital auxiliaries
Hospital bed capacity	Hospital administrators	Hospital communication systems
Hospital costs	Hospital charges	Hospital design and construction
Hospital distribution systems	Hospital departments	Hospital mortality
Hospital patient relations	Hospital information systems	Hospital planning
Hospital records	Hospital–physician joint ventures	Hospital shared services
Hospital shops	Hospital restructuring	Hospital volunteers
Hospitalization	Hospital units	Hospitals, chronic disease
Hospitals	Hospitals	Hospitals, county
Hospitals, community	Hospitals, convalescent	Hospitals, general
Hospitals, district	Hospitals, federal	Hospitals, military
Hospitals, group practice	Hospitals, maternity	Hospitals, packaged
Hospitals, municipal	Hospitals, osteopathic	Hospitals, proprietary
Hospitals, pediatric	Hospitals, private	Hospitals, religious
Hospitals, psychiatric	Hospitals, public	Hospitals, special
Hospitals, rural	Hospitals, satellite	Hospitals, university
Hospitals, state	Hospitals, teaching	Hospitals, voluntary
Hospitals, urban	Hospitals, veterans	

health behavior, sexual and social behavior, and life events), and evaluation of intervention. The *Abstract* is prepared by the International Medical Abstracting Service (Excerpta Medica, P.O. Box 548, 1000 AM Amsterdam, the Netherlands). *Public Health, Social Medicine and Epidemiology* is now also available via Elsevier (http://www.elsevier.com/wps/find/journaldescription .cws_home/505986/description#description).

National Technical Information Service (NTIS) Health Collection covers such areas as community and population characteristics, data and information systems, economics and sociology, environmental and occupational factors, health care delivery organization and administration, measurement methodology, needs and demands, technology, delivery plans, projects and studies, education and personnel training, and health-related costs, resources, and services. This publication is prepared by the National Technical Information Service, U.S. Department of Commerce, Technology Administration (Springfield, VA 22161; 703-467-4650). The NTIS Health Collection is now also available online (http://www.ntis.gov/products/families/health.asp?loc=4-3-3).

The federal government, through its many agencies, also publishes numerous research reports and bibliographies. Most government documents are printed by the U.S. Government Printing Office, which issues a monthly catalog indexing recently published documents. The publication *Guide to U.S. Government Publications* provides an excellent introduction to potential reviewers. State governments have likewise published many research works that may be obtained from libraries or state agencies. The 2005 edition of *Guide to U.S. Government Publications* was published by Gale (P.O. Box 9187, Farmington Hills, MI 48333-9187).

There are also many abstracting services that focus on general social science disciplines rather than exclusively on health. Many relevant HSR publications may be retrieved from these popular sources. For example, the *Social Sciences Citation Index* covers 50 different social science disciplines and carries more than 1,500 journals. It categorizes studies based on the work cited in them as well as their topical focus. Thus, reviewers can retrieve studies that cite principal researchers in an area and screen them for topic relevance. *Social Sciences Citation Index* is available online via the Web of Science (http://www.isinet.com/products/citation/ssci). *Psychological Abstracts* is frequently used in the behavioral sciences. Published monthly, the abstracts are generally written by authors of the articles themselves, although indexing terms are applied by the staff. All psychology-related journals are covered. *Psychological Abstracts* is included in the online database PsycINFO (http://www.apa.org/psycinfo). *Dissertation Abstracts International* focuses exclusively on abstracts of dissertations regardless of discipline. Table 4.2 displays a range of medical and health services–related search engines.

Although abstracting and indexing services are the major sources for literature searching, they are by no means the only ones used. Browsing through library shelves, obtaining topical bibliographies compiled by others, and making formal requests of scholars active in the field are some of the other methods of obtaining literature relevant to the topic at hand. Some circumstances require consultation with a librarian or other person skilled in research retrieval techniques. Many researchers have the habit of keeping personal libraries where they keep track of publications related to the topics of interest to them. Most scholars follow particular journals and keep abreast of information in the field with the current publications. Also, professional conferences provide excellent opportunities for scholars to exchange research experience and keep informed of what others are doing.

Another popular retrieval method is to track the bibliographies in already obtained studies. These methods, while convenient, share a potential bias: a lack of

Table 4.2. Online medical/health services research search engines

Resource	Internet Address	Content	Dates	Cost
PubMed (includes MEDLINE)	www.nlm.nih.gov/ hinfo.html	Premier database for searching biomedical literature; over 15 million citations	1966–present	Free
Cochrane Library	http://www.cochrane .org/reviews/ clibintro.htm	Reviews of evidence for and against effectiveness and appropriateness of health care services	1988–present	Abstracts are free, individual subscription (online or CD-ROM) is $265; free in some libraries
PsycINFO	http://www.apa.org/ psycinfo	Abstract (not full-text) database of psychological literature	1887–present	$11.95 for 1 day of unlimited access; free in some libraries
Dissertation abstracts online	http://library.dialog.com/ bluesheets/html/ bl0035.html	American and Canadian doctoral dissertations in several disciplines, including health sciences	1861–present	Small fee per abstract; free in some libraries
EMBASE	http://embase.com	Similar to PubMed; different navigational tools	1966–present	Quotes available upon request; free in some libraries
Biosis	http://www.biosis.com	Life sciences abstracts	1969–present	Quotes available upon request; free in some libraries
National Information Center on Health Services Research and Health Care Technology, National Library of Medicine	http://www.nlm.nih.gov/ nichsr/index.html	HSR search filters for PubMed; databases on current HSR projects	1993–present	Free
ABI/INFORM	http://www.proquest .com/products_pq/ descriptions/ abi_inform.shtml	Business and management journals	1971–present	Quotes available upon request; free in some libraries

representativeness. The number of journals individuals can follow is limited. Locating bibliographies from available studies is likely to overrepresent publications that appear in particular journals. Another bias, one that affects those relying on abstracting services as well as other methods, is that published studies may be significantly different from unpublished studies. Studies get published not solely because of scientific merit but also because of the significance of the findings. The tendency of many journals to favor significant findings is harmful to the truthful representation of scientific facts. Practitioners may be disheartened to find their efforts fail even though they have followed the steps of reported research without knowing that many similar attempts have been unsuccessful and unpublished. Researchers have the duty to caution readers about this flaw in the publication media, if they are not capable of overcoming it.

While it is good to be comprehensive, investigators should also be prepared to complete the search process. The number of studies reviewed can vary significantly, depending partly on the topic and partly on the researchers' assiduity in tracking down relevant literature. The adequacy of literature search is not so much determined by the sheer number of studies retrieved as by the representativeness of those studies. Since abstracting services contain most journals in the field, they are believed to generate more representative studies than other methods. A proper protection against inadequate collection would be to include at least one major computer-based retrieval system (e.g., MEDLINE) and a couple of informal methods, such as reviewing personal collections and bibliographies from available studies. Regardless of the search methods employed, investigators should be explicit about how their search was conducted, including a discussion of the sources used, years covered, and key terms applied. Such information enables others to retrieve similar studies, thus assuring replicability. The validity of the review can also be judged against the source materials covered in the search.

Upon completing the literature search, the researcher has a list of titles and abstracts of studies related to the topic of interest. The next step is to obtain copies of the full-length articles and reports. Generally, the investigator's institutional library is the first place to start. However, it is possible that some articles and reports cannot be located there. A number of approaches may then be used to retrieve these studies. The researcher can use an interlibrary loan service, available in most libraries. Contacting original authors directly to request reprints of studies and reports is another option. Dissertations may also be purchased from University Microfilms International in Ann Arbor, Michigan. Time and cost are important factors affecting the extent of the retrieval effort. If some studies are deemed unretrievable either because they are too expensive or time-consuming to obtain, the researcher needs to document the search effort and the percentage of studies unable to be retrieved for various reasons.

After copies of the original studies are obtained, the investigator will have an opportunity to judge whether these studies are truly relevant to the review being conducted. Both inclusion and exclusion criteria must be explicitly stated. Commonly used exclusion criteria include wrong subject matter (i.e., title and abstract may not fully reflect the contents of the paper), flawed design (e.g., questions untestable by the methods adopted; study instrument, target population, or data sets cannot provide answers to the questions posed; samples poorly chosen; comparison groups inappropriate; sample size too small), and flawed analysis (e.g., statistical procedures not described, statistical tests unsuitable for the data, results not presented, or presented results inconsistent). Such information will be valuable in reporting reviews. If researchers work as a team, all should be involved in setting up the inclusion and exclusion criteria but should apply the criteria to the articles independently before comparing the outcome and reconciling the differences.

Synthesizing Research Publications

There is a close relationship between synthesizing and coding studies. Before studies can be synthesized, they need to be properly coded. The proper coding of studies relies on knowledge about how the studies will eventually be analyzed and synthesized. Thus, even though analysis and synthesis are performed much later, the strategy needs to be delineated before the coding sheet is designed.

Coding accuracy is important, especially when a large number of studies are involved and the coders have limited research backgrounds. A codebook that provides definitions of the codes may be necessary to accompany the coding sheet. Coders need to be trained and monitored. Intercoder reliability may be checked by having different coders code the same studies. Coding may not start until a high level of coding reliability is established.

Synthesizing research publications entails categorizing a series of related studies, analyzing and interpreting their findings, and summarizing those findings into unified statements about the topic being reviewed. The traditional approach that focuses on a few selected studies places little or imprecise weight on the volume of available studies and fails to portray accurately the accumulated state of knowledge. Lack of standardization in how researchers arrive at specific conclusions calls into question the validity of the review. Properly conducted, synthesizing research publications is a systematic process that integrates both quantitative and qualitative strategies.

Quantitative Procedures

The application of quantitative procedures in research review serves a number of purposes. Quantitative approaches tend to be more standardized, less subjective, and hence less subject to bias. The application of the quantitative review is also a response to the ever-expanding literature base. Researchers' understanding of a topic can be improved by analyzing and synthesizing the results of many studies. Appropriately used, quantitative research review provides an integrated summary of research results on a specific topic and enables the investigator to capture the findings of all relevant studies in an objective fashion.

The term that describes quantitative approaches to reviewing related studies is **meta-analysis** (Bangert-Drowns, 1995; Fitz-Gibbon and Morris, 2002; Glass, 1977; Glass, McGaw, and Smith, 1981; Preiss and Alien, 1995; Soeken, Bausell, and Li, 1995). Meta-analysis refers to statistical analyses that combine and interpret the results of independent studies of a given scientific issue for the purpose of integrating the findings. The approach in essence treats each study in the review as a case within a sample of relevant studies and applies statistical analysis to all the cases. For example, to assess whether the fact that two-thirds of all the studies reviewed found a particular (statistically significant) association is itself a statistically significant finding. It allows the researcher to synthesize the results of numerous tests so that an overall conclusion can be drawn. Generally, meta-analytic procedures are appropriate for research syntheses of studies based on experimental and quasi-experimental designs. At a minimum, for meta-analysis to be feasible, study results should be quantitative so that they can be subject to statistical analysis. Meta-analysis is an important tool to learn not only because it facilitates quantitative review but also because of its increasing popularity (Bausell, Li, Gau, and Soeken, 1995). Investigators are likely to find that meta-analyses have been conducted in almost all areas of social inquiry. Therefore, an investigator needs to be familiar with the meta-analytic technique to interpret the review literature.

There are some fundamental assumptions related to meta-analysis (Rosenthal, 1991). First, the same conceptual hypothesis or research question is assumed for all studies combined in the analysis. Second, the separate studies included in the analysis should be independent of each other. Third, the assumptions used by primary researchers in computing the results are believed to be correct. If any of these assumptions may be challenged, then the use of meta-analysis can be problematic. The techniques described below are chosen because of their simplicity and broad applicability. Readers who want more in-depth coverage of these and many more techniques should consult a meta-analysis textbook from the suggested references at the end of this chapter. For example, see Eddy (1992), Fleiss and Gross (1991), Hedges and Olkin (1985), Hunter and Schmidt (2004), Petitti (2000), Slavin (1984), and Wolf (1986).

The first thing researchers can do is to summarize the information abstracted from the studies reviewed based on the coding sheets (see Figure 4.2). The summary permits the investigator as well as readers to quickly compare the studies in terms of their design, measurement, and results. It is a starting point for further in-depth analysis and discussion by the researcher.

Next, the investigator may conduct a more refined subgroup analysis; that is, group the studies into comparable categories based on a number of criteria. Examples include: (1) same or similar hypotheses being tested, (2) comparable study design, (3) comparable population even though actual samples are different, and (4) similar statistics presented in the reports or available to the investigators. Studies that share similar characteristics can then be summarized and analyzed together. The results of the subgroup analysis can be compared with the analysis done on the total studies. Such a comparison enables researchers to evaluate whether sources and quality of research are significantly related to differences in results. If they are, investigators can present the meta-analytic results separately for different sources of information and different levels of quality of research.

If the findings with respect to particular variables are mixed, that is, some studies indicate a positive impact whereas others show a negative impact, the researcher may conduct a simple vote counting using a sign test to assess whether observed differences are significant (Cooper, 1989a). In Formula 4.1, z_{sign} is a

Studies   1   2   3   4   ...   N

1. Background Information
First author
Journal
Year

2. Design Information
Primary/Secondary study
Random/Nonrandom
Control/No control
Matching/Statistical control
Pretest/No pretest
Intervention(s)
Population
Sample size
Response rate
Sample characteristics
Sample representativeness
Sample biases

3. Measurement Information
Research question or hypothesis
Dependent variable(s)
Independent variable(s)
Validity of measures
Reliability of measures
Statistical measures
Model specifications

4. Outcome Information
Hypothesis supported or refuted
Significant variable(s)
Insignificant variable(s)
R^2

Figure 4.2. Summary presentation of studies reviewed

z score for the sign test, N_p refers to the number of studies with positive findings, and N_t refers to the total number of studies, including both positive and negative findings. The z score can be referred to a standard z table to find the associated probability.

Formula 4.1

$$z_{sign} = \frac{(N_p) - (\tfrac{1}{2}N_t)}{\tfrac{1}{2}\sqrt{N_t}}$$

For example, if 20 among 25 studies find results in the positive direction, the z score will be 3 {[20 − (¹⁄₂ × 25)] ÷ ¹⁄₂√25)} and the associated probability is less than .01, indicating the probability that the positive and negative directions have an equal chance of occurring in the population is highly unlikely. Thus, we are more confident about the positive impact of the variable of interest. The researcher needs to be aware that the assumption in the sign test is that the studies are comparable. Otherwise, weighting is necessary to take into account different sample sizes and/or qualities of study.

The most popular as well as important meta-analysis procedure is called effect size analysis (Fitz-Gibbon and Morris, 2002). **Effect size** may be defined as the size or strength of the impact of one factor on another. There are many ways to calculate effect size. The examples cited here may be used to summarize the results of studies in which there was some kind of control or comparison group so that an effect size can be calculated for each study. The concept of an effect size implies that there is a "true" population value for the effect of something and each time we run an experiment we obtain one sample of this effect. A researcher can expect the obtained effect size to fluctuate around the population value just as sample means fluctuate around the "true" population mean.

The first step in computing an effect size is to identify the effect size to be investigated. An example is weight loss due to exercise in the experiment group but not in the control group. The second step is the actual computation of an effect size for each study reviewed. The following formulas (4.2–4.4) may be used depending on what information is available in the published reports.

Formula 4.2 $\text{Effect Size} = \dfrac{(\text{mean } y \text{ for } E\text{-group}) - (\text{mean } y \text{ for } C\text{-group})}{SD \text{ of } y}$

Formula 4.3 $\text{Effect Size} = t\sqrt{(1/n_{\text{E}}) + (1/n_{\text{C}})}$

Formula 4.4 $\text{Effect Size} = \dfrac{2r}{\sqrt{1 - r^2}}$

In Formula 4.2, y stands for the outcome measure (weight) that is affected by the program or the treatment received (exercise) by the experimental group (E-group), but not by the control group (C-group). SD of y stands for the pooled standard deviation of y (or the average standard deviation of the two groups), which may be retrieved directly from the reports.

In situations where data have already been processed, the effect size can be computed based on the given information. Formula 4.3 assumes that t values are calculated and presented. In the formula, n_{E} is the sample size for the experiment group, and n_{C} for the control group. Formula 4.4 uses correlation between y (weight change) and group membership (experiment versus control).

The substantive interpretation of the size of the effect may be made by reference to other information. For example, have there been previous meta-analyses with which findings of this study can be compared? At the time of the study, what is in the literature about this intervention? The most informative interpretation occurs when an effect size is compared with other effect sizes using similar variables. Cohen (1988) has suggested that effect sizes of about 0.20 are small, 0.50 are medium, and 0.80 are large. The practical significance needs to be taken into account in interpreting effect size. The same effect size of life saved is certainly more significant than number of pounds lost. Effect size may also be converted into dollar figures to highlight the significance. For example, 0.3 hospitalization days averted may translate into hundreds of dollars saved per person.

The standard error measures how accurately the effect size has been measured. Formula 4.5 may be used to calculate the standard error. The smaller the standard error, the more accurate is the measurement. The 95 percent confidence interval of an effect size may be calculated using Formula 4.6. The researcher may graphically display effect sizes calculated for different studies, with effect sizes displayed on the vertical axis and studies on the horizontal axis. The graphical display presents an informative summary of the distribution of effect sizes.

Formula 4.5 ES for Effect size $= e = \sqrt{ES^2/2(n_E + n_C) + [(1/n_E) + (1/n_C)]}$

Formula 4.6   Effect size $+ 1.96e$ and Effect Size $- 1.96e$

Once the researcher has calculated effect sizes for all studies, he or she then averages these effects to obtain the mean. A mean effect size based on all studies calculated may also be computed using Formula 4.7, where ES refers to the effect size, and w is a weight. Since effect sizes likely come from studies with very different sample sizes, it is a common practice to weigh individual effect sizes based on the number of subjects in their respective samples.

Formula 4.7   Mean of $ES = \dfrac{\sum w \times ES}{\sum w}$ where $w = \dfrac{1}{e^2}$

To test for homogeneity of effect sizes (H), that is, whether obtained effect sizes were random samples estimating a single effect size (appearing homogeneous) or coming from different populations (appearing heterogeneous), researchers use Formula 4.8. The result of the homogeneity test will be compared with a chi-square for $df = k - 1$, where k is the number of studies. If the value is larger than the critical value in the chi-square table, the result becomes significant and suggests the effect sizes did not come from a single population value (i.e., are heterogeneous). The homogeneity statistic indicates whether an intervention has a consistent impact on an outcome variable.

Formula 4.8 $H = \sum (ES - \text{Mean of } ES)^2 \times w$ where $w = \dfrac{1}{e^2}$

Table 4.3 applies the above formulas to a research review example about the impact of a health promotion exercise intervention on weight loss among overweight adults. The example uses five studies and assumes only sample size and t statistic information are available from the reports.

Meta-analysis is proposed as a more rigorous approach to research reviews, but it does not entirely resolve the question of partial or selective coverage. Further, different quantitative procedures employed by investigators may create variations in the conclusions of reviews. Meta-analysis is merely a useful tool. Its successful application hinges on an extensive and systematic literature search

Table 4.3. Example of effect size analysis

Studies	1	2	3	4	5	Total
n (Experiment)	100	150	200	250	300	
n (Control)	100	150	200	250	300	
$(1/n_E) + (1/n_C)$	0.02	0.01	0.01	0.01	0.01	
t	4.86	2.32	5.14	3.50	10.20	
ES	**0.69**	**0.27**	**0.51**	**0.31**	**0.83**	
$ES/2$	0.47	0.07	0.26	0.10	0.69	
$2(n_E + n_C)$	400	600	800	1000	1200	
$(1/n_E) + (1/n_C)$	0.02	0.01	0.01	0.01	0.01	
SE for ES $= e$	**0.15**	**0.12**	**0.10**	**0.09**	**0.09**	
$ES + 1.96e$	0.97	0.50	0.71	0.49	1.00	
$ES - 1.96e$	0.40	0.04	0.32	0.14	0.67	
95% CI of ES	**(0.97,** 0.40)	**(0.50,** 0.04)	**(0.71,** 0.32)	**(0.49,** 0.14)	**(1.0,** 0.67)	
w	47.21	74.33	96.80	123.49	138.03	**479.87**
$w \times ES$	32.45	19.91	49.76	38.66	114.96	255.73
Mean of ES						**0.53**
$(ES - $ Mean of $ES)$	0.15	−0.27	−0.02	−0.22	0.30	
$(ES - $ Mean of $ES)^2$	0.02	0.07	0.00	0.05	0.09	
$(ES - $ Mean of $ES)^2 \times w$	1.13	5.22	0.04	5.97	12.42	
Homogeneity						**24.77**

and the presence of sufficient quantitative information in published reports. To make computations possible, authors should routinely report the exact test statistics (e.g., r, t, F, z) along with their degrees of freedom and sample sizes. Editors and researchers should also require the reporting of these statistics.

A common criticism of meta-analysis is that poor studies are summarized together with good ones. To adjust for study quality, a system of weighting can be used. A weight of zero can be assigned to a study of extremely poor quality. A study twice as good as the average can be weighted twice as heavily. However, weighting itself may introduce bias if researchers assign heavier weight only to studies whose results they favor and lower weights to those they oppose. A more objective way would be to have each study weighted by outside experts who do not have a vested interest. Or, if investigators were to do the weighting themselves, they could weight each study twice, once after reading only the design section of the study, the other after reading both the design and results. The reason for the first weighting is to ensure that one weighting is made uninfluenced by the results of the study. If both weightings are comparable, there is less likelihood for bias to be introduced associated with weighting.

Qualitative Procedures

Even though quantitative approaches are preferred in research reviews, there are circumstances in which the use of quantitative procedures is inappropriate. A basic premise of quantitative approaches is that the studies reviewed address an identical conceptual hypothesis. If studies address different hypotheses, although related to the same topic, quantitative methods may not be appropriate.

Quantitative approaches are likely to gloss over details, ignoring idiosyncrasies related to differences among studies. The researcher should be aware that not all studies are of the same quality. Studies can be incomplete in their description of design, measurement, and results. Incomplete description of statistical values will affect the performance of quantitative synthesis. Reporting errors may be found in statistical analyses. Inconsistency may be noted between results reported in the tables and in the text. When studies present insufficient statistical information or when there are obvious errors in the choice of statistical procedures as well as in calculations, the investigator cannot use quantitative approaches.

The qualitative approach to research review aims at overcoming the deficiencies associated with the quantitative approach. Specifically, qualitative narratives provide an opportunity for the researcher to address the nonquantifiable features of the study, such as settings and background or interesting anecdotes and cases, as well as the historic evolution of the topic. The qualitative approach is frequently used in theoretical reviews where relevant theories are compared and summarized. The implications of the results and their policy relevancy may be analyzed using a qualitative approach. In sum, a complete research review should integrate both quantitative and qualitative approaches.

Reporting Previous Research

In reporting the findings of a research review, the investigator may follow a format similar to that used in reporting empirical research, including such sections as introduction, methods, results, and discussion. The introduction section presents an overview of the theoretical and conceptual issues related to the topic and summarizes previous reviews on the topic and issues left unresolved. The methods section describes specific steps in the literature search and specific approaches adopted in analyzing and integrating study results. The results section provides a sense of the representativeness of the sampled reviews and presents cumulative findings on the literature reviewed. The discussion section serves to summarize the major findings, draw implications of the findings, and suggest directions for future research.

Specifically, in the introduction section, the researcher reports: (1) the research topic or problem and its significance, (2) a historical overview of the theoretical issues related to the topic, (3) a historical overview of the methodological issues related to the topic, (4) historical debate surrounding the topic, (5) a summary of previous reviews on the topic and highlights of the findings, and (6) the need for the current review as a result of unresolved controversies surrounding the topic, new developments in issues related to the topic, and/or significant increases in recent studies on the topic. For instance, in Stevens and Shi (2003), "Racial and Ethnic Disparities in the Primary Care Experiences of Children: A Review of the Literature," the introduction states why racial and ethnic disparities in primary care experiences among children are a major public health problem, how this problem has been identified as a priority for elimination by the Institute of Medicine and other public health leadership organizations, how the topic has been approached by researchers in the past, and how the current article is a new and needed critique and synthesis of the literature relevant to racial and ethnic disparities in children's primary care experiences.

In the methods section, the researcher reports: (1) the sources from which studies were retrieved, including which abstract and indexing services were used, which bibliographies were consulted, which years were covered in the search, which key terms were used to assist the search, which other informal sources were consulted, and the percentage distribution of materials selected from each of the sources; (2) the inclusion and exclusion criteria for selecting studies to be reviewed, an assessment of the impact of these criteria (e.g., how many studies were excluded by each criterion), and how these criteria were actually applied (e.g., how many studies were included and excluded from reading the titles, abstracts, and full texts, respectively); (3) a summary of the different hypotheses or research questions related to the topic; (4) a systematic review of the different prototypes of studies reviewed, including descriptions of designs, population and sample characteristics, variables, models, and statistics applied; and (5) a discussion of specific approaches (e.g., meta-analytic techniques) used in analyzing, integrating, and synthesizing study findings, the statistics needed for applying these techniques, whether weights were assigned, and if so, how, and how missing information was handled. For instance, a review of the literature on income inequality and health included a methods section detailing when the search was conducted (between October 2001 and January 2002), electronic databases searched (PubMed, OVID, and dissertation abstracts), search terms used ("income inequality AND health"), languages of articles searched (English, French, and Spanish), number of articles initially retrieved ($N = 327$), number of articles eventually abstracted ($N = 47$), inclusion and exclusion criteria, and a conceptual framework describing how the literature was organized for review (Macinko, Shi, Starfield, and Wulu, 2003).

In the results section, the researcher records: (1) descriptive results of the studies reviewed, including types of studies, sources of studies, publication dates, hypotheses or research questions, population and samples, measurement characteristics, and the like; (2) the results of each hypothesis and/or research question tested, along with a breakdown of the relationship between results and different types of studies (e.g., published versus nonpublished, experiment versus non-experiment, random versus nonrandom, and so on); (3) results of other tests conducted (e.g., vote counts and effect size analysis); and (4) a qualitative summary of findings not captured in the quantitative analysis. The structure of the results section may vary depending on the review topic, space limitations, and authors' preferences. For instance, the results section of a literature review on the effect of patients having a regular source of medical care described all of the studies included in the review, organized by specific topic and geographical area (Starfield and Shi, 2004). The review of literature on income inequality and health (described previously) presented its results in a similar fashion, but also included an appendix to organize the relevant information from each article (Macinko, Shi, Starfield, and Wulu, 2003).

In the discussion section, the researcher records: (1) a summary of major findings of the research review; (2) a comparison of current findings with previous reviews, if available; (3) a discussion of the theoretical and practical implications of the findings; (4) a summary of the limitations of the current review; and (5) a discussion of the directions for future research surrounding the topic reviewed.

STRENGTHS AND WEAKNESSES

The principal strength of research review is its contribution to the advance of scientific knowledge. Scientific knowledge is cumulative knowledge and research review provides a critical assessment of the state of research related to a given topic, thus suggesting fruitful directions for future research. Research review based on a systematic rather than an idiosyncratic approach is important to maintaining the credibility of conclusions, particularly at a time when research review plays an increasing role in the definition of knowledge.

Research review also has the advantage of being efficient. Money spent in retrieving studies is usually far less than in collecting primary data. The staff necessary to carry out the review is far less than in most primary studies. The time requirement for research review is also significantly less demanding than for primary research. In addition, the schedule is more predictable and less subject to outside factors.

The principal disadvantage of research review is that it is constrained by the materials available for review. Inconsistencies, missing information, and many other quality variations among published reports invariably create problems for the investigator. Assumptions have to be made and compromises sought to make use of current studies. Research review on some topics may not be feasible if a limited number of studies have been conducted on these topics.

Some of the limitations of research review represent pervasive concerns in primary research as well. For example, when the researcher encounters access problems, particularly to unpublished studies, that could have a significant bearing on the outcome of the review, the representativeness of the research review is threatened. The cost of data collection, even though significantly less than most primary studies, would be much higher based on the approaches specified in this chapter than based on the traditional approach. Should a researcher with limited funding be discouraged from undertaking research review? Certainly not. Just as primary research can never be perfect, the perfect review is merely an ideal. The steps are presented as guidelines, not prerequisites, for conducting research review. They may also assist us in assessing reviews conducted by others.

SUMMARY

Research review is an efficient method of synthesizing existing knowledge on a topic. It can be used both as part of an empirical investigation or independently, focusing on theories, methodology, or policies. The integrative research review, the most commonly used, consists of five integrated steps that include identifying the topic, preparing a coding sheet, searching for research publications, synthesizing research publications, and reporting previous research on the selected topic. Properly used, these steps will make research review systematic and replicable, contributing to the advancement of scientific knowledge.

REVIEW QUESTIONS

1. What are the types of research reviews and their respective purposes?
2. Identify commonly used computerized abstracting and indexing services used in health services research.
3. What are the strengths and weaknesses of research review as a scientific inquiry?
4. Do the following exercise as a way to learn the process of research review. The purpose of this exercise is to conduct an integrative research review on a health services research topic of interest to you. Your review should follow the five-step process delineated in this chapter. It is possible that the class may be divided into groups, with each member responsible for one step of the process.

   ■ First, conduct a preliminary review to identify the topic to be reviewed.

   ■ Second, prepare a coding sheet based on the preliminary review, pilot-test the coding sheet using additional studies, and then revise the coding sheet.

   ■ Third, ascertain the key terms used in your search. You may want to consult *Index Medicus* or other index publications for verification. Identify a computer-based abstracting service available in your library (e.g., MEDLINE) and conduct the search using the MeSH terms that coordinate best with your key terms. You may want to limit your initial search to a few years. Perform a parallel manual search and compare the differences between the two approaches.

   ■ Fourth, record relevant study information on the coding sheets. If feasible, have different coders code the same studies and compare the results. If there are too many differences between the coders, you may want to revise the coding sheet or design a code book that accompanies the coding sheet. Then recode the articles.

■ Fifth, based on the information abstracted on the coding sheets, prepare a summary table of the major variables of interest. If applicable, conduct an effect size analysis using the formulas and the example from Table 4.2 as a reference. Make qualitative assessments of the studies being reviewed, focusing particularly on the uniqueness of study settings, interventions, and sample characteristics.

■ Finally, prepare a formal report of your review using the following sections: introduction, methods, results, and discussion. Consult the relevant sections for contents to be included in the review.

REFERENCES

American Hospital Association Resource Center. (1994). *Hospital Literature Index.* Chicago: American Hospital Association.

Bangert-Drowns, R. L. (1995). Misunderstanding meta-analysis. *Evaluation and the Health Professions, 18,* 304–314.

Bausell, R. B., Li, Y. E., Gau, M. L., and Soeken, K. L. (1995). The growth of meta-analytic literature from 1980 to 1993. *Evaluation and the Health Professions, 18,* 238–251.

Cohen, J. (1988). *Statistical Power Analysis for the Behavioral Sciences* (2nd ed.). New York: Academic Press.

Cooper, H. M. (1982). Scientific guidelines for conducting integrative research reviews. *Review of Educational Research, 52,* 291–302.

Cooper, H. M. (1989a). *Integrating Research: A Guide for Literature Reviews* (2nd ed.). Newbury Park, CA: Sage.

Cooper, H. M. (1989b). The structure of knowledge synthesis: A taxonomy of literature reviews. *Knowledge in Society, 1,* 104–126.

Eddy, D. M. (1992). *Meta-analysis by the Confidence Profile Method: The Statistical Synthesis of Evidence.* Boston: Academic Press.

Fitz-Gibbon, C. T., and Morris, L. L. (2002). *How to Analyze Data* (2nd ed.). Thousand Oaks, CA: Sage.

Fleiss, J. L., and Gross, A. J. (1991). Meta-analysis in epidemiology, with special reference to studies of the association between exposure to environmental tobacco smoke and lung cancer: A critique. *Journal of Clinical Epidemiology, 44,* 127–139.

Glass, G. (1977). Integrating findings: The meta-analysis of research. *Review of Research in Education, 5,* 351–379. Itasca, IL: F. E. Peacock.

Glass, G., McGaw, B., and Smith, M. (1981). *Meta-analysis in Social Research.* Newbury Park, CA: Sage.

Harper, R., Weins, A., and Matarazzo, J. (1978). *Nonverbal Communication: The State of the Art.* New York: Wiley.

Hedges, L. V., and Olkin, I. (1985). *Statistical Methods for Meta-analysis.* New York: Academic Press.

Hunter, J. F., and Schmidt, F. L. (2004). *Methods of Meta-analysis: Correcting Error and Bias in Research Findings* (2nd ed.). Thousand Oaks, CA: Sage.

Macinko, J. A., Shi, L., Starfield, B., and Wulu, J. T. (2003). Income inequality and health: A critical review of the literature. *Medical Care Research and Review, 60*(4), 407–452.

National Library of Medicine. (2006a). *Fact Sheet: Medical Subject Headings (MeSH)*. Retrieved July 2, 2007, from http://www.nlm.nih.gov/pubs/factsheets/mesh.html

National Library of Medicine. (2006b). *Fact Sheet: The National Library of Medicine.* Retrieved July 2, 2007, from http://www.nlm.nih.gov/pubs/factsheets/nlm.html

Petitti, D. B. (2000). *Meta-analysis, Decision Analysis, and Cost-Effectiveness Analysis: Methods for Quantitative Synthesis in Medicine* (2nd ed.). New York: Oxford University Press.

Preiss, R. W., and Alien, M. (1995). Understanding and using meta-analysis. *Evaluation and the Health Professions, 18*, 315–335.

Rosenthal, R. (1991). *Meta-analytic Procedures for Social Research.* Newbury Park, CA: Sage.

Slavin, R. E. (1984). Meta-analysis in education: How has it been used? *Educational Researcher, 13*, 6–15, 24–27.

Soeken, K. L., Bausell, R. B., and Li, Y. E. (1995). Realizing the meta-analytic potential: A survey of experts. *Evaluation and the Health Professions, 18*, 336–344.

Starfield, B., and Shi, L. (2004). The medical home, access to care, and insurance: A review of the evidence. *Pediatrics, 113*(5), 1493–1497.

Stevens, G. D., and Shi, L. (2003). Racial and ethnic disparities in the primary care experiences of children: A review of the literature. *Medical Care Research and Review, 60*(1), 3–30.

Wolf, F. M. (1986). *Meta-analysis: Quantitative Methods for Research Synthesis* (QASS Series 07-059). Newbury Park, CA: Sage.

CHAPTER 5

Secondary Analysis

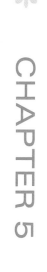

KEY TERMS

cohort study
content analysis
ecological fallacy
historical analysis

individualistic fallacy
panel study
primary research
reactive effect

records
secondary analysis
trend study

LEARNING OBJECTIVES

■ To become familiar with the types of secondary analysis.

■ To identify the general categories of secondary data sources.

■ To describe administrative records research analysis, content analysis, published statistics analysis, and historical analysis.

■ To understand the strengths and weaknesses of secondary analysis.

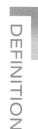

DEFINITION

Secondary analysis is any reanalysis of data or information collected by another researcher or organization, including the analysis of data sets collated from a variety of sources to create time-series or area-based data sets (Singleton and Straits, 2005; Stewart and Kamins, 1993). Secondary analysis is commonly applied to quantitative data from previous studies. However, it can also be used for archival information (typically words and text) prepared by others (e.g., documents, historical materials, letters, diaries, or records). When applied to archival information, secondary analysis often employs qualitative methods. Secondary analysis can also be used to study the quantitative information from published studies. When applied to published quantitative studies, secondary analysis is often called meta-analysis (see Chapter 4).

Secondary analysis differs from **primary research** in that primary research involves firsthand collection of data or information by the researcher or research team. The data are gathered through the research and did not exist prior to the study. By contrast, secondary analysis uses available data or information collected by others for completely different purposes, whether research-oriented or not (e.g., administrative records or archival information). Since secondary analysis does not require researchers to have contact with subjects, it is sometimes referred to as nonreactive or unobtrusive research.

TYPES

There are several ways to classify the types of secondary analysis. The classification may be based on the number of databases used (both cross-sectionally and longitudinally), the sources of data, or the methods adopted to analyze the secondary data.

Number of Databases Used

The simplest approach is to use a single data set, either to replicate the original researcher's results or to address entirely different research questions. A second approach is to use a single data set that is extended by the addition of data from other sources, thus providing a richer and more comprehensive basis for the secondary analysis. More complex secondary analysis involves the use of multiple data sets to provide an overall assessment of findings on a topic.

Secondary data sets may be cross-sectional, capturing one moment in time, or longitudinal, recording data elements over a series of time periods. Most secondary data sets are designed to study some phenomenon by taking a cross section of it at one time and analyzing that cross section carefully. Exploratory and descriptive studies are also often cross-sectional. Many explanatory studies are also cross-sectional, but this poses an inherent problem. Typically, their aim is to understand causal processes that occur over time, yet their conclusions are based on observations made at only one point in time.

Longitudinal studies are designed to permit observations over an extended period. Three special types of longitudinal studies are trend, cohort, and panel studies. A **trend study** is one that investigates changes within some general population over time. Examples would be a comparison of U.S. health care expenditure, utilization, and outcomes over time, showing the extent of compatibility. A **cohort study** examines more specific subpopulations (cohorts) as they change over time. Typically, a cohort is an age group, such as those people born during the same year, but it can also be based on some other time grouping, such as people discharged from the same hospital, having the same insurance coverage, and so forth. A **panel study** is similar to a trend or cohort study, except that the same set of people is investigated each time.

In general, it is more difficult to find multiple data sets over a series of time periods than to find one such data set. Longitudinal studies have an obvious advantage over cross-sectional ones in providing information describing processes over time. But often this advantage comes at a heavy cost in both time and money, especially in a large-scale survey. Panel studies, which offer the most comprehensive data on changes over time, face a special problem: panel attrition. Some of the respondents studied in the first wave of the survey may not participate in later waves. The danger is that those who drop out of the study may not be typical, thereby distorting the results. Another potential problem occurs when questions have been altered from one study to the next so that the questions for different waves may not be entirely comparable. The problem does not always disappear even when questions remain constant. Because the meaning of a concept may have changed over time, the same question may not be measuring the same concept. A good example is the reduced buying power of the U.S. dollar. Comparisons of total national health expenditures across different years would be less meaningful if the dollars were not adjusted for inflation. In using published time-series data, researchers need to be aware that the earliest points in their series may be composed of corrected data, while more recent points in their series may be uncorrected or partially corrected. Greater errors may be contained in the latter than in the former.

Sources of Data

The variety of secondary data is tremendous. A secondary data source may be classified as produced either specifically for a research purpose or not for a research purpose.

Research-Oriented Secondary Data

Research-oriented secondary data include all data sets collected by others for research rather than other purposes. There are numerous examples of such secondary data sets. Chapter 3 enumerated some data sets regularly collected by government agencies, including the Area Resource File, National Ambulatory Medical Care Survey, National Health Interview Survey, National Hospital

Discharge Survey, and Medical Expenditure Panel Survey, to name just a few. These data sets are stored on CD-ROMs that are available for public use, often for a fee. Another excellent resource for locating secondary data sources is the Inter-University Consortium for Political and Social Research website (http://www.icpsr.umich.edu/). Table 5.1 describes several additional research-oriented secondary data sources.

The fundamental difference between research- and nonresearch-oriented secondary data has to do with quality both in terms of data collection and documentation. Research-oriented data sets are generally collected according to strict scientific procedures of sampling and measurement. To the extent errors occur, they are more likely to be properly documented. Nonresearch-oriented data sets are comparatively less strict on both accounts. The sampling procedures may be inaccurate and measurement may be idiosyncratic rather than tested. Incomplete or missing data are also more common. Documentation of data collection procedures and measurement is less refined. Thus, extra caution needs to be exercised when researchers use secondary data that were not collected for research purposes.

Nonresearch-Oriented Secondary Data

Nonresearch-oriented secondary data include public documents, official records, private documents and records, mass media, and physical, nonverbal materials. **Records** are systematic accounts of regular occurrences. Examples of public documents and official records include proceedings of government bodies, court records, state laws, city ordinances, directories, almanacs, and publication indexes such as the *New York Times Article Archive* and *The Reader's Guide to Periodical Literature* (Singleton and Straits, 2005; Stewart and Kamins, 1993). Private documents and records refer to information produced by individuals or organizations about their own activities, including diaries, letters, notes, personnel and sales records, inventories, tax records, and patient records. Examples of mass media include television, newspapers, radio, periodicals, movies, and so on. Examples of physical, nonverbal materials consist of works of art (paintings and pictures), artifacts, and household collections.

Of particular interest to health services researches, with regard to government documents, are the numerous volumes of official statistics, such as vital statistics from birth, death, marriage, and divorce certificates and population demographics from census data. State laws require that all births and deaths be recorded. The variables in birth records include demographic information about the newborn child, as well as information about the parents (e.g., names of mother and father, address, age, and occupation). Death records contain biographic information of the deceased, cause of death, length of illness, cause of injury (accidental, homicidal, or self-inflicted), and time and place of death. These data make possible research ranging from, for example, a study of fertility patterns in an area to epidemiological investigations into the incidence and prevalence of disease. Census data, collected and maintained by the U.S. Bureau of the Census, provide

Table 5.1. Selected research-oriented secondary data sources

Source	Owner	Contents	Unit of Observation
HRSA Geospatial Data Warehouse	HRSA	Report and mapping tools, demographics, HRSA program information	State/territory, county, city, zip code, HHS region, congressional district
Uniform Data System (UDS)	BPHC	Patient demographics, staffing, financial information	Community health centers, migrant health centers, health care for the homeless sites
Pregnancy Risk Assessment Monitoring System (PRAMS)	CDC	Maternal attitudes and experiences before, during, and after pregnancy	Individual
National Survey of Children with Special Healthcare Needs	NCHS, CDC	Prevalence and impact of special health care needs among children	Parents of children with special health care needs
Medical Expenditure Panel Survey (MEPS)	AHRQ	Health status, insurance coverage, health care service utilization, sources of payment, characteristics of facilities and services	Households, nursing home residents, employers, hospitals, physicians, home health care providers
Healthcare Cost and Use Project (HCUP)	AHRQ	Diagnoses and procedures, LOS, patient demographics, total charges, hospital characteristics	Inpatient sample (nationwide and in participating states)
Medicare Current Beneficiary Survey (MCBS)	CMS	Use of health services, medical care expenditures, health insurance coverage, sources of payment, health status and functioning, demographic and behavioral information	Medicare beneficiaries
National Health Care Survey (NHCS)	NCHS	Includes National Ambulatory Medical Care Survey, National Hospital Ambulatory Medical Care Survey, National Survey of Ambulatory Surgery, National Hospital Discharge Survey, National Nursing Home Survey, National Home and Hospice Care Survey, National Employer Health Insurance Survey, National Health Provider Inventory	Health care facilities, providers, patients
National Health Interview Survey (NHIS)	NCHS	Health status, health care service utilization, health behaviors	Households and sample individuals within households

(continues)

Table 5.1. Selected research-oriented secondary data sources (continued)

Source	Owner	Contents	Unit of Observation
Cardiovascular Health Study (CHS)	National Heart, Lung, & Blood Institute	Quality of life, social support, social network, physical activity, medication, assessment of physical functioning	Medicare-eligible individuals
National Sample Survey of Registered Nurses	HRSA	Number of RNs, education and training, employment status, salaries, geographic distribution, demographics	Individual RNs
Medicaid Analytic eXtract	CMS	Medicaid eligibility, health care service utilization	Medicaid claims

detailed information about the demographic characteristics of the populations of states, counties, metropolitan areas, cities and towns, and neighborhood tracts and blocks. The most recent official population census of the United States was conducted in April 2000. In addition, the Bureau of Census conducts regular censuses of businesses, agriculture, and other institutions, as well as conducting the *Current Population Survey*, a monthly survey of a representative sample of households throughout the 50 states. These data, when used with other health-related data sets such as health services utilization, enable researchers to examine many topics central to health services research (e.g., the relationship between population characteristics and health services use).

Of particular interest to health services researchers, with regard to private records, are administrative records kept by hospitals and other health institutions. Health-related administrative records are collections of documents containing mainly factual information compiled either directly, from those concerned, or indirectly, from employers, doctors, and agencies acting as informants. These records are used by health organizations to document the development and implementation of decisions and activities that are central to their functions. Examples are health service records, insurance membership and payment records, organizational accounts and personnel records, and hospital revenues and expenditures.

The potential for research analysis of health administrative records is expanding as more organizations are transferring such records from manual systems of files, forms, and cards to computerized systems, including CD-ROMs (Stewart and Kamins, 1993). In the process, these collections of records are being redesigned as health information systems that can be analyzed quickly and routinely to produce summaries of particular aspects of the data. This conversion also makes it easier to provide suitably anonymous extract tapes for health services research purposes. The computerization of many record systems facilitates linkages of different databases, such as hospital patient records, population censuses, and sample surveys. In linking different databases or extracting the required information from records or computer files, it is essential that sufficient time and resources be allocated to the tasks of familiarization with content, preparation of documentation (with reference to the specific questions addressed by the study and pertinent data items), and, in some cases, determination as to whether missing values can reliably be imputed or estimated. Perhaps the most common mistake is to think of data from records as ready-to-use research data, whereas they usually require more preparation, care, and effort than an equivalent secondary analysis of a research-oriented data set.

There are several potential conceptual and structural problems with administrative data. First, because administrative databases are not specifically designed for the needs of researchers, there may be issues with inconsistent data collection and quality. Coding may lack standardization and may change over time. In addition, there may be large gaps in administrative data, especially across time periods, as populations included in the data shift (Connell, Diehr, and Hart, 1987).

Before using administrative data, it is important that the researcher determines the data set's sampling frame, inclusion/exclusion criteria (and whether exclusion or refusal rates differed among subgroups), methodology and time frame for data collection and processing, whether the records are aggregated or disaggregated, and whether the use of more than one dataset will be necessary. If so, it is necessary to determine whether and how these datasets are linked (Connell et al., 1987).

Another important step in using administrative data is establishing an appropriate strategy for querying. As discussed, changes in administrative data sets over time (which may include changes in the database structure or vendor software) can affect the content of the data. In addition, these changes may affect how the data should be queried in order to produce meaningful and accurate results. Enlisting the assistance of a person familiar with the administrative data at hand is at times necessary to ensure one's querying strategy is appropriate.

Methods of Secondary Analysis

Methods used to analyze available data take many forms. The type of analysis chosen is usually a function of the research purpose, the design, and the nature of the data available. For example, descriptive accounts of a topic differ from tests of general hypotheses. Longitudinal designs entail different analytic methods than cross-sectional surveys. The quality of available data also dictates the proper analytic procedures to be used. When data are collected by some nonrandom means, no statistical estimates of sampling errors are possible, and the use of analytical statistics is limited. For the most part, health services researchers use quantitative methods to analyze available data. For a glimpse of some of these methods, refer to Chapter 14. In addition to these commonly used quantitative methods, there are some qualitative methods that are less frequently used by health services researchers but commonly used by other social scientists, especially in performing secondary analysis on archival records.

Content analysis is a research method appropriate for studying human communication and aspects of social behavior (Carney, 1972; Holsti, 1969; Krippendorff, 1980). It is typically used with archival records. The basic goal is to take a verbal, nonquantitative document and transform it into quantitative data. The usual units of analysis in content analysis are words, paragraphs, books, pictures, advertisements, and television episodes. Contents can be manifest or latent. Manifest content refers to characteristics of communication that are directly visible or objectively identifiable, such as the specific words spoken or particular pictures shown. Latent content refers to the meanings contained within communications that have to be determined by the researcher. For example, what constitutes sexual harassment in the workplace? Or, what is the process of implementing informed consent in health services organizations? Coding may be used to transform raw data into more quantitative forms that can then be counted and analyzed. The results of content analysis can generally be presented in tables containing frequencies or percentages, in the same way as survey data. Content analysis has the advantage of economy in terms of both time and money and with regard to unobtrusiveness and safety. It also has the benefit of permitting study over a long period of time. Its primary disadvantage is that it is limited to the study of recorded communications only. Content analysis is frequently used to analyze the symbolic content of communication, especially verbal materials from the media. Content analysis can also be used in health services research. For example, the study of health legislation may enhance our understanding of why U.S. health care delivery has evolved into its current form.

Analyzing published statistics is another way researchers use available data (Jacob, 1984). The analysis of published statistics is different from the use of secondary data because published statistics are aggregate information and cannot be traced to the individual level from which the aggregation is made. For confidentiality and privacy reasons, aggregate data may be the only available information for studying a particular topic. At minimum, published statistics should always be used as supplemental evidence to the research. Examples of published statistics include the reference work *The U.S. Fact Book: The American Almanac Demographic Yearbook*, available through the United Nations; the countless data series published by various federal agencies; chamber of commerce reports on business; and public opinion surveys published by George Gallup. The unit of analysis involved in the analysis of published statistics is often not the individual but rather some aggregate element, such as country, region, state, county, or city.

In using aggregate statistics, researchers should guard against committing the **ecological fallacy**, which refers to the possibility that patterns found at a group level differ from those that would be found on an individual level. Thus, it is usually not appropriate to draw conclusions at the individual level based on the analysis of aggregate data. Conversely, in analyzing individual data, researchers should guard against committing an **individualistic fallacy**, which attributes study outcome to individual measures only and ignores community and area effects on the study outcome. A more appropriate approach is to consider both individual and context predictors and avoid committing either individualistic or ecological fallacies.

Researchers need to be assiduous in tracking down important information that may not be available in the published reports. For example, the data found in published sources are often extracted from other studies that include more information about sampling error. Consequently, the investigator needs to go to the original source cited in the report to track down more information.

The principal advantage of using published statistics is economy in terms of time and money. The main disadvantage is the limitations of the existing data. The proper analysis of existing statistics relies heavily on the quality of the statistics themselves. Often existing data do not cover everything the researcher is interested in, and the measurements may not be exactly valid representations of the concepts the researcher wants to draw conclusions about.

Examples of research based on published statistics include studies of rates of crimes, accidents, diseases, and mortalities. Health services researchers may find data of great interest and relevance from such publications as the annual *Statistical Abstract of the United States*, published by the U.S. Department of Commerce, and *Health United States*, published by the U.S. Department of Health and Human Services. These sources facilitate comparative studies of health indicators across countries. Examples of data provided include physician–population ratios, hospital beds–population ratios, days of hospitalization per capita, death rates (number of deaths per 1,000 population), and, more specifically, infant mortality rates (the number of infants who die during their first year of life among every 1,000 births).

Historical analysis

Historical analysis involves attempts to reconstruct past events (descriptive history) and the use of historical evidence to generate and test theories (analytical history) (Babbie, 2006). The basic evidence primarily consists of authentic documents, such as testimony, and organizational records, including charters, policy statements, and speeches. These are considered secondary sources because they originate from other, firsthand, documents. Since historical research is largely a qualitative method, there are no easily listed steps to follow in the analysis of historical data. Generally, *verstehen* (translated loosely as "understanding") is necessary. In other words, in interpreting historical data, researchers need to mentally take on the circumstances, views, and feelings of the participants and compare and critically evaluate the relative plausibility of alternative explanations. Examples of historical analysis include the study of health-seeking patterns by different cultures, and the account by Marmor (2000) of the evolution of the Medicare program for the elderly.

STRENGTHS AND WEAKNESSES

The principal advantage of secondary analysis is economy, achieved through money, time, and personnel saved in data collection and management. For example, administrative records can be used for research and evaluation without additional demand for data collection. The savings vary depending on the quality of the data set, including proper documentation, format compatibility, and ease of access.

With the development of computer-based analyses, it has become relatively easy for health services researchers to share their data with one another. The multiple sources of secondary data enable researchers to conduct inquiries into many areas of interest. Vast quantities of information are collated and recorded by organizations and individuals for their own purposes, well beyond the data collected by researchers purely for research purposes. The information is typically extensive and is often available for a considerable span of time.

Because of the economy and availability of secondary data, secondary analysis is fast becoming one of the most popular methods of health services research. For example, research in health economics is largely based on the secondary analysis of macro-level, time-series data consisting of a large number of national statistical indicators and measures collated from a variety of official surveys and statistical series.

In addition to savings on time, cost, and personnel, the use of available data may afford the opportunity to generate significantly larger samples than primary research, such as surveys and experiments. The federal government and major foundations spend millions annually to collect a variety of health-related information, which provides a rich source of secondary analyses. Large sample size is important to researchers because it allows more sophisticated multivariate analysis and enhances confidence in research results. Studies performed on large data sets generally provide more reliable estimates of population parameters.

Secondary data, particularly administrative records, may be viewed as more objective and, therefore, more credible because the purpose of data collection is not research-oriented and personal biases are less likely to be introduced. A particular problem with research is the **reactive effect**, changes in behavior that occur because subjects are aware they are being studied or observed (see reactivity and Hawthorne effect in Chapter 1). Research using available data may still encounter this problem if the sources of data are surveys. But many available data sources such as administrative records are nonreactive.

Secondary analysis affords the opportunity to study trends and changes over a long period of time. Available data often are the best and only opportunities to study the past as well as trends. Studying the evolution of health care delivery and financing, for example, necessitates the use of data collected in the past.

Because of the commitment and cost involved, researchers rarely conduct longitudinal surveys over a long span of time. Longitudinal studies for the most part rely on available data.

Secondary analysis is also the general approach used to carry out area-based research, especially cross-national comparative studies. Secondary analysis of existing data is likely to remain by far the most common approach to carrying out international comparative studies, especially for studies that seek to cover large numbers of countries and/or trends over time. Aggregate national statistics from each country derived from official statistics and censuses, for example, enable the conducting of international macro-level comparative studies. Secondary analysis of multisource data sets is also employed to study geographical patterns and variations within countries, sometimes using existing compilations of area-based statistics, sometimes using data sets specially collated for counties, cities, or other areas. Thus, when the units of analysis are countries or social units rather than individuals or groups, secondary analysis may be the only viable research option.

The principal weakness of secondary analysis is the extent of compatibility between the available data and the research question. Secondary data such as surveys, records, and documents must be found rather than created to the researcher's specification. Searching for relevant data sources is by no means easy. While the material to study a given topic may exist, how does the researcher know where to look for it? To a large extent, identification of relevant data hinges on the general knowledge of the investigators.

Once identified, the value of available data will depend on the degree of match between the research questions to be addressed and the data that happen to be available. Often, available data will not be ideally suited to the purposes the researcher has in mind. Creativity is needed to reconstruct original measures that approximate the variables of interest.

Because of potential compatibility problems, the design of secondary studies may have to be started from back to front. Instead of designing the study and then collecting the necessary data, the researcher obtains details of the contents and characteristics of a set of secondary data and then identifies the corresponding research model. One key disadvantage is that the scope and content of the studies are constrained by the nature of the data available. Even when relevant secondary data exist, they may not provide the particular items of information required to address the question at issue. In other words, information may be present but the definitions and classifications applied may be incompatible with those the researcher wishes to use.

Accessibility to available data may pose a challenge to investigators. Some data sets extracted from government records are routinely released for public use. Data compiled by government agencies are mandated for public use without restrictions. In other cases, access may need to be specially negotiated, and there may be constraints on access due to confidentiality and ethical concerns. In yet others, laws specifically prohibit the release of such data for confidentiality reasons.

Another limitation of secondary data, particularly administrative records that were not collected for research purposes, is that records are frequently incomplete or inaccurate. There may be large blocks of missing data as a result of nonrigorous data recording. This may not matter for administrative purposes, but it presents serious problems for a research analysis. In the pressures of the day, recorders may forget to keep track of all the relevant information.

The decision to accept or reject a data set based on quality concerns hinges on several factors. First, is there an alternative data set that might have superior quality and that is available or accessible to the researcher at a reasonable cost? If such an alternative exists, it should be used. A second factor is the magnitude of errors and their significance to the research outcome. If the errors are large and significant, the data set may not be tolerated. If the errors are minor or inconsequential toward study findings, the data set may still be used with the limitations duly stated. A third factor has to do with the purpose of the study. Is it an exploratory study that may tolerate larger measurement errors, or is it a causal modeling that seeks to confirm or disconfirm a set of hypotheses? A study from which important theoretical or policy implications are to be drawn requires a data set of acceptable quality. It may be wise to abandon such a study rather than conduct it with flawed data.

Another disadvantage or caution is that the process of examining secondary data can be time consuming. Some researchers may think that because the data are already collected and stored on computer, they can begin analysis immediately. This may not always be the case. When an investigator gathers the data firsthand, he or she is aware of their limitations and errors and can adjust the analyses accordingly. In contrast, if the investigator has not participated in data collection, he or she may have to spend hours getting familiar with the documentation and data structures.

There are also several ethical issues to consider regarding secondary data analysis. First, it is necessary for the researcher to obtain informed consent to use secondary data. Authorship and acknowledgment issues must also be worked out between the researcher and the owner of the data. It is important that the researcher make his or her intentions for the use of the data clear at the start of the project and that he or she maintains the subjects' confidentiality in the data throughout the project. Finally, careful citation is critical so as to avoid plagiarism (Daly, Kellehear, and Gliksman, 1998).

SUMMARY

Secondary analysis is any reanalysis of data collected by another researcher or organization. Secondary analysis may be based on the number of databases used both cross-sectionally and longitudinally, the sources of data, and the methods adopted to analyze the secondary data. The principal advantage of secondary analysis is economy, achieved through money, time, and personnel saved in data collection and management. Its principal weakness is the extent of compatibility between available data and the research question.

REVIEW QUESTIONS

1. What is the difference between secondary analysis and primary research?
2. What are the major types of secondary analysis?
3. What secondary data sources can you identify?
4. What are the strengths and weaknesses of secondary analysis as a scientific inquiry?
5. Do the following exercise as a way to learn the process of conducting secondary analysis. Choose an available data set, either from published sources or other researchers, and study the measurements carefully. Based on the measurements available, try to conceptualize a research topic of interest to you. Describe, in detail, what measures will be used by you to study your topic. Describe any limitations you might encounter (e.g., missing variables or inaccurate approximates).

REFERENCES

Babbie, E. (2006). *The Practice of Social Research* (11th ed.). Belmont, CA: Thomson/Wadsworth.

Carney, T. F. (1972). *Content Analysis: A Technique for Systematic Inferences from Communications*. London: Batsford.

Connell, F. A., Diehr, P., and Hart, L. G. (1987). The use of large databases in health care studies. *Annual Review of Public Health*, 8, 51–74.

Daly, J., Kellehear, A., and Gliksman, M. (1998). Secondary analysis, Chap. 9 in *The Public Health Researcher: A Methodological Guide*. Oxford: Oxford University Press.

Holsti, O. R. (1969). *Content Analysis for the Social Sciences and Humanities*. Reading, MA: Addison-Wesley.

Jacob, H. (1984). *Using Published Data*. Beverly Hills, CA: Sage.

Krippendorff, K. (1980). *Content Analysis: An Introduction to Its Methodology*. Beverly Hills, CA: Sage.

Marmor, T. R. (2000). *The Politics of Medicare* (2nd ed.). Somerset, NJ: Aldine Transaction.

Singleton, R. A., and Straits, B. C. (2005). *Approaches to Social Research* (4th ed.). New York: Oxford University Press.

Stewart, D. W., and Kamins, M. A. (1993). *Secondary Research: Information Sources and Methods*. Newbury Park, CA: Sage.

Qualitative Research

KEY TERMS

case study
constant comparative analysis
ethnographic
extreme case sampling
field research
focus group study
heuristics
in-depth interview

intensity sampling
narrative analysis
observational research
participant observation
phenomenological inquiry
qualitative research
saturation
sociography

stratified purposeful
    sampling
symbolic interactionism
time sampling
triangulation
typical case sampling

LEARNING OBJECTIVES

- To understand the major purposes of conducting qualitative research.

- To differentiate various terms related to
  qualitative research.

- To explain the major types of qualitative
  research, including participant observation,
  focused interview, and case study.

- To describe the process of qualitative
  research.

- To identify the strengths and weaknesses of
  qualitative research.

PURPOSE

Qualitative research serves four major purposes: it can be used as an exploratory study method, a complement to large-scale systematic research, a method for certain research purposes, and an alternative when other approaches cannot be properly used. Qualitative research is particularly oriented toward exploratory discovery and inductive logic. Inductive analysis begins with specific observations and builds toward general patterns. The objective is to let important analytic dimensions emerge from patterns found in the cases under study without presupposing what these dimensions are.

Qualitative research is often used to complement quantitative approaches, such as surveys and experiments. Qualitative research may be used when investigators know little about the subject, because the less they know, the more they can be open to other possibilities. It is often conducted first, providing leads and feedbacks for more structured or large-scale quantitative explanatory research. Quantitative research, on the other hand, generally requires a certain amount of prior knowledge about the topic to provide guidance for instrument design or intervention manipulation and control. In areas where measurements have not been developed and tested, it is appropriate to first gather descriptive information about the subject areas and then develop measures based on the gathered information. Qualitative research also plays confirmatory and elucidating roles. It adds depth, substance, and meaning to survey and experimental results.

Beyond its role in exploratory or preliminary analysis, qualitative research often stands on its own as a valuable tool of health service research. The qualitative research method is more appropriate for certain objectives, topics, problems, and situations than other methods. These include the study of: (1) complete events, phenomena, or programs; (2) developmental or transitional programs and events; (3) attitudes, feelings, motivations, behaviors, and factors associated with the changing processes; (4) complex events with interrelated phenomena; (5) dynamic or rapidly changing situations; (6) relationships between research subjects and settings; and (7) processes, or how things happen, rather than outcomes, or what happens. Qualitative research can produce results that would be unattainable using quantitative research. For instance, qualitative research may elucidate the experiential process of living with AIDS, or provide a picture of the atmosphere, culture, and interaction dynamics of a health care setting—these research outcomes are not quantifiable but nevertheless provide valuable insight and improve our understanding of health and health services.

Qualitative research may be used as an alternative when methodological problems and ethical concerns preclude the use of other methods. For example, qualitative research is more appropriate and less intrusive in situations where experimental designs and the administration of standardized instruments would affect normal operations. When subjects are unable (e.g., in the case of illiterates, the mentally ill, or young children) or unwilling (e.g., as with social deviants) to participate in a formal survey or experiment, qualitative research may be used as a viable alternative. From an ethical standpoint, the control and manipulation necessary for experiments (e.g., creating certain medical conditions such as disabilities) are not always feasible, and qualitative research is often a preferred alternative.

Table 6.1 compares several aspects of qualitative and quantitative research, which this chapter explores in some depth. As the table displays, qualitative and quantitative research have distinct purposes and are associated with different scientific disciplines. They are different in the way they advocate relationships with research subjects, use instruments, and collect data. However, both forms of research are valuable and should complement each other rather than be mutually exclusive.

DEFINITION

The term *qualitative research* is used to serve as a contrast to quantitative research, because qualitative research embodies observations and analyses that are generally less numerically measurable than methods typically considered as quantitative research (e.g., surveys and experiments). This classification does not mean there are no quantitative elements in qualitative research. Qualitative research may also involve counting and assigning numbers to observations. The term is used simply because qualitative statements and concepts, rather than quantitative numbers, represent the bulk of qualitative analysis.

Although the term *qualitative research* has been used thus far, several other terms are often applied to the methodological approach examined here (Patton, 2002). The term **field research** is often used because qualitative researchers observe, describe, and analyze events happening in the natural social setting (i.e., field). Indeed, fieldwork is the central activity of qualitative inquiry. Going into the field means having direct and personal contact with people under study in their own environments (Babbie, 2006). Qualitative approaches emphasize the necessity and importance of going to the field and getting close to the people and situations under study so that researchers become personally aware of the realities and details of daily life. The term *field* is not used in this book because qualitative research may also take place in the field (e.g., in the form of an interview survey).

Another often-used term is **observational research**, or participant observation. The term is used because observation is a primary method of qualitative research. Qualitative researchers observe for the purpose of seeing the world from the subject's own perspective. The word *observation* is not used because the term is basic to all scientific inquiry rather than limited to qualitative research. However, qualitative observation differs from other forms of scientific observation in two important ways. First, qualitative observation emphasizes direct

Table 6.1. Comparing Qualitative and Quantitative Research

	Qualitative	Quantitative
Associated scientific disciplines	Anthropology History Sociology	Economics Political science Psychology
Purposes	Explore multiple phenomena Develop concepts and questions Improve understanding Develop theories	Establish facts Make predictions Show relationships between variables Provide statistical description Test theories
Relationship with subjects of research	Egalitarian In-depth contact Long-term	Distant Detached and objective Short-term
Instruments and tools	Tape recorder Interview guide Transcriber Coding software	Questionnaires Scales Indices Statistical software
Types of data	Descriptive Field notes Official statistics Personal documents Photographs Quotations from subjects	Counts, measures Operationalized values Numerical Statistical
Data analysis occurs	Inductive Occurs throughout data collection Development of themes, concepts	Deductive Occurs at end of data collection Statistical
Design	Flexible, evolving plan Semistructured or unstructured	Detailed plan of operation Structured
Sample	Small Nonrepresentative	Large Representative
Methods	Participant observation Focused interview Case study	Experiments Quasi-experiments Data sets Surveys Structured interviews

Source: Adapted from Neutons & Robinson (1997).

observation, usually with the naked eye, rather than indirect observation, for example, the type represented in questionnaires or interviews. Second, qualitative observation takes place in the natural setting rather than a contrived situation or laboratory.

Case study is another term often associated with qualitative research because qualitative research typically examines a single social setting (i.e., case), such as an organization, a community, or an association. However, while case studies may use qualitative approaches, they may also use quantitative methods such as surveys and quasi-experiments. In addition, not all qualitative studies are concerned with detailed description and analysis of study settings.

Qualitative studies may also be termed **ethnographic**, which refers to the description of a culture after extensive field research. The primary method of ethnographers is participant observation. However, qualitative research is not limited to the study of culture. There are large numbers of additional topics pertinent to qualitative research, including the physician–patient relationship, the experience of dying, living through HIV/AIDS, building a regional health-delivery network, and so on.

Qualitative research is also related to **phenomenological inquiry**, focusing on the experience of a phenomenon by particular people. The phenomenon being experienced may be an emotion (e.g., loneliness, jealousy, or anger), a relationship, a marriage, a job, a program, an organization, or a culture. In terms of subject matter, phenomenological inquiry holds that what is important to know is what people experience and how they interpret the world. In terms of research methodology, phenomenological inquiry believes the best way for researchers to really know what another person experiences is to experience it through participant observation.

Heuristics, a form of phenomenological inquiry, focuses on intense human experience from the point of view of researchers. It is through the intense personal experience that a sense of connectedness develops between researchers and subjects in their mutual efforts to elucidate the nature, meaning, and essence of a significant event. Qualitative research encompasses both the research subject and the method of phenomenological inquiry but is much broader in both areas. In addition to individuals, qualitative research may focus on a group, organization, community, or any social phenomenon or entity. Qualitative research may include, along with participant observation, focused interviews, case studies, or other methods suitable for qualitative fieldwork.

The field of **symbolic interactionism** contributes to qualitative observation and analysis. The importance of symbolic interactionism to qualitative research is its special emphasis on a common set of symbols and their interpretations by those who use them in explaining human interactions and behaviors.

Qualitative research may be defined as research methods used to provide detailed descriptions and analyses of issues of interest in terms of how and why things happen the way they do. It aims at gaining individuals' own accounts of their actions, knowledge, thoughts, and feelings. Qualitative analysis provides rich descriptions of individuals' perspectives, focusing on meanings, interpretations, attitudes, and motivations. By capturing an insider's view of reality, qualitative researchers can understand the substance and logic of views that may seem to be implausible to outsiders. Qualitative research is an excellent way of gaining an overview of the process of a complicated event or problem.

TYPES

There are many types of qualitative research methods. Three widely used approaches are participant observation, in-depth interview, and case study (Babbie, 2006; Bailey, 1994; Denzin and Lincoln, 2005; Patton, 2002; Rubin, 1983; Singleton and Straits, 2005; Sterk and Elifson, 2004; Yin, 2003).

Participant Observation

To fully understand the complexities of certain phenomena, merely relying on surveying what people say is limiting because people may be unwilling to share important details, especially if they are sensitive. Direct participation in and observation of the phenomena are critical. Observations enable researchers to go beyond the selective perceptions of others and experience the setting firsthand. In **participant observation**, researchers study a group or organization by becoming part of that group or organization (e.g., by joining a hospital or managed care organization). Participation may be open or disguised. In open participation, investigators make their role as researchers known to group members. However, the group leader or head of the organization always needs to be informed and his or her collaboration sought. The choice of open versus disguised participation depends on whether knowledge of the study by members will significantly affect their normal behavior.

As participants, researchers pay close attention to the physical, social, and human environment surrounding the topic under study; the formal and informal interactions; and the unplanned activities. Informal interactions in the research setting include activities, hierarchy of command, span of control, channels of communication, and languages used and their meanings from the perspective of those being observed. Qualitative analysis must be faithful to facts and enable readers to understand the situation described. The goal is to describe the problem under study to outsiders based on an understanding of the insiders' perspectives.

Participant observation has many advantages. It sensitizes researchers to the research setting and the members within. By becoming part of the group, researchers are more likely to see events from the perspective of insiders. By directly observing operations and activities within the setting, researchers gain a better understanding of the context and process of activities. The firsthand experience acquired through participant observation helps address the whys and hows of research questions.

In-Depth Interview

The **in-depth interview** is made up of three types of qualitative interviews: the informal conversational interview, the standardized open-ended interview, and the general interview guide approach (Patton, 2002). In an informal conversational interview, neither specific questions nor general topics are predetermined. Rather, they emerge naturally. Questions are spontaneously asked based on the natural flow of conversation. Informal conversational interviews take place most often in participant observation.

The standardized open-ended interview consists of a questionnaire instrument with a set of questions carefully worded and sequenced. Each respondent is asked the same set of questions in the same sequence. Instructions on probing accompany the questionnaire so that probing is used consistently by different interviewers toward different respondents. The standardized open-ended interview is used when it is important to minimize variation in the questions posed to interviewees, particularly when studies involve many interviewers. The downside of this approach is that it is less flexible or spontaneous.

The general interview guide approach has an outline of issues to be explored during the interview. The issues are unstructured and open-ended (i.e., there is no formal questionnaire) and of variable length (e.g., interviews may take up to several hours). The issues in the outline are prepared before the interview but need not be addressed in any particular sequence. The wording of the issues can be changed during the interview so long as their essence is maintained. Their sequence can also be altered to fit in with the actual flow of the interview. The outline of issues simply serves as a basic interview guide, or checklist, to make sure that no relevant issues are left out. Often, new findings during the interview may determine subsequent questions. Respondents are free to answer in their own words, either briefly or at length. Respondents' answers are written or typed by hand or, with their permission, can be recorded electronically. This approach is most frequently used during in-depth interviews.

In-depth interviews may be conducted with one individual or a group of individuals. The latter is often referred to as focus group study, or focus group (Morgan, 1997). **Focus group study** involves interviewing a small group of people on a particular topic. A focus group typically consists of six to twelve people who are brought together in a room to engage in a guided discussion of some topic for up to two hours. Focus group participants are selected on the basis of relevancy to the topic under study; they are not likely to be chosen through probability sampling methods. This means that participants are not statistically representative of any meaningful population. The purpose of the study is to explore rather than to describe or explain in any definitive sense. For instance, in Dayton, Ohio, a focus group study gathered a group of school nurses to discuss barriers to optimal asthma care for children in an urban school system (Forbis,

Rammel, Huffman, and Taylor, 2006). Because school nurses spend a great deal of time caring for children with asthma, their perspectives on how better to manage this chronic illness are highly relevant to advancing knowledge in this area of health services research.

At least two investigators should be present during focus group study, one serving as moderator and the other as recorder. The moderator, guided by the interview checklist, facilitates and controls the discussion to make sure it is not dominated by one or two highly verbal people and that everyone has an opportunity to talk and share their views. Facilitating and conducting a focus group study requires considerable group process skill. Recording can be done in the same room or in an adjacent room where the focus group activities can be observed. Focus group study can also be videotaped and analyzed later.

Participants talk about their perceptions of the issues raised by the facilitator, hear one another's views, and provide additional comments. Although there will be less detail about individual motivations and views than in individual in-depth interviews, group discussions can yield valuable information about group interactions and dynamics as people react to views they agree or disagree with. Participants are not required to reach any consensus on any issues. The objective is to allow people to provide their own views on the topic of interest in the context of other people's views. A given study may consist of one or more focus groups.

In in-depth interview studies, the final number of participants included depends on the point at which the interviewer starts to hear the same ideas repeated and no new information being shared. This point is called **saturation**. Qualitative researchers have increasingly called for a more rigorous definition of what saturation entails, as this concept has been invoked to justify small samples with inadequate data (Charmaz, 2005). Thus, saturation as a criterion of adequacy continues to evolve, but its basic premise remains a central concept of qualitative research.

The in-depth interview has several advantages (Patton, 2002). It is flexible, has high face validity, and is low in cost. The focus group study is an efficient data collection method, because during one setting investigators can gather information from six to twelve people instead of only one person. The process also enhances data quality as participants provide checks and balances on each other that reduce inaccurate information and extreme views. Further, it allows investigators to assess whether views are shared relatively consistently among participants on certain issues.

The in-depth interview has several weaknesses, however. The number of questions to be asked or issues explored is limited since it takes time for respondents to think about each open-ended question and then to say what they think. This is particularly true in focus group study, where each participant responds to the same questions. Focus group study also affords the researcher less control than individual interviews do. When participants share opposing views and are nonconciliatory, the interview may be difficult to conduct. The in-depth interview requires greater facilitating skill on the part of investigators. Another weakness of the in-depth interview is the difficulty of taking notes while also facilitating the interview. Usually, the interview is tape-recorded and transcribed later. And the transcription of notes is time consuming. Finally, data resulting from in-depth interviews are usually a challenge to analyze.

Case Study

A **case study** may be defined as an empirical inquiry that uses multiple sources of evidence to investigate a real-life social entity or phenomenon (Yin, 2003). It is particularly valuable when the research aims at capturing individual differences or unique variations from one setting to another or from one experience to another.

The case study method is flexible and diverse. It may be a small project carried out by a single researcher or a large one carried out by a team of investigators over several years. It may focus on a single case or multiple cases. A single case often forms the basis for research on typical, deviant, or critical cases. Multiple case designs can be limited to two or three settings or extend to dozens of cases, either to achieve replication of the same study in different settings or to compare and contrast different cases.

A case can be a person, an event, a program, an organization, a time period, a critical incident, or a community. Regardless of the unit of analysis, a case study seeks to provide a richly detailed portrait of a particular unit so that an in-depth and comprehensive understanding can be achieved.

When the case study focuses on one individual, that individual is interviewed over an extended period of time to obtain detailed accounts of his or her personal history and the events he or she has experienced. The individual case study is commonly used to study ethnic or cultural groups who are difficult to locate and whose experiences are more distinctive and less well known. For example, an individual case study can be conducted on health-seeking patterns of ethnic groups. To complement and substantiate the individual's personal account, the researcher refers to a variety of other sources of evidence, such as interviews with other people (family, friends, and colleagues who have had contact with the subject), documentary sources (records), and observations of relevant social settings and events.

A case study may focus on a particular social entity, such as a single local community, to describe and analyze certain aspects of community life that could include politics, religious activities, crime, health, and the like. For example, a community case study could be performed to investigate a community-based health care network, including community organizing, needs assessment, restructuring, and evaluation (e.g., the Robert Wood Johnson Foundation's Community Tracking Study). The term **sociography** may be used for community-based studies to denote the social mapping of a community's institutions, structure, and patterns of relationships. A community case study can focus on one or more communities.

A case study may be conducted for social groups, such as families, work units, or interest groups. This group investigation might focus on typical as well as deviant groups. For example, such a study could research health interest groups in terms of their influences on national health policy and regulations.

A case study may be conducted for organizations or institutions such as health services organizations, schools, regulatory agencies, or, say, the World Health Organization. For example, a case study of a health maintenance organization (HMO) can reveal its impact on cost containment and quality care.

In a case study, the type and quantity of data collected and analyzed can also vary enormously. Researchers usually use several methods of data collection, including the analysis of administrative records and other existing documents, in-depth interviews, structured surveys, and participant observation. Data obtained through multiple sources enable researchers to get a more complete account of the relevant issues under study. The costs and timetables for case study designs thus vary significantly. A case study may be extended into a longitudinal study with periodic follow-up data collection and analysis.

PROCESS

Qualitative research may be considered a process consisting of a number of essential components: preparation, access, design, data collection, analysis, and presentation. It must be emphasized that qualitative research rarely proceeds smoothly, in a sequence of steps, although each step is a necessary part of the process.

Preparation

As is true with other research methods, qualitative research starts with a review of all relevant literature related to the topic. Such a review enables the researcher to ascertain the current knowledge on the topic and the existing gaps. Since qualitative research is likely to be concerned with exploratory issues, relevant existing literature could be limited. However, researchers may still gain an understanding as to the problems likely to be encountered in this kind of study. If the investigator seeks to study a particular organization, a relevant literature source would be that organization's charts, mission statements, annual reports, and other pertinent statements. Researchers should avoid going in cold. Familiarity with relevant literature and background materials will prepare them well during the field study.

Access

The choice of a research setting hinges on a number of considerations, including whether the site is consistent with the researcher's interests, whether it is accessible, and whether a rapport with informants is possible. It is also possible that several sites may be selected in order to obtain enough informants for the study. In other situations, the site is predetermined and is linked with the problem of investigation.

Gaining access to the group or setting an investigator wishes to study depends on the nature of the group or setting. If the setting is a public place, the researcher may not need to negotiate for access. If it is a formal organization, permission is critical. If researchers are to conduct a study in a hospital, they need to approach the administrator to obtain permission and cooperation. The general purpose of the study as well as its significance should be explained. Strict confidentiality should be guaranteed.

However, investigators may want to be ambiguous about the detailed research objectives for several reasons. The revelation of the detailed study objectives may distort the outcome of the research if the host agency is able to alter its normal course of action. In addition, at the beginning of a qualitative research study, researchers may not know exactly what they are looking for. They should not commit themselves too narrowly, because when research questions are changed along the way, the host agency may perceive researchers as being dishonest. Further, if the study objectives are contrary to the interests of the organization or group within, investigators' access may be hindered or denied outright. While most often the administrator has formal control over access to patient populations, persons dealing with the patient on a day-to-day basis, such as physicians, nurses, technicians, and receptionists, can be critically important in facilitating or hindering real access (Grady and Wallston, 1988).

One approach often used to obtain entry is the known-sponsor approach (Patton, 2002). Investigators rely on the legitimacy and credibility of another person or agency to establish their own legitimacy and credibility. Before using this approach, researchers need to be certain that the known sponsor is indeed a reliable source.

In identifying informants, researchers should recognize informal leadership. The help of group leaders is often critical. Investigators should also try to select a representative cross section of people, including different sociodemographic groups, organizational units, and tasks. Atypical individuals should also be sought. To select the ideal mix of informants, researchers need to be familiar with the setting. Familiarity may be gained through a background reading of the organizational literature.

Access may also be gained with a snowball strategy, which locates additional contacts through informants. Once researchers have established trust and rapport with the informants, these informants may be able to reveal additional names of people who can provide more information about the questions of interest.

Regardless of which methods are used to gain access, researchers should be clear about the actual reasons people allow themselves to be interviewed. Some commonly encountered reasons are:

- interest (respondent interest in the research topic or in participating in research)

- legal/agency requirement (as part of the contract, compliance with agency's policy)

- public information (public officials, politicians, agencies that spend tax dollars)

- coercion or disincentive (superior–inferior relations, to avert penalties and other problems)

- reward or incentive (financial and nonfinancial benefits associated with participation)

- clarification (to tell his or her side of the story, to change an opinion or perception)

- seeking support (to look for assistance)

- pique or pleasure (whistle-blower, an opportunity to praise something)

- catharsis (to vent feelings from a traumatic experience)

- sociability (fond of conversation)

- courtesy (being polite and cooperative)

Design

In qualitative research, investigators do not attempt to manipulate the research setting. This naturalistic characteristic makes qualitative research design rather flexible. In general, the design features (e.g., operational measurement, hypotheses, and sampling methods) cannot be completely specified prior to entering the research setting. Qualitative design needs to remain open to permit adjustment as warranted by the fieldwork. The design unfolds after investigators have become familiar with the major issues to be studied and the opportunities and obstacles afforded by the research setting. Once specified, qualitative design may also change during the course of the study as a result of new or unforeseen events.

The flexibility of research design does not mean qualitative researchers should not think about design. On the contrary, researchers will be better prepared if they know what they are looking for and how to look for it ahead of data collection. One important way to strengthen the validity and reliability of qualitative research is through **triangulation**, or the use of a combination of several methods in the study of the same topic, including both quantitative and qualitative. Examples of triangulation types include data (i.e., the use of a variety of data sources in a study), investigator (i.e., the use of several different researchers or evaluators), theory (i.e., the use of multiple perspectives to interpret a single set of data), and methodology (i.e., the use of multiple methods to study a single problem or program) (Yin, 2003).

Specifically, design considerations include the unit of analysis, the preliminary sampling procedures, the researchers' roles in the study, and the ethical implications of the fieldwork. Other aspects of the design phase include methods of data collection (through observations and interviews), primary questions to be explored, and analysis strategy, which will be covered in detail in later chapters.

Unit of Analysis

In qualitative research, the unit of analysis varies significantly depending on the research purposes or what investigators intend to accomplish at the end of the study. The same study may also use several units of analysis. Examples include individuals, groups, cultures, brief actions such as incidents, longer actions such as events and activities, meanings and relationships, and the research setting itself. The choice of the unit of analysis determines the ensuing strategies for data collection, analysis, and reporting.

Sampling

In qualitative research, typically both the research sites and subjects are predetermined based on their availability and accessibility. Random sampling is usually not possible. Rather, small nonrandom sampling characterizes the selection of research sites and subjects. In these situations, attempts should be made to be as representative as possible in the selection of sites and subjects. For example, if qualitative research is conducted to investigate statewide hospital conditions, one may be able to study only one or two sites because of the time constraints. Therefore, the representativeness of the choice of hospitals becomes significant. A purposive, or quota, sampling technique may be relied on to ensure the hospitals chosen share certain important characteristics with the average hospitals in the state, such as an urban or rural location, socioeconomic status of the patients in the community, and hospital size. Even when probability sampling methods are impossible or inappropriate, the logical link between representativeness and generalizability still holds for qualitative research. Later in this chapter, strategies for ensuring the rigor of qualitative research are described in detail.

Other commonly used qualitative sampling methods include time sampling, typical case sampling, extreme (deviant) case sampling, intensity sampling, and stratified purposeful sampling (Patton, 2002). **Time sampling** is based on sampling periods (e.g., months of the year) or units of time (e.g., hours of the day). It is used when activities are believed to vary significantly at different time periods or units. **Typical case sampling** provides a detailed profile of one or more typical or usual cases to demonstrate the major features of the topic under study. **Extreme**, or deviant, **case sampling** focuses on cases that are different from typical cases to provide examples of unusual or special situations. **Intensity sampling** focuses on information-rich cases that strongly demonstrate the topic under investigation. Intensity cases are not unusual because they are not extreme cases. **Stratified purposeful sampling** is a combination of typical case sampling and extreme case sampling. Cases are first stratified into different categories of interest (e.g., above average, average, and below average), and then samples are selected from each.

Roles

Investigators need to be clear about their roles during research and about how much they will reveal themselves as researchers. At one extreme, investigators are observers only, watching events and activities but never participating. At the other extreme, they may participate in all of the events and activities as if they were members of the group. In between, a researcher can combine observation and participation by adopting the role of either participant observer, with the emphasis on participation, or observer participant, with the emphasis on observation.

Researchers should also determine whether to make known their role as investigators. If they choose to reveal their true identities, they need to build a rapport with and gain trust and cooperation from the subjects. They must also consider whether the subjects' behavior will be affected by their presence. If researchers hide their true identities, they must consider the ethical consequences of such deception.

Ethical Implications

In designing and implementing qualitative research, investigators should consider several ethical issues that might be relevant to their studies. The first concern is the potential risk to the subjects. Examples of risk include bodily harm, side effects, undue stress, legal liabilities, loss of benefits, and ostracism by colleagues. When researchers are unsure about potential ethical or legal implications, they should consult with the institutional review board (IRB) for clarification. A large project usually has an ethical counselor on staff to deal with both anticipated and unanticipated ethical issues.

Before data are gathered, investigators should obtain informed consent from the subjects. During the study, the subjects should be given the opportunity to ask questions and decline involvement. After the study, confidentiality should be maintained in data storage, processing, analysis, and reporting. If researchers have made any promises to the study subjects, either financial (e.g., cash) or nonfinancial (e.g., copies of the study report), they should live up to their promises in in a timely fashion so that the subjects' cooperation continues.

Data Collection

In general, qualitative researchers use multiple sources of evidence to address a broad range of issues related to a topic, and to validate study findings. The most common methods of data collection are observations, interviews, and case studies. Observations consist of detailed descriptions of the subjects' activities, behaviors, actions, interactions, and organizational processes and dynamics. Interviews reveal the subjects' experiences, ideas, perceptions, feelings, and knowledge. Case studies include a variety of relevant information about the setting under study.

Qualitative investigators also rely heavily on existing data sources, including media publications (e.g., newspaper clippings and articles), administrative documents (e.g., proposals and project reports), formal studies (e.g., consulting reports and previous evaluations), figures (e.g., organizational charts, diagrams, and maps), service records (e.g., clients' for major services), personnel records (e.g., directories and telephone listings), financial records (e.g., budgets), personal records (e.g., diaries, calendars, and appointment books), communications (e.g., letters and memoranda), survey data (e.g., census records), and administrative records (e.g., previously collected site data).

There are three major ways to record data during a field study: relying simply on memory, taking notes by hand or using a computer, or recording the data electronically. Relying on memory is used in informal interviews. It permits an informal conversation without interruptions so that the interview will appear more natural. However, an individual's memory is usually faulty. Typically, only an approximation of the actual interview can be reproduced.

Note taking is used in more formal interviews. It enables researchers to record the subjects' responses verbatim. It is also flexible in that investigators may ignore repetitions and digressions by subjects. Laptop computers can be used to facilitate note taking. In recording field notes, researchers should assign a code and date to each interview so that notes can be easily sorted. In addition to recording the subjects' perceptions on the issues under study, researchers can also jot down their own feelings, reactions, insights, interpretations, and reflections to facilitate later analysis. However, they should clearly indicate which are the subjects' responses and which are their own. The downside of note taking is that it can be distracting, tends to slow down the interview, and reduces the spontaneity of the conversation.

Tape recording provides complete coverage of an interview without interrupting the flow. However, respondents may be uneasy about providing forthright answers if they are perceived to be "on record." In addition, transcribing tapes is a time-consuming process. It may take five hours to transcribe one hour of tape. Also, nonverbal behavior cannot be tape-recorded. A camera or videotape recorder may be used to make a visual record of an interview.

Recording is not limited to interviews. Qualitative researchers also take notes of things they observe and of their thoughts related to the observation. Some researchers use a Stenomask to facilitate note taking. A Stenomask is a sound-shielded microphone attached to a portable tape recorder. Researchers can dictate to the recorder during observation without attracting the attention of the subjects.

To collect data properly, researchers need to hone their interviewing skills. They should have an inquiring mind and not be trapped by their personal perceptions and preconceived ideologies. Before the interview, they should have a general idea of the topic and issues being studied as well as the type of information to be collected. Such an understanding allows the research to be conducted with focus.

During the interview, researchers should be good listeners. They must maintain neutrality and not ask leading questions or offer personal opinions. Probing when necessary should be kept neutral. They should be sensitive and responsive to the subjects. Investigators should understand that the interview setting may affect responses. For example, interviews conducted in an office setting are more formal than those conducted in a public place, such as a cafeteria or the subjects' own homes. The method of recording interviews can also affect responses. Subjects are most self-conscious when they are being tape-recorded and most relaxed during informal conversation.

Analysis

There are few guidelines and procedures that govern all types of qualitative analysis. However, several major steps are common to most analyses of qualitative data, whether the data are derived from observation, interviews, or case studies. These steps include becoming familiar with the relevant literature in the field in order to develop hypotheses and analytic frameworks, reading one's research notes carefully, coding important topics of conversation or observation, and developing classification schemes based on major themes. In general, researchers should be watchful for biases and seek multiple sources of evidence to corroborate research findings.

One major objective of qualitative analysis is description. Researchers provide detailed descriptions of insiders' views of the issues of interest. Qualitative descriptions use anecdotes, examples, and quotes from subjects. Descriptions may be organized in one of several ways: chronologically, covering various periods and processes of the program and the events within those periods; in terms of importance, focusing on critical events and major activities relevant to primary research questions; or around major units of analysis, such as research sites, individuals, or groups. Qualitative descriptions aim at answering the "how" questions.

Based on detailed descriptions, a qualitative analysis then integrates concepts and ideas to help explain and interpret the actions, activities, and beliefs described. The underlying meanings are explored, guided by existing theoretical frameworks. Significance is attached to the results and this is generated into patterns. Themes and concepts are identified and become the components of grounded theories. This level of qualitative analysis answers the "why" questions.

To assist qualitative analysis, researchers think about analysis at the very start of data collection. The frequent review and editing of field notes is the beginning of qualitative analysis. As soon as data are collected, they are coded and organized in different categories to facilitate later analysis. Coding is an iterative process. One way to approach coding is to begin with a small segment of data (e.g., with interview or observational notes), identifying each unique response, theme, or concept. This initial set of coding categories acts as a foundation for analyzing the next segment of data. Categories may be added and refined as the investigator's understanding of the data improves. Examples of these categories are background information, bibliographies, settings, biographies, issues, relationships, concepts, examples, supporting data, and quotes. When no new categories present themselves, the researcher is ready to develop instructions for coding, as well as a framework that links the codes typologically. After this step, all of the data should be re-coded, using the same instructions and framework. If more than one person is performing the coding, it is important to periodically check inter-coder reliability.

Computers can be used to facilitate the filing and analysis process. Word processing allows the investigator to set up a filing system with relative ease.

Software programs designed for qualitative data analysis can be used to help analyze field notes. For instance, there are numerous computer programs that act as text retrievers (e.g., Metamorph, Orbis, Sonar Professional, Text Collector, Word Cruncher, and ZyIndex). In addition, there are several code-and-retrieve programs (e.g., HyperQual2, Kwalitan, Martin, QualPro, and Ethnograph) and code-based theory-builders (e.g., Aquad, Atlas/ti, HyperResearch, Nud.ist, QCA) that may facilitate qualitative analysis.

Specific Qualitative Analytic Strategies

While an exhaustive description of the myriad approaches used to analyze qualitative data is outside the scope of this chapter, some central methods of qualitative data analysis are described below.

Constant Comparative Analysis

Glaser and Strauss (1967) first developed constant comparative analysis in their seminal text, *The Discovery of Grounded Theory*. **Constant comparative analysis** is a process that involves comparing one piece of data (such as one interview or one statement) to others to develop an understanding of the relationships among the different pieces of data (Thorne, 2000). Through constant comparative analysis, the researcher may identify similarities and differences across the data and begin to develop theories about relationships, patterns, and themes. Through this process, the researcher develops a better understanding of a human phenomenon within a particular context. The products of constant comparative analysis are theories about basic social processes (such as coping with grief or with disease) and factors that may account for variations in people's experience of these processes (Thorne, 2000).

One example of this type of analysis is a study conducted at the Washington Diabetes Care Center in Seattle by researchers who used constant comparative methods to explore issues of trust and collaboration in the health care setting (Ciechanowski and Katon, in press). First, 27 diabetic patients completed a self-report measure of "attachment style," which captures the level of trust patients feel toward the health care system. A wide range of attachment styles were identified in this group of patients, allowing for comparisons within the group. Researchers interviewed the patients, asking questions about their experiences in the health care setting and about their interactions with providers. By comparing the interview results of patients with varying levels of attachment style, the investigators were able to develop theories about how patients with different levels of trust in the health care system can be better served.

Narrative Analysis

Another central method of qualitative analysis is narrative analysis. As the name implies, **narrative analysis** involves generating, interpreting, and representing people's stories (Thorne, 2000). A narrative may be spoken during an interview, in the course of conversation, or in the field, or it may be written (Chase, 2005). A narrative may take on any number of different forms. It can be a long life story, a short anecdote, or a description of a particular event or time in one's life. As Chase (2005, p. 657) explains, narrative analysis as a method of qualitative research is distinguished by its ability to "highlight the uniqueness of each human action and event rather than their common properties." Narrative analysis is distinct from constant comparative analysis in that the goal is not to identify patterns and themes across data, but rather to concentrate first on patterns and themes within each narrative. The goal of narrative research is not to create generalizations for a certain population. Rather, it is to emphasize the particularity of each narrative and to place each narrative into a broader frame (Chase, 2005).

In health services research, narrative analysis can help improve knowledge in areas such as patients' personal experiences with disease. For instance, noting that there was very little information in the literature on what it is like to live with lupus (a chronic autoimmune disease), one researcher conducted a narrative analysis on interview data from lupus patients to learn more (Mendelson, 2006). Seven women with lupus participated in three interviews, one month apart, and maintained a daily symptom journal. Additional narrative accounts were gathered from 23 women who were recruited from the Internet. Using narrative analysis, the researcher identified patterns and themes within each narrative and identified many overlapping themes across the narratives, such as feelings of uncertainty, a shifting sense of identity, and experiences of financial stress related to living with lupus.

Presentation

There are many ways to present the results of qualitative research. Results may be published as a book or journal article or as a report submitted to the funding agencies. A summary of the findings may be presented at conferences or published by the media. The styles of writing also vary significantly, from a narrative style to a format with tables, graphs, and pictures. A more structured format is suggested below and is composed of six major sections: introduction, setting, design, findings, discussion, and bibliography.

In the introduction section, the author describes the issue or problem being studied and its significance. He or she also presents a review of the relevant theoretical and practical literature. In the section about research setting, the author provides a brief account of the historical development, current characteristics (both qualitative and quantitative), and major problems or issues related to the setting that the author studied, as well as a discussion about why this setting was selected. In the design section, the author summarizes the methods adopted for entering the site, sampling subjects, establishing rapport, and collecting and analyzing data. In the findings section, the author gives an overview of the major results of the study, with many pertinent examples as supporting evidence. The raw data drawn from field notes and other sources are organized into meaningful subsections reflecting the major themes and research questions. Illustrative examples and quotes are provided throughout the presentation of results. The qualitative findings are presented in combination with quantitative data. In the discussion section, the author analyzes the findings in terms of the underlying meanings, patterns, alternative perspectives, and policy or theoretical implications. The bibliography section can be drafted at the beginning of the study and augmented later with new citations when necessary.

The presentation of study results is tied to the intended audience. For example, if the primary audience involves professional colleagues in the same field, the contribution to theory development is likely to be important. If the audience consists of policy makers or practitioners, the policy and practical implications become more important. If the audience is the funding agency, the fulfillment of the research objectives and the rigor of the research become important concerns. Because of potential differences among audiences, a successful presentation may need more than one version of the study report.

Ensuring Rigor in Qualitative Research

Devers (1999) and Bowling (1997) suggest several criteria for ensuring the rigor and quality of qualitative research. First, the research question, the theoretical framework, and the methods used throughout the research process should be clearly stated. The context of the research (including how the investigator's role was defined, how the setting and the researcher might have influenced the nature and types of data collected, and how events over time may have affected results) should also be thoroughly described. The research study design should reflect that the researcher considered the implications of choosing a particular sample. Generalizability of qualitative research is enhanced if the sample includes a diverse range of individuals and settings, if appropriate. Data collection methods, data types and sources, and analysis methods must be described and justified. Ideally, an independent investigator should be able to repeat the data collection and analysis, based on the researcher's description, and produce similar results. Credibility of the data is enhanced if the researcher uses triangulated methods, as described earlier in the chapter. Other strategies for enhancing the rigor of qualitative research include searching for evidence that may disprove the results, carrying out data archiving, conducting a peer review, and engaging in reflective journal keeping. Finally, presenting adequate amounts of raw data (e.g., transcripts of interviews) in a systematic fashion in the final report also helps convince readers that the researcher's interpretation of the data is based on the evidence and is not impressionistic.

STRENGTHS AND WEAKNESSES

The main strength of qualitative research is the validity of the data obtained: individuals are interviewed in sufficient detail for the results to be taken as true, correct, complete, and believable reports of their views and experiences. The question "why" can usually be answered through qualitative research. However, validity largely hinges on the skill, competence, and rigor of the researchers conducting the investigation.

Qualitative research is more effective for studying topics that are difficult to analyze quantitatively. Qualitative methods are better suited for the study of attitudes, meanings, perceptions, feelings, behaviors, motivations, interrelations among factors, changes, complexities, idiosyncrasies, and contextual background.

Qualitative research is also a less expensive approach both in terms of money and personnel required. Other research methods may require expensive equipment or a large staff, but qualitative research can typically be undertaken by one or a few researchers. For example, survey research generally incurs greater expenses in sampling, data collection, and analysis. Similarly, experiments, while generally on a smaller scale than surveys, can be more complex and expensive to conduct.

Flexibility is another strength of qualitative research. The design and scope of a study may be modified at any time to account for changing situations or conditions.

The major weakness of qualitative research has to do with its lack of generalizability. Its depth and detail typically derive from a small number of respondents or case studies that cannot be taken as representative, even if great care is taken to choose a cross section of the type of people or sites. With its qualitative rather than quantitative focus, qualitative research rarely yields descriptive statements about the characteristics of a large population. The conclusions reached through this method of study are generally regarded as less definitive.

Reliability is another potential problem. Even though qualitative measures are detailed and comprehensive, they are also personal and idiosyncratic. Another researcher studying the same topic may use entirely different measures or analysis strategy, and may come to a different conclusion.

When a case study is carried out by an active participant (in a social group or an organization, for example), ethical issues may arise, and there may be practical difficulties in combining the sometimes conflicting roles of group member and researcher.

Also, qualitative research places great demands on research skills. The in-depth interview requires researchers to demonstrate adequate prior knowledge of the subject and sufficient sensitivity to research subjects. Other important skills for qualitative researchers include the ability to observe details and conduct analysis and interpretation based on direct observation as well as on available data. Qualitative research benefits from good writing and presentation skills more than other research methods. Capable qualitative researchers must have keen observational, interviewing, interpretive, and writing skills.

SUMMARY

Qualitative research may be used as an exploratory study method, as a complement to large-scale systematic research, as a method for specific nonquantitative kinds of research, or as an alternative when other methods cannot be properly used. Other terms often employed to denote qualitative research include field research, observational research or participant observation, case study, ethnographic study, phenomenological inquiry, and heuristics. Three of the major types of qualitative research methods are participant observation, focused interview, and case study. The process of qualitative research consists of a number of essential elements: preparation, access, design, data collection, analysis, and presentation. The strengths of qualitative research include its relative high validity, its appropriateness for topics that are difficult to analyze quantitatively, its relatively low cost, and its flexibility. Its major weaknesses include the lack of generalizability and reliability.

REVIEW QUESTIONS

1. What purposes does qualitative research serve?
2. Draw distinctions among the various terms used to denote qualitative research.
3. Why and how do researchers conduct a focus group study?
4. What are the components in qualitative research? What does each component entail?
5. What are the various methods of data collection in qualitative research? Assess their pros and cons.

REFERENCES

Babbie, E. (2006). Field research. Chap. 11 in *The Practice of Social Research* (11th ed.). Belmont, CA: Thomson/Wadsworth.

Bailey, K. D. (1994). Observation. Chap. 10 in *Methods of Social Research* (4th ed.). New York: Free Press.

Bowling, A. (1997). *Research Methods in Health: Investigating Health and Health Services*. Buckingham, UK: Open University Press.

Charmaz, K. (2005). Grounded theory in the 21st century. Chap. 20 in N. K. Denzin and Y. S. Lincoln (Eds.), *The Sage Handbook of Qualitative Research* (3rd ed.). Thousand Oaks, CA: Sage.

Chase, S. E. (2005). Narrative inquiry: Multiple lenses, approaches, voices. Chap. 25 in N. K. Denzin and Y. S. Lincoln (Eds.), *The Sage Handbook of Qualitative Research* (3rd ed.). Thousand Oaks, CA: Sage.

Ciechanowski, P., and Katon, W. J. (In press). The interpersonal experience of health care through the eyes of patients with diabetes. *Social Science and Medicine*.

Denzin, N. K., and Lincoln, Y. S. (Eds.). (2005). *The Sage Handbook of Qualitative Research* (3rd ed.). Thousand Oaks, CA: Sage.

Devers, K. J. (1999). How will we know "good" qualitative research when we see it? Beginning the dialogue in health services research. *Health Services Research*, *34*(5, Pt. 2), 1153–1187.

Forbis, S., Rammel, J., Huffman, B., and Taylor, R. (2006). Barriers to care of inner-city children with asthma: School nurse perspective. *Journal of School Health*, 76(6), 205–207.

Glaser, B. G., and Strauss, A. L. (1967). *The Discovery of Grounded Theory*. Hawthorne, NY: Aldine.

Grady, K. E., and Wallston, B. S. (1988). *Research in Health Care Settings*. Newbury Park, CA: Sage.

Mendelson, C. (2006). Managing a medically and socially complex life: Women living with lupus. *Qualitative Health Research, 16*(7), 982–997.

Morgan, D. L. (1997). *Focus Groups as Qualitative Research* (2nd ed.). Thousand Oaks, CA: Sage.

Neutens, J. J., and Rubinson, L. (1997). Qualitative research. Chap. 8 in *Research Techniques for the Health Sciences* (2nd ed.). Needham Heights, MA: Allyn & Bacon.

Patton, M. Q. (2002). *Qualitative Evaluation and Research Methods* (3rd ed.). Thousand Oaks, CA: Sage.

Rubin, H. J. (1983). *Applied Social Research*. Columbus, OH: Charles E. Merrill.

Singleton, R. A., and Straits, B. C. (2005). *Approaches to Social Research* (4th ed.). New York: Oxford University Press.

Sterk, C. E., and Elifson, K. W. (2004). Qualitative methods in community-based research. Chap. 7 in D. S. Blumenthal and R. J. DiClemente (Eds.), *Community-Based Health Research: Issues and Methods*. New York: Springer.

Thorne, S. (2000). Data analysis in qualitative research. *Evidence Based Nursing, 3*, 68–70.

Yin, R. K. (2003). *Case Study Research: Design and Methods*. Thousand Oaks, CA: Sage.

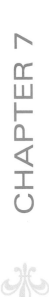

❖ CHAPTER 7 ❖

Experimental Research

KEY TERMS

attrition
comparison group
contamination
control group
demonstration
double-blind experiment
ecological validity
experimental group
experimental research
external validity
field experiment
history
instrumentation

interaction between selection
  bias and the intervention
interaction effect of testing
internal validity
laboratory experiment
matching
maturation
midtests
model
multiple-treatment
  interference
natural experiment
population validity

posttests
pretests
quasi-experimental
random sampling
randomization
reactive effects of the
  experimental arrangements
selection
simulation
statistical regression
testing
time-series tests

LEARNING OBJECTIVES

- To describe the major elements of experimental research.
- To understand the major types and designs of experimental research.

- To identify major threats to validity in research designs.
- To explain the strengths and weaknesses of experimental research.

164

PURPOSE

The major purpose of experimental research is to study causal relationships (Broota, 1989; Campbell and Stanley, 1966; Cochran, 1957; Kirk, 1994). A causal relationship may be established when the independent variable is associated with and influences the dependent variable, and when rival explanations about this relationship have been eliminated. The simplest experimental study seeks only to ascertain whether there is a direct link between two factors (i.e., whether changes in a given factor produce changes in another factor). A more complex experimental study seeks to assess the importance or magnitude of the changes caused (i.e., the size of the effect). Still more complex experimental research examines the relative effects of a host of relevant factors on the dependent variable of interest. Experimental research is believed to be better suited than other research methods for explanatory studies whose goal is to provide more definitive answers to questions about causal relationships.

DEFINITION

Experimental research tests a hypothesis through planned interventions carried out so that explicit comparisons can be made between or across different intervention conditions. The term **demonstration** is sometimes used to indicate interventions carried out primarily to extend or test the applicability of already existing knowledge rather than to add to scientific knowledge. In experimental research, the unit of analysis may be individuals, families, small groups, organizations, or communities. The essential elements of experimental research in the natural as well as social sciences are experimental and control groups, randomization, pretest and posttest, and the application of the intervention factor.

Experimental and Control Groups

The word *group* refers to individuals defined by the service or program (i.e., intervention) they receive or do not receive. The **experimental group** includes those individuals or other units of analysis that receive the intervention, such as a particular health care service or program. The **control group** includes those individuals or other units of analysis that do not receive the intervention or that receive an alternative form of intervention (e.g., an existing service or program rather than a new one).

Ideally, the control group consists of subjects or other units who are as similar as possible to those in the experimental group except that they do not receive the experimental intervention. In reality, the degree of similarity between the experimental and control groups varies for each study. There are two types of control groups: those made equivalent by random assignment, which generally assures a nonbiased distribution of the various characteristics; and those that do not employ random assignment and are termed *nonequivalent* (Fitz-Gibbon and Morris, 1987). The former are also referred to as true control groups, and the latter, comparison groups. **Comparison groups** are control groups selected through nonrandom methods and are so called to distinguish them from true control groups. If random assignment into experimental and control groups is not possible, then researchers should try to find a group as similar as is practical to the experimental group in terms of the key characteristics.

The use of control groups allows researchers to account for the effects of the experiment itself. Participation in an experimental intervention or program can sometimes impact the outcome independent of the experiment itself. A classic example in medical research is when patients who participate in experimental treatment appear to improve or get better. But it is not clear how much of the improvement has resulted from the treatment and how much from participation. The use of a control group that does not receive the treatment would allow researchers to assess the true impact of the treatment.

In social science experiments, control groups are used not only as a guard against the effects of participation, but also to account for events that occur outside the experimental setting in the course of experiments. To the extent that both experimental and control groups are subject to the effects of outside events, the biases experienced will likely cancel out, and the true effect of the experiment can still be determined.

Experimental research is not limited to using one experimental group and one control group, although they are the minimum groups required. Often an experimental design uses more than one experimental and/or control group. When using multiple experimental and control groups, researchers should clearly specify the differences among the groups. In analysis, the impact of each level of intervention should be examined separately, and the combined intervention effect should also be assessed.

Randomization

Randomization means taking a set of units and allocating them to an experimental or control group by means of some random procedure. Randomization is not equivalent to **random sampling**, which consists of selecting units in an unbiased manner to form a representative sample from a population of interest.

In a pure experimental design, random sampling is first used to select a representative number of units, such as people or groups, for study from a target population. This process is needed to ensure that study results are externally valid or generalizable to the population of interest. Randomization procedures are then used to allocate each member of the sample to experimental or control groups, regardless of individual characteristics or preferences. This process aims at ensuring internal validity of the study by eliminating self-selection. When people voluntarily participate in the intervention, they are likely to be different from those choosing not to. Through selection effects, these volunteers serve to confound the impact of the experimental factor.

The best way to accomplish randomization is to use a random procedure to assign subjects to experimental or control groups. The random procedure ensures that each individual unit has an equal chance of being assigned to either the experimental or control group. From a sampling frame composed of all the units in the population under study, researchers can select subjects by numbering all units and picking numbers based on a random number table. The odd-numbered subjects are then assigned to the experimental group and the even-numbered subjects to the control group. Tossing a coin is another way of assuring that subjects have an equal chance of being selected in either group.

Randomly selected subjects are more likely to resemble the population from which they are selected. Since both experimental and control groups are randomly selected, they will likely resemble each other. Randomization is the most effective way of eliminating alternative explanations. It automatically controls for factors that might have been neglected but that might influence results. Individual characteristics or experiences that might confound the results will be almost evenly distributed between the two groups. In addition, randomization allows the proper application and accurate interpretation of inferential statistics to analyze the experimental results.

Use of Placebo

In addition to randomly selecting subjects from the population and randomly assigning them to the experimental and control groups, sometimes it is necessary to administer a placebo to the control group. A placebo, from the Latin for "I shall please," is an inactive substance (e.g., a pill or liquid) that is administered as if it were a therapy but that has no therapeutic value. In testing the effects of new drugs, for example, medical researchers frequently administer a placebo, such as sugar pills, to the control group so that members of the group believe they, like the experimental group, are receiving an experimental treatment. Often their health may improve due to the placebo effect or the belief in the presence of a promising treatment even though it is in fact an inert placebo. However, if the new drug is effective, those receiving the drug will improve more than those receiving the placebo.

Sometimes, knowledge of the experiment can make researchers and experimenters become biased in assessing outcomes. In medical research, the experimenters, especially those who developed the experimental drug, may be more likely to "observe" improvements among patients receiving the drug than among those receiving the placebo. Similarly, in HSR, opponents of a particular cost-saving program are more likely to "note" quality deterioration among patients using new programs. This bias could be reduced if researchers responsible for administering the drug or assessing program outcomes were not told which subjects were receiving the intervention and which were receiving the placebo. Conversely, researchers who have knowledge about which subjects are placed in experimental or control groups are not given the responsibility for administering the experiment or evaluating the outcomes. Such **double-blind experiments** reduce prejudice because neither subject nor researcher nor experimenter knows which is the experimental group and which is the control group. Another way to reduce experimenter bias is to make the operational definitions of the outcome measures more precise. For example, researchers make fewer errors in reading patients' temperatures than in assessing how lethargic patients are.

Quasi-experiment

Although randomization is crucial for experimental results to be valid, in many practical situations, as in HSR, it is not always feasible for both practical and ethical reasons. For example, people might object to being randomly assigned to interventions that last a long time and that are likely to significantly affect their lives. Also, it can be unethical to withhold certain interventions or programs from those in the control group. These studies are quasi-experimental because they lack the element of random assignment that is essential for true experimentation (Rossi, Lipsey, and Freeman, 2004). Often subjects in the experimental group are predetermined. Researchers then have to use alternative methods to ensure comparability between the experimental and control groups. Fitz-Gibbon and Morris (1987, pp. 28–29) have illustrated that the following approaches may be used instead.

One approach is called the *two new interventions* or *two new programs approach*. Because new programs are often more attractive, researchers may use a second new program as a control for the main intervention program. Subjects can be randomly assigned to one new program or the other. The second new program can be a version of the main intervention without the more costly components. It can also be a true competitor to the intervention program that is used by others in the community.

Another approach is the *borderline control-group strategy*. This strategy is appropriate when the people most in need must be given a particular program (e.g., Medicaid recipients or people with a special need). The measure of who is most needy is not always accurate. The borderline group refers to those who are immediately above the cutoff point. Many of them are also in need of the program. For example, if low income is used to decide who gets the program, the borderline people will be those whose income is slightly higher than the cutoff point. In such a case, the nonborderline, most needy people must be assigned to the intervention program, but the borderline group can be randomly assigned to the intervention program or the control group. This approach allows for a comparison to be made within a similar population, that is, the borderline group. Information regarding the value of the program is also valuable for policy decisions on whether or not to expand the program.

A further example is the *taking turns*, or *delayed program*, *approach*. Sometimes groups can take turns receiving the intervention or program. For instance, a workplace health promotion program may be introduced to company employees from different divisions at different time periods. Because divisions can be randomly assigned to their turn, a true control group is achieved even though all people will eventually be given the program. Starting out on a small scale is a cautious strategy in implementing new programs.

One commonly used nonrandom assignment method is called **matching**, which involves attempting to make the control group as similar to the experimental group as possible. The matching process can be efficiently achieved through the creation of a quota matrix that includes all the relevant characteristics to be matched. For example, if demographic similarities between experimental and control groups are important, researchers should select control group subjects based on the demographics of the predetermined experimental group. As a result, the average demographic characteristics of the experimental group will be comparable to those of the control group. They should have, say, the same average age, gender, racial composition, and so forth. If the experimental group is selected by means of a pretest, then the pretest should also be introduced to the control group so that subjects from both groups are exposed to the same outside stimuli other than the experimental intervention or program. Finally, researchers should record the similarities and differences between control and experimental groups. To the extent that subjects from both experimental and control groups can be demonstrated to be similar in all important characteristics except for the intervention, the validity of the findings will be enhanced.

Random sampling cannot always generate representative samples. When the sample size is small and the population heterogeneous, random sampling may produce a nonrepresentative sample, and matching may be the only viable alternative. Matching and randomization can sometimes be combined to produce more comparable groups. Beginning with a pool of subjects, researchers first create strata of subjects similar in characteristics that need to be matched. Then, from each of the strata, subjects are randomly assigned to experimental and control groups. This procedure is called the *stratified random sampling procedure.* See Chapter 11 for additional random sampling procedures.

Before using the matching process to assign subjects to experimental and control groups, researchers should understand the conditions of matching. First, the variables being matched should be truly critical and are expected to affect the outcome of the intervention if not taken into account. Second, since most of the statistics used to evaluate experimental results are based on randomization, nonrandom sampling will limit the choice of statistics for data analysis.

Testing

Both experimental and control groups are tested or observed before and after the intervention and at the same points in time (Fitz-Gibbon and Morris, 1987). Tests given before an experimental intervention or program are called **pretests**, which stands for preprogram or preexperiment tests. Similarly, tests given after the experimental intervention or program are called **posttests**. Comparisons of the "before" and "after" information for experimental and control groups are used to assess the impact of the intervention or program. In the simplest experimental design, subjects are pretested on a dependent variable (e.g., weight), exposed to an intervention (e.g., weight control program), and then posttested in terms of the dependent variable (e.g., weight). Differences noted between pretests and posttests on the dependent variable are then attributed to the influence of the intervention.

Researchers may wish to make some measurement during the time the intervention or program is being implemented. These tests are termed **midtests**, or *midprogram tests*, and indicate the impact of the intervention or program over time. Likewise, a series of measurements or tests may be conducted well after a program finishes, thus allowing the assessment of the long-term impact of the intervention or program. A series of tests given at equal intervals before and after the program are called **time-series tests**. Generally, at least three measures are desirable in order to draw a trend line. These three measures must be on the same instrument, for example, the same test or questionnaire. A series of tests administered systematically before a program starts may reduce the need for a control group because the results of these pretests can be used to project the outcome when there is no intervention.

Intervention

An experiment essentially examines the effect of an intervention factor (i.e., independent variable) on a dependent variable. The independent variable is the cause and the dependent variable the effect. Typically, the independent variable takes the form of an experimental stimulus that is either present or absent. This is known as a dichotomous variable because it has two attributes.

It is essential that both independent and dependent variables be operationally defined for the purpose of the experiment. Such operational definitions might involve a variety of observation methods. Taking a drug, being subjected to a treatment, becoming eligible for a service, participating in a workshop, undergoing exercises, receiving certain information, undergoing a particular experience or event, responding to a questionnaire, and the like, are some common health-related interventions. More complex experimental designs are also available, for example, using several levels of intensity in the intervention treatment or carrying out repeated follow-ups of the two groups in order to differentiate the immediate, short-term impact from the longer-term impact, which may differ in strength and in character.

TYPES

Many types of experiments may be conducted, including laboratory (or controlled) experiments, field experiments, natural experiments, and simulations.

Laboratory Experiment

Traditionally, the terms *experiment* and *laboratory experiment* tend to be equated with each other. **Laboratory experiments** may be defined as experiments conducted in artificial settings where researchers have complete control over the random allocation of subjects to treatment and control groups and the degree of well-defined intervention. They represent the ideal prototype of a true experiment. However, the laboratory experiment is rarely used in HSR due to the practical constraints on random assignment as well as the manipulation of intervention. Another reason for its limited use in HSR is the highly interactive health services environment where a multiplicity of social and economic as well as health-related factors interact. This environment is very difficult to recreate in an artificial setting.

Field Experiment

Health services and many social scientific experiments often occur outside laboratories or the controlled environment, typically in real-life settings. **Field experiments** are experiments conducted in a natural setting. The experimental observations are unobtrusive and take place as subjects are going about their normal activities. For example, one may observe the interaction or lack thereof between physicians and patients in clinical encounters or study the triage system at work in the emergency departments of urban hospitals. Field experiments have high external validity and are particularly suitable for applied research that focuses on problem solving.

The major weakness of field experiments is the low level of control compared with laboratory experiments. Researchers may not be able to assign subjects randomly to the various treatment conditions or to control groups due to ethical considerations or subject preferences. Consequently, in the field experiment, it is usually more difficult to ensure that there are no systematic differences between experimental and control groups. In addition, because of the unobtrusive nature of field experiments, it may be inappropriate to obtain prior informed consent. The lack of informed consent can have both legal and ethical consequences.

An example of a health policy field experiment is the Rand Health Insurance Experiment (HIE), one of the most important health insurance studies ever conducted. The HIE provides a good example of true experiments carried out in real-life settings and with samples sufficiently large and representative for the results to be extrapolated to the national level. The HIE was started in 1971 and funded by the Department of Health, Education, and Welfare (now the Department of Health and Human Services). It was a 15-year multimillion-dollar effort that to this day remains the largest health policy study in U.S. history. It addressed two key questions in health care financing: How much more medical care will people use if it is provided free of charge? What are the consequences for their health? The study concluded that cost sharing reduced care but had little effect on health (Keeler, 1992). These conclusions encouraged the restructuring of private insurance and helped increase the stature of managed care. Since the study, conventional health insurance plans have increased front-end cost sharing to restrain spending on health care.

Natural Experiment

Experiments in real-life settings, however, are still somewhat artificial in that they occur purely for research purposes and researchers have control over the random allocation of subjects to treatment and control groups. Many times, practical and ethical considerations may rule out experiments on some topics, such as the effects on health status of lack of access to care, so that research (if done at all) must rely on truly naturally occurring events in which people have different exposures that resemble an actual experiment. This type of **natural experiment** may also be called a social experiment, where, in the course of normal social events, nature designs and executes experiments that researchers may observe and analyze.

Simulation

Simulation, or modeling, is a special type of experiment that does not rely on subjects or true intervention (Stokey and Zeckhauser, 1978). A **model** is a representation of a system that specifies its components (variables in health services models) and the relationships among the components. Simulation is a special kind of model—a model in motion, and one that is operating over a period of time to show not only the structure of the system (what position each variable or component occupies in the system and the way components are related or connected), but also the way change in one variable or component affects changes in the values of the other variables or components. The validity of the predictions depends on the validity of the model. Simulation is an imaginative "acting out" of how a program is supposed to be implemented and achieve its effects. It is a powerful method that enables researchers to observe as an artificial world moves forward into the future, giving the user the opportunity to intervene and attempt to make improvements to performance (Dooley, 2002). It is a laboratory for testing out hypotheses and making predictions, safe from the risks of the real environment. Whereas other research methods help researchers answer questions such as "What happened?" "Why?" and "How?" simulation is best used to answer the question "What if?" Because of the increasing access to computers and the availability of sophisticated software for the analysis of research data, a great deal of simulation and modeling can be done with the use of computer software. Examples include various simulation studies concerning the scheduling of patients and coordinating patient referrals; designing critical paths or clinical pathways for patient care that maximize efficiency and quality; and managing hospital ancillary services. Simulation is common in health services organizations because large-scale change in organizations (e.g., of human resources or information systems) is difficult, and one wants to be relatively sure of a change's potential before investing greatly in the change effort.

The major advantages of simulation are economy, visibility, control, and safety. Operation of a simulation may not only be much cheaper than operation of the real event, but it can also provide trial runs that will help avoid costly mistakes in the real operation. Simulation can heighten the visibility of the phenomenon to be studied by making the phenomenon more accessible to the investigator. It clarifies the phenomenon by separating the essential components of the system from irrelevant or less relevant features. Researchers often have a greater level of control over the simulation of an intervention than over the actual intervention itself. Another feature of control is the possibility that certain conditions can be manipulated in order to observe the difference in the results of the simulation. Simulations have potential use in situations that are theoretically important but will cause harm, embarrassment, or other moral and ethical problems if human subjects are used in a natural environment. It is a substitute for experimentation when such experimentation is too dangerous, costly, untimely, or inconvenient.

The major disadvantage of simulation is its artificiality. By its very definition, a simulation is merely an imitation or copy of the real event. As a working model or substitute, there is always the possibility that the simulation is so inaccurate or incomplete that conclusions gained from it are not applicable to the phenomena being modeled, and thus that the findings will be invalid. Particularly in social modeling, in which the social system may be highly complex, researchers may have little assurance that all the essential components are included in the model or that the relationships between components are specified correctly. Since simulation is only as good as the assumptions used in its construction, it is a useful approach when a significant amount of empirically based knowledge is available. It is less useful or even misleading in areas in which little knowledge is available.

The requirement of a high level of quantitative skills may present problems for some researchers. A complex simulation, particularly a computer simulation, may require not only costly computers and other machines but also complicated program (software) writing and complex mathematical computing. Researchers unable to solve complex mathematical problems or do sophisticated computer programming, and who do not have consultants available to solve these problems, may be unable to perform the simulation.

VALIDITY THREATS

For any experiment to be valid, researchers should guard against potential threats to validity. The two types of validity researchers are most concerned with are external validity and internal validity (Campbell and Stanley, 1966). **External validity** is related to the generalizability of the experimental results. An experiment is considered externally valid if its effect can be generalized to the population, setting, treatment, and measurement variables of interest. External validity can be divided into **population validity and ecological validity.** Population validity refers to the representativeness of the sample of the population and the generalizability of the findings. A study has high population validity if the sample closely represents the population and study findings work across different kinds of people. Ecological validity refers to the degree that study results can be generalized across settings. A study has high ecological validity if it generalizes beyond the laboratory to more realistic field settings. The development of many clinical practice guidelines was based on the experience of doctors serving large metropolitan teaching hospitals (which typically get the NIH grants for clinical trials). The experience of physicians serving other markets, especially vulnerable populations such as racial/ethnic minorities and the uninsured or underinsured, was typically underrepresented. Thus, current clinical practice guidelines may lack external validity when applied to the U.S. population as a whole.

An experiment maintains **internal validity** if it shows that the study outcome is caused by the hypothesized independent variables alone, rather than any extraneous variables. In an internally valid study, one can conclude that changes in the independent variables caused the observed changes in the dependent variables and that the evidence for such a conclusion is good. Alternatively, a study is not internally valid if changes in the dependent variable or outcome can be attributable to other causes than the independent variable or intervention. For example, health promotion studies using self-selection typically attract people already self-motivated. Results of their achievements in risk reduction can often be attributable to self-initiated health practices, in addition to interventions. Therefore, health promotion interventions typically lack internal validity.

Threats to External Validity

The factors that might affect representativeness or external validity of the research include the interaction effect of testing, the interaction between selection bias and intervention, the reactive effects of the experimental arrangements, and multiple-treatment interference. **Interaction effect of testing** occurs when a pretest increases or decreases the subjects' sensitivity or responsiveness to the experimental variable, thus making the results unrepresentative of the population who have not received any pretest. **Interaction between selection bias and the intervention** involves the selection of subjects who are not representative of the population and may respond better or worse than the general population to the intervention. The **reactive effects of the experimental arrangements** refers to control group subjects getting exposed to part of the experimental intervention, thus limiting the generalizability of the true experimental effect. **Multiple-treatment interference** occurs when multiple treatments are applied to the same subjects, largely because the effects of prior treatments are not usually erasable. It then becomes difficult to determine the true cause of the outcomes.

Threats to Internal Validity

The factors that might affect causal explanation or internal validity of the research include history, maturation, testing, instrumentation, statistical regression (or regression toward the mean), selection, attrition, and contamination.

History refers to events happening in the course of the experiment, other than the manipulated independent variable, that may affect the outcome of the experiment. These events are termed extraneous variables; they may compete with the independent variable in explaining the outcome of the study. When extraneous variables do in fact influence the independent variable or outcome, they become confounders. With a single-group design, where a control group is absent, a confounder is an extraneous event that occurs at the same time as the program and might be expected to influence the program's outcome measures. With an experimental design, a confounder is something extraneous to the program that happens to only one group (either the experimental or control group), not to both groups, and this can influence the outcome measures for the program.

Maturation represents any changes to research subjects due to the passage of time rather than to the experimental intervention. In the course of an experiment, particularly one of long duration, subjects may change psychologically (e.g., become more knowledgeable) or physically (e.g., become stronger or weaker). Although these changes can affect experimental outcome, the experiment did not cause them.

Testing, a frequent rival explanation for research findings, involves changes caused by measurement rather than by the experiment. For example, individuals having repeated measurements generally improve their score because each measurement serves as a practice opportunity.

Instrumentation refers to changes in study outcomes due to characteristics of the measuring instrument or procedure rather than the experiment itself. For example, if not properly trained, different interviewers may conduct interviews differently. The results of the interviews may differ because of the manner in which they are conducted. Another example of instrumentation is when the time spent on the intervention or program varies significantly between the experimental and control groups. This can cause biases. A program that provides lengthy contact periods with subjects may turn out better results independent of the actual quality of that program. In analyzing program results, therefore, researchers need to take into account the actual time allocated to the program and the participation records of subjects.

Statistical regression is another threat to internal validity. It is the tendency for extreme subjects to move (regress) closer to the mean or average with the passage of time. This phenomenon is most likely to affect experimental results when subjects are selected for an experimental condition because of their extreme conditions or scores. The more deviant the score, the larger the error of measurement it probably contains. On a posttest, it is expected the high scorers will decline somewhat on the average and the low scorers will improve their relative standing, regardless of the intervention.

A further threat to internal validity, **selection**, occurs when there are systematic differences in the selection and composition of subjects between the experimental and control groups. Selection bias often occurs when the assignment of subjects to experimental or control groups is not determined by chance but by other mechanisms. Obvious forms of selection bias occur when studies use subjects who are volunteers or nonvolunteers (i.e., captive audiences). Selection bias can take more subtle forms. For example, a researcher assessing the impact of a community-wide smoking cessation program finds, as its control, a nearby community that does not have the program. However, there are many personal, cultural, and economic factors that influence where a person lives. To the extent these factors are different for the two communities and may also influence smoking patterns, there will be selection bias in the estimate of the effects of the smoking cessation program.

Attrition, the withdrawal of subjects from an experiment, is another threat to internal validity. Attrition poses the greatest threat to internal validity when there is differential attrition, that is, when the experimental and control groups have different dropout rates. Invariably, those subjects who drop out differ in important ways from those who remain so that the experimental conditions are no longer equivalent in composition. The reasons subjects withdraw from an experiment include dissatisfaction with the experience, illness, a loss of interest, and geographic relocation. Differential attrition usually defeats the purpose of random assignment. Differential attrition rates also offer another cause for concern. The loss of subjects will lead to loss of data, which may affect program results. If subjects who performed less well or were less motivated dropped out of a new program, for example, the new program would obtain higher average results simply because of the loss of certain participants.

Contamination is another potential problem during the implementation stage. It occurs when the control group uses, to some extent, the methods or components of the intervention program. Contamination may be less of a problem when experimental and control groups are at different sites so that control groups are less likely to be aware of the experiment.

DESIGNS AND THREATS TO VALIDITY

There are many configurations of experimental and quasi-experimental designs as summarized by numerous authors over the years (Black, 1993; Broota, 1989; Campbell and Stanley, 1966; Cochran, 1957; Cook and Campbell, 1979; Creswell, 2002; Finney, 1955; Fitz-Gibbon and Morris, 1987; Gliner and Morgan, 2000; Kirk, 1994; Miller, 1984; Singleton and Straits, 2005). In implementing these designs, researchers must guard against potential threats to validity as summarized above. This section, based on previous researchers' work, introduces the more commonly used designs and evaluates potential threats to their validity.

Quasi-Experimental Designs

Quasi-experimental, or nonequivalent comparison, group designs often are used when the experimental treatment is administered to intact groups, such as work units, making random assignment of individual subjects impossible. The simple notation employed in the classic work by Campbell and Stanley (1966) is used here to diagram the various designs. Specifically, the diagrams use the following symbols:

R indicates random assignment

O indicates an observation or a measurement being made

X indicates the experimental intervention or program

Design 1: The Single Group Case Study

Figure 7.1 illustrates the simple single group case study experimental design. The experiment or intervention is represented by *X* (i.e., the independent variable), and O_1 stands for the outcome measurement of the experiment or intervention (i.e., the dependent variable). Time moves from phase 1 (pre-intervention) to phase 2 (post-intervention).

An example of this type of design is the evaluation of a disease-management training program for nurses working in a clinic. The clinic administrator is interested in determining whether the nurses learned the new skills the training program was intended to teach, so she asks the nurses to take a quiz at the end of the program. The nurses' skills prior to the training program were not assessed, so there is no basis for before-and-after comparison. In addition, all of the nurses in the clinic received the training. Thus, there is no group of untrained nurses that can take the quiz for comparison purposes.

The fatal flaw of this design is that there is no baseline measurement to provide comparison with the intervention outcome; nor is there any comparison

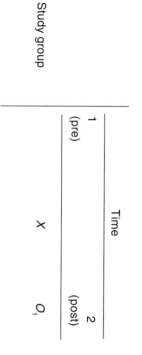

	Time	
	1 (pre)	2 (post)
Study group	*X*	O_1

Figure 7.1. Design 1: The single group case study

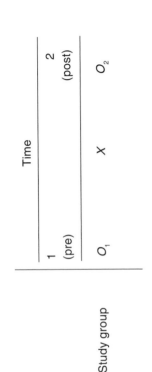

	Time	
	1 (pre)	2 (post)
Study group	O_1	X	O_2

Figure 7.2. Design 2: The single group before-and-after

group. Thus, it is impossible to tell whether there is an improvement in outcome. Other threats to the internal validity of the simple case study design are attrition, maturation, and history.

Design 2: The Single Group Before-and-After

A second quasi-experimental design, the single group before-and-after design (see Figure 7.2), consists of measuring or making observations of one group of subjects (the pretest), implementing an intervention or a program (the independent variable), and measuring the subjects at the end of the intervention or program (the posttest). The pre-intervention observations are represented by O_1, the independent variable by X, and the post-intervention observations by O_2. Using the same example as Design 1, the clinic administrator using the before-and-after design would give the nurses a pretraining quiz as well as a post-training quiz.

This is an improvement over Design 1 because it at least provides a basis for comparison. The attrition threat is controlled in the Design 2 study because the pre-intervention observation makes it possible to determine whether those who dropped out before the second observation differed initially from those who remained. Only the data from those subjects observed both before and after the intervention would be used in analyzing the effects of the independent variable.

However, Design 2 is still subject to major threats to its validity. Two of the threats found in Design 1, maturation and history, also affect the single group before-and-after design. The longer the period of the experiment, the more likely that these two threats will happen and confound the results. Other potential threats to internal validity include testing, instrumentation, and, statistical regression. Unless objective reference or norm groups are available for comparison, considerable problems will occur when researchers try to make any judgments about program X on the basis of this design.

Design 3: The Comparison Group Posttest-Only

As symbolized in Figure 7.3, the rows represent separate groups. The intervention or program is represented by X and the blank space under X stands for the no-intervention comparison group. The outcome of the dependent variable is measured by O, and each group is measured just once (i.e., post-intervention).

Figure 7.3. Design 3: The comparison group posttest-only

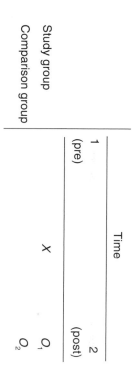

	Time	
	1 (pre)	2 (post)
Study group	X	O_1
Comparison group		O_2

This third quasi-experimental design, the posttest-only design, like Design 2, is an improvement over the simple case study design in that it provides a set of data from the comparison group with which to compare the post-intervention results. While Design 2 provides pre-intervention results on the same group, Design 3 provides the results of a comparison group. Continuing with the nurse training program example, in this case there would be two groups of nurses: one group that receives the training program, and the other group that does not. Both groups of nurses take the quiz at the end of the training program.

Design 3 is an improvement over the previous two quasi-experimental designs also in terms of controlling threats to internal validity. The threat of history is largely controlled, as subjects in the two groups should experience the same major external events. The absence of a pretest avoids testing bias. Instrumentation can be controlled if the same instrument or measurement is consistently administered to both groups. Selection bias is the most serious threat to internal validity. Without the random assignment of subjects to the study and comparison groups, there is no control of possible pre-intervention differences. Indeed, there is no formal way to tell whether the two groups are comparable.

Another threat to internal validity is attrition, which is uncontrolled because no pretest data exist by which the investigator may find out whether subjects who drop out of a study are comparable to those who remain. To the extent differences exist between those who drop out and those who remain in the study, study results may not be generalized to the population with confidence. Differential attrition rates between study and comparison groups can also bias the study results. Maturation may become a problem if the study is of long duration and if maturational factors are operating differently in the two groups. Contamination may also be a concern with Design 3 if the study group interacts with the comparison group and shares information that may change outcomes.

Design 4: The Nonequivalent Comparison Group Pretest–Posttest

Design 4 is a pretest–posttest design with a nonequivalent (nonrandomized) comparison group (see Figure 7.4). Prior to intervention, measurements are made in both study and comparison groups. Continuing with our example of the nurse study, in this type of design, both groups of nurses (i.e., the group receiving

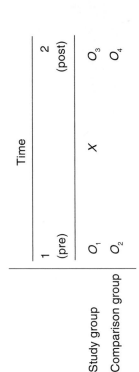

Figure 7.4. Design 4: The nonequivalent comparison group pretest–posttest

	Time		
	1 (pre)		2 (post)
Study group	O_1	X	O_3
Comparison group	O_2		O_4

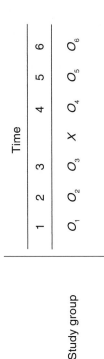

Figure 7.5. Design 5: The single group time series

	Time					
	1	2	3	4	5	6
Study group	O_1	O_2	O_3	X	O_4	O_5	O_6

the training and the group not receiving the training) take a quiz before and after the intervention. This design is an improvement over Design 3 as it adds pretests for both the study and comparison groups. The pretest results provide the opportunity to examine the similarity of the two groups, which is crucial to assessing the impact of the intervention. Except for the lack of randomization in sample selection, this design is similar to the classic-experiment true-control group pretest–posttest design (Design 7). It is frequently used in health services research when random assignment is not possible. The inclusion of a comparison group, especially one highly similar to the study group in known respects, makes it superior to previously introduced quasi-experimental designs. If the groups are similar in important characteristics, then the design controls for history, maturation, testing, and regression to the mean.

Design 5: The Single Group Time Series

Design 5 uses the subjects in the experimental intervention or program as their own control group (see Figure 7.5). The same measurement is made on intervention or program subjects at regular intervals several times before and after the intervention. In this case, the nurses from the previous examples are tested several times before the training program, and several times after the training program. The impact of the intervention or program can be assessed by comparing the trend of measurement before the intervention with that after the intervention. If the intervention has any impact, the two trends will be significantly different. This design is a much better one than the before-and-after design, because obtaining a series of measurements before and after the intervention provides a more accurate picture of the intervention effect. The essence of the time-series design is the presence of a periodic measurement process and the introduction of an experimental change into this time series of measurements.

However, history may represent a potential threat to internal validity in Design 5. Even if a clear change is noted in the observations following the implementation of program X, it is difficult to know for certain whether X caused the change or whether X just happened to occur at about the time that the measures would have changed anyway because of some other outside events. Such coincidences, however, may be ruled out by obtaining additional contextual information. Testing may also pose a threat to internal validity in this type of design. Individuals with repeated measurements may improve their scores due to practice rather than the intervention.

Design 6: The Time Series with a Nonequivalent Control Group

Design 6 is like Design 5 except with the addition of a nonequivalent control group (see Figure 7.6). It also incorporates the pretest–posttest nonequivalent control group design (Design 4). Two groups of subjects (e.g., the nurses undergoing training and the nurses not undergoing training) are measured regularly both before and after the intervention or program, which is available to one group but not the other. The addition of a comparison group makes it possible to control for external events that might take place during the course of the study. In other words, subjects from both groups are subject to the same external influence. The alternative explanation for the results due to external influence or history can often be ruled out. In addition, the selection–maturation interaction is controlled to the extent that, if the study group generally showed a greater rate of gain, it would be seen in the pre-intervention observations as well.

			Time			
	1	2	3	4	5	6
Study group	O_1	O_3	O_5	X	O_7	O_9 O_{11}
Comparison group	O_2	O_4	O_6		O_8	O_{10} O_{12}

Figure 7.6. Design 6: The time series with a nonequivalent control group

Experimental Designs

The single most important difference between experimental and quasi-experimental designs is randomization, or the random assignment of subjects to experimental or control groups. Randomization is present in experimental designs but absent in quasi-experimental designs. Randomization is represented by the letter R (see Figure 7.7). The other symbols are joined by R, with the study period shown as time moves from left to right. The rows represent study or experimental and control groups. Observation or measurement of the dependent variable is indicated by O. The intervention or program of the independent variable is represented by X.

Design 7: The True Control Group Pretest–Posttest

Design 7 is the classic true experimental design (see Figure 7.7). It is like Design 4 except that the control group is formed by random assignment. Research subjects are randomly assigned to either the experimental or control groups. Subjects assigned to the experimental group receive experimental intervention or program X. Subjects assigned to the control group do not receive experimental intervention or program X. However, they may get an alternative program (X). The pretest–posttest control group design involves measuring both the experimental and control groups at approximately the same time before and after the intervention or program. The pretest results can be used to assess the similarities or equivalencies between the two groups. The posttest results are used to assess the impact of the intervention or program (X). For example, if subjects from the experimental group performed significantly better than those from the control group, as reflected in the posttest–pretest difference, the difference may be attributed to the effect of the intervention, or program X.

This is a very good design and permits a powerful test to be made between program X and the alternative. Generally, threats to internal validity are dealt with successfully. For example, comparison of O_1 and O_2 provides a check on the randomization procedure with regard to initial differences in the dependent variable between the experimental and control groups. Given sufficient sample size, the randomization procedure should eliminate biases associated with selec-

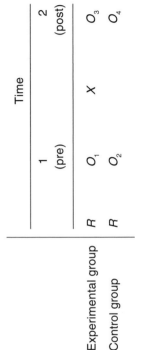

	Time	
	1 (pre)	2 (post)
Experimental group	R O_1	X O_3
Control group	R O_2	O_4

Figure 7.7. Design 7: The true control group pretest–posttest

Figure 7.8. Design 8: The true control group posttest-only

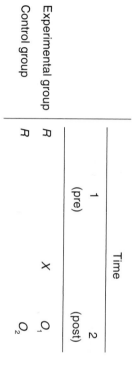

	Time		
	1 (pre)		2 (post)
Experimental group	R	X	O_1
Control group	R		O_2

tion and regression to the mean. In terms of history, any event in the external environment that would produce a difference between the pretest and posttest in the experimental group (O_1-O_3) would also do so in the control group (O_2-O_4). Likewise, this design effectively controls for other potential threats to internal validity, including maturation, testing, and instrumentation, because they will affect both groups and not affect differences between the posttests, O_3 and O_4. This design permits the assessment of possible attrition effects by comparing the pretest results of those who drop out for both groups. However, even though Design 7 adequately controls the threats to internal validity, it is still susceptible to threats to external validity, which reflects the extent to which the experimental results may be generalized.

Design 8: The True Control Group Posttest-Only

Design 8 is a simple true experimental design. Subjects are randomly assigned to experimental or control groups. No pretest or measurement is given. Instead, the intervention or program is administered to the experimental group. The control group does not receive any intervention. Measurement is made after the intervention for both groups (see Figure 7.8). It is like Design 7 except that no pretest is used. Except for the use of subject randomization, Design 8 resembles the quasi-experimental comparison group posttest-only design (Design 3). Unlike Design 3, however, Design 8 controls for the common threats to internal validity adequately (e.g., testing, maturation, regression to the mean, and instrumentation). This design effectively eliminates the possibility of an interaction between the pretest and the experimental manipulation. It is therefore useful when a pretest, such as attitude measures, might interfere with the program effects in some way. It may also be used when a pretest is not available or would take too much time. The random assignment of subjects to either the experiment or control groups, especially if numbers in the groups are large enough, is generally sufficient to ensure approximate equivalence.

Design 9: The Solomon Four-Group

The Solomon four-group design is another true experimental design. It is relatively complex and integrates both Designs 7 and 8 (see Figure 7.9). There are

		Time		
		1 (pre)		2 (post)
Experimental group 1	R	O_1	X	O_3
Control group 1	R	O_2		O_4
Experimental group 2	R		X	O_5
Control group 2	R			O_6

Figure 7.9. Design 9: The Solomon four-group

two experimental groups and two control groups. A randomization procedure is used in assigning subjects to each of the four groups. Pretest measurement is used for one pair of experimental control groups but not for the other. The same intervention is implemented in both groups. Posttest measurement is used for all four groups at about the same time.

The Solomon four-group design combines the strengths of the two previous experimental designs and enables the researcher to make additional comparisons. For example, the effectiveness of randomization may be assessed by comparing the pretests between Experimental Group 1 and Control Group 1 (O_1 and O_2). A positive result will build confidence in the random assignment of Experimental Group 2 and Control Group 2 where no pretest is conducted. A comparison between the outcome of Experimental Group 1 and Experimental Group 2 (O_3 and O_5) shows the extent of interaction between pretesting and intervention. A comparison between the outcome of Control Group 1 and Control Group 2 (O_4 and O_6) indicates the extent of testing effects. The effect of the intervention or independent variables can be examined by: (1) comparing O_3 and O_4, (2) comparing O_5 and O_6, and (3) comparing the net effect between (1) and (2), which may be used to tease out the effect of the pretest. This design also effectively controls for threats to internal validity. However, the design may be twice as expensive due to the addition of two extra groups.

Design 10: The Time Series with an Equivalent Control Group

Design 10 is like Design 6 except with the addition of random assignment (see Figure 7.10). Two groups of subjects are randomly selected, measured regularly before the program, and then only one group gets program X; the other might get an alternative program or no program. This is a very powerful design effectively controlling for all threats to internal validity. However, it is also a very expensive design and is seldom used.

Figure 7.10. Design 10: The time series with an equivalent control group

		Time				
		1	2	3	4	5	6
Study group	R	O_1	O_3	O_5	X O_7	O_9	O_{11}
Comparison group	R	O_2	O_4	O_6	O_8	O_{10}	O_{12}

STRENGTHS AND WEAKNESSES

The principal advantage of a controlled experiment lies in its validity in studying causal processes. Because the experiment reflects the direction of influence among variables and controls for extraneous variables, it has strong internal validity and provides relatively accurate inferences about cause and effect.

Experimental research is longitudinal in that observations are required for at least two points in time (before and after the intervention). The experiment therefore provides the opportunity for studying change over time. In an experiment, investigators generally observe and collect data over a period of time and measure at more than one interval. The intervention itself may have a duration time of a few hours, or many months. Even a short intervention period provides a greater opportunity to study change than does a cross-sectional study, such as survey research.

For many decades, the randomized controlled experiment was presented in textbooks as the norm or ideal to strive for in the design and conduct of social research. However, because of the applied nature of HSR, the utility of experiments cannot be taken for granted. Researchers must critically evaluate whether an experimental research design is more appropriate than other designs for the particular issue or question under study.

The principal disadvantage of the experimental approach has to do with its limitations in generalizability or external validity. For example, the health behavior or social process observed in an artificial environment (i.e., laboratory) will be drastically altered, or simply not occur at all, if examined out of its natural social setting. If the stringent requirements of experimental research designs are to be met, the design often becomes feasible only with small and atypical groups, in which case the conclusions cannot be generalized with any certainty. An experiment is designed to show the effect of a particular factor, not all other factors that may produce or moderate the same effect. But there may be little practical

185

value in seeking a precise separation of these factors if, in the real world, they operate together. For example, in a controlled medical experiment, patients are generally not representative of all patients with a particular condition. Therefore, it cannot be known how the treatment being evaluated will work within the larger population of patients. Moreover, treatment in such an experiment is usually not at varying levels of intensity or in combination with other interventions. A narrower range of outcomes typically is considered.

Experimental designs may simply not be feasible for many of the topics and questions addressed by social scientists, including health services researchers. For example, it is not appropriate or ethical to randomly assign people to an experiment in which they will experience poor health outcomes. Experiments are appropriate for research on unidirectional causal processes (i.e., where the influence works one way only). But when reciprocal causal processes (i.e., where a change in X produces a change in Y, and a change in Y also produces a change in X) are expected, other types of study (e.g., qualitative research) may be more appropriate and effective. Apart from practical constraints on the type of treatment that can be tested, feasibility problems arise also in relation to people's willingness to be experimental guinea pigs. Many people are simply not available for participation in experiments, and volunteers may not be representative. This tends to limit experimental research to captive populations, such as students in schools and other educational institutions, recipients of a government benefit program (e.g., Medicaid or WIC), employees in a company, and so on.

Many of the controls required in experimental research may be difficult or impossible to realize in health services or other social science research, especially when a natural setting is used. When a double-blind process cannot be implemented, the experimenter's expectations may affect the results of the experiment either through cues given (perhaps subconsciously) to the research subjects, who then conform to the experimenter's wishes, or through the misinterpretation of the experimental results in an effort to more closely approximate the study's hypothesis. In other instances, ethical and time considerations make it unfeasible to study behavior in artificial settings. In addition, conducting true experiments with large and representative samples is typically more complex and costly than other designs. Because of these limitations, quasi-experimental designs are more widely used in HSR.

SUMMARY

Experimental research involves planned interventions carried out so that explicit comparisons can be made between or across different intervention conditions to test research hypotheses. Its essential elements consist of experimental and control groups, randomization, pretest and posttest, and the application of the intervention factor. Experiments may be conducted in the laboratory, or in the natural environment with or without controls. Simulation is a special type of experiment that does not rely on subjects or true intervention. The principal strength of experimental design lies in its validity in studying causal processes.

Its principal weakness has to do with the limit in generalizability, or that it tends to be low in external validity.

There are also many configurations of experimental and quasi-experimental designs. Examples of quasi-experimental designs are the simple case study; the before-and-after design; the comparison group posttest-only design; the non-equivalent comparison group pretest–posttest design; the single group time series design; and the time series with a nonequivalent control group design. Examples of experimental designs include the true control group pretest–posttest design; the true control group posttest-only design; the Solomon four-group design; and the time series with an equivalent control group design.

For any experiment to be valid, researchers should guard against threats to both external and internal validity. Threats to external validity include interaction or the reactive effects of testing, the interaction between selection bias and the experimental variable, the reactive effects of the experimental arrangements, and multiple-treatment interference. Threats to internal validity include history, maturation, testing, instrumentation, statistical regression or regression toward the mean, selection, and attrition.

REVIEW QUESTIONS

1. What are the essential elements of an experiment?
2. In designing studies, if randomization is not feasible, what can researchers do to ensure comparability between the experimental and control groups?
3. Describe commonly used experimental and quasi-experimental designs. What potential threats to validity must be guarded against for each of these designs?

REFERENCES

Black, T. R. (1993). *Evaluating Social Science Research*. Thousand Oaks, CA: Sage.

Broota, K. D. (1989). *Experimental Design in Behavioral Research*. New York: Wiley.

Campbell, D. T., and Stanley, J. C. (1966). *Experimental and Quasi-experimental Designs for Research*. Chicago: Rand McNally.

Cochran, W. G. (1957). *Experimental Designs*. New York: Wiley.

Cook, T. D., and Campbell, D. T. (1979). *Quasi-experiment: Design and Analysis Issues for Field Settings*. Chicago: Rand McNally.

Creswell, J. W. (2002). *Research Design: Qualitative, Quantitative, and Mixed Methods Approaches* (2nd ed.). Thousand Oaks, CA: Sage.

Dooley, K. (2002). Simulation research methods. Chap. 4.6 in J. Baum (Ed.), *Companion to Organizations*. London: Blackwell.

Finney, D. J. (1955). *Experimental Design and Its Statistical Basis*. Chicago: University of Chicago Press.

Fitz-Gibbon, C. T., and Morris, L. L. (1987). *How to Design a Program Evaluation*. Newbury Park, CA: Sage.

Gliner, J. A., and Morgan, G. A. (2000). *Research Methods in Applied Settings: An Integrated Approach to Design and Analysis*. Mahwah, NJ: Lawrence Erlbaum Associates.

Keeler, E. B. (1992). Effects of cost-sharing on use of medical services and health. *Journal of Medical Practice Management, 8*(2), 317–321.

Kirk, R. E. (1994). *Experimental Design: Procedures for the Behavioral Sciences* (3rd ed.). Belmont, CA: Wadsworth.

Miller, S. H. (1984). *Experimental Design and Statistics*. London: Methuen.

Rossi, P. H., Lipsey, M. W., and Freeman, H. E. (2004). *Evaluation: A Systematic Approach* (7th ed.). Thousand Oaks, CA: Sage.

Singleton, R. A., and Straits, B. C. (2005). *Approaches to Social Research* (4th ed.). New York: Oxford University Press.

Stokey, E., and Zeckhauser, R. (1978). *A Primer for Policy Analysis*. New York: W. W. Norton.

Survey Research

KEY TERMS

cold-deck imputation
cross-sectional survey
deductive imputation
hot-deck imputation
interview survey

longitudinal survey
multiple imputation
panel study
random digit dialing (RDD)

self-administered
    questionnaire survey
statistical imputation
survey research
trend study

LEARNING OBJECTIVES

■ To describe the major elements of survey
    research.

■ To understand the process of conducting
    survey research.

■ To appreciate the major types of survey
    research.

■ To explain the strengths and weaknesses
    of survey research.

PURPOSE

Survey is the most commonly used method of data collection (Converse, 1987). It
is extensively used both inside and outside the scientific community for different
purposes (Bailer and Lamphier, 1978; Dillman, 2000; Fowler, 2002; Miller and

Salkind, 2002; Singleton and Straits, 2005). Social scientists, including health services researchers, use surveys for both descriptive and explanatory research purposes. Survey research is used primarily to describe a population of interest, by showing the distribution of certain characteristics, attitudes, opinions, feelings, or experiences within a population. Surveys offer an effective means of description and provide detailed and precise information about large heterogeneous populations. Survey research may also be used to examine the causal relationships among variables and explain how these variables are related. Guided by theories and using multivariate statistics, researchers can also examine factors associated with the problems of interest.

Outside the scientific community, survey is widely used by both the public and private sectors. The federal government conducts or sponsors many major surveys (including health-related surveys) each year for the purpose of gathering information, planning, and decision making. The news media conduct opinion polls to gauge public reactions to important events, policies, programs, and political candidates. Businesses (including health services organizations) conduct surveys to test-market new products and services, assess consumer satisfaction with current products and services, and compile consumer profiles.

Survey is most popular with researchers because it enables a wide range of topics to be covered. It may be used to discover factual information, such as age and income, as well as to ascertain attitudes, beliefs, opinions, and values. Knowledge questions are often surveyed as well. Survey can record reports of past behavior as well as future intentions. Properly constructed, survey can explore factors associated with a phenomenon of interest and thus test a particular hypothesis.

Indeed, survey is such a basic method that it can be found in many other types of research. A research review of existing studies may show that many of the findings are the result of surveys. Similarly, in secondary analysis, many of the secondary data sets may originate from surveys. Qualitative research, particularly case studies, may integrate the survey component in its data collection. Experiments commonly use surveys to collect data measuring the impact of intervention. Evaluation research may also use survey findings to assess program impact.

DEFINITION

Survey research can be defined as the use of a systematic method to collect data directly from respondents regarding facts, knowledge, attitudes, beliefs, and behaviors of interest to researchers, and the analysis of these data using quantitative methods.

Typically, survey research consists of the following characteristics: large and randomly chosen samples, systematic instruments, and quantitative analysis

(Bailer and Lanphier, 1978; Cox and Cohen, 1985; Fowler, 2002; Miller and Salkind, 2002; Singleton and Straits, 2005). A large sample of respondents randomly chosen from the population of interest will make the survey findings more representative and generalizable. Usually, probability sampling procedures are used to select the survey sample to ensure precise estimates of population characteristics. Chapter 11 examines probability and nonprobability sampling methods.

Survey research uses a systematic questionnaire or interview guide to ask questions of respondents. Regardless of whether a survey obtains information through an interview or a questionnaire, the data collection instrument and procedures tend to be standardized for all respondents. Questions are written beforehand and presented or asked in the same order for all respondents. During the interview, since changes in the wording of questions or in the behavior of interviewers (e.g., tone of voice, friendliness, appearance) may influence responses, interviewers are trained to present questions with exactly the same wording and in the same order and manner. They are also trained in the use of introductory and closing remarks, transitions from topic to topic, and supplementary questions or probes to gain more complete responses. Such standardization is necessary to enhance data reliability by minimizing measurement error and to facilitate hypothesis testing. If the purpose is to acquire preliminary data in an area in which little research has been done in order to generate hypotheses, a less structured approach, such as unstructured interviewing, is generally used.

Surveys may be cross-sectional (capturing one point in time), or longitudinal (providing a series of observations). The cross-sectional survey (one survey for one sample) is by far the most commonly used survey design. In a **cross-sectional survey**, data on a sample or cross-section of respondents representing a target population are collected within a short period of time. Data collection may be through interviews or self-administered questionnaires. Although a cross-sectional survey may ask prospective (future), contemporaneous (now), or retrospective (past) questions, it is limited by the amount and accuracy of the information that individual respondents can capably report due to memory and recall capability. Because the cross-sectional survey collects data at one point in time, it does not adequately show the direction of causal relationships or rule out alternative rival explanations.

As an example, the 2002 Community Health Center User Survey, conducted by the Bureau of Primary Health Care (BPHC) of the Health Resources and Services Administration, provides a snapshot of health center patient demographics and health status, health care utilization, and quality of services received. The survey was designed to match as closely as possible the content and the sampling strategy used to produce the nationally representative data of the National Health Interview Survey. It was carried out with the assistance of the National Center for Health Statistics. All health centers that received BPHC funding and provided primary care were included in the sampling frame of the User Survey. The survey excluded temporary clinics, clinics open for less than one year, school-based health centers, and specialized clinics. Nine strata were formed based on census region and urban/rural designation, and a tenth was formed for health centers with large proportions of managed care patients. Selection was carried out using probability-proportional-to-size methodology within a stratum. Of the 581 eligible health centers in 2002, 70 centers (or 12 percent of total eligible centers) were randomly selected for inclusion in the study, and all participated.

The **longitudinal survey** follows a single sample or another similar sample with repeated (at least two) surveys, over a period of time. Unlike cross-sectional surveys, where all respondents are asked the same questions, longitudinal surveys may be designed as multipurpose surveys. In addition to a set of core questions that are asked in each survey, noncore questions or topics may be included on an ad hoc basis to take into account the latest developments and interests.

Longitudinal surveys may be carried out at predetermined intervals: quarterly, annually, or biannually. Or they may be conducted on a continuous basis, that is, with interviews spread out evenly across the calendar year so that the data are not affected by seasonal variations.

The two major types of longitudinal surveys are trend studies and panel studies. A **trend study** refers to conducting a series of cross-sectional surveys to collect data on the same items or variables with randomly selected samples of the same population. Even though different samples are selected, they all represent the same population of interest. A trend study can also be designed as a cohort study when the impact of a development, such as aging or health behavior, is to be studied. A cohort consists of persons (or other units, such as households or organizations) who experience the same significant event (e.g., a particular illness) within a specified period of time, or who have some characteristic in common (e.g., same date of birth or marriage, same illness or symptom, membership in the same organization).

Most of the national health surveys sponsored by the federal government are longitudinal trend surveys. For example, the National Health Interview Survey mentioned above is an annual probability survey of the U.S. noninstitutionalized population. It includes detailed questions on health conditions, doctor visits, hospital stays, household characteristics, and personal characteristics. See Chapter 3 for a more detailed description of this survey as well as other well-known government-sponsored longitudinal surveys.

A **panel study** takes as its basis a representative sample of the group of interest, which may be individuals, households, organizations, or any other social unit, and follows the same unit over time with a series of surveys. Whereas trend studies focus on variables and their changes over time, panel studies focus on individuals and their changes over time. The same individuals are repeatedly studied. In a panel study, a more personalized relationship with study members is needed to promote their active interest and reduce sample attrition and nonresponse rates.

As an example, the Medical Expenditure Panel Survey (MEPS), conducted by the Agency for Healthcare Research and Quality and the National Center for Health Statistics, is a well-known longitudinal panel survey on financing and use of medical services in the United States. The MEPS consists of three major components: the Household Component Survey, which collects medical expenditure data at the personal and household levels; the Medical Provider Component Survey, which surveys medical providers and pharmacies identified by household respondents; and the Insurance Component Survey, which collects data on health insurance plans obtained through private- and public-sector employers.

A longitudinal survey is initiated when cross-sectional surveys or other sources of data reveal new trends that these tools cannot fully describe or explain. A longitudinal survey provides strong inferences about causal direction and more accurate studies of processes of change. Thus, it is unique in its ability to answer questions about causes and consequences and hence to provide a basis for substantiated explanatory theory.

However, the longitudinal survey, especially the panel study, represents a small component of survey research, mainly for economic reasons and given the problem it poses with respect to follow-up. The continued implementation of a longitudinal survey requires the commitment of both long-term funding and a secure organizational base. However, both are difficult to maintain. There are substantial practical problems associated with sample attrition and nonresponse. The failure to trace sample members at each subsequent wave of the study and members' inclination to drop out of the study are likely to increase over time. Therefore, the subgroup that is successfully covered up to completion of the study may no longer be fully representative.

Change presents another obstacle to longitudinal surveys. In a prolonged longitudinal survey, the methods of data collection and the instrument itself may change over time, to take account of maturation and aging. For example, children may be interviewed directly as they reach maturity, whereas personal interviews pose greater problems as people reach old age. The questions addressed at the start of the study may be overtaken by events, or simply cease to attract the same degree of interest. However, questions that change from one study to the next may affect the comparability of information obtained over time. Even when questions remain constant, particular concepts may have changed meaning over time so that the same variable may not be measuring the same construct. Changes in research staff are also likely and may produce discontinuities in the approach or methods adopted for the study.

Finally, the inadequate development of a theoretical framework and methodologies to be used for analyzing longitudinal data presents another obstacle. The analysis of data from a longitudinal survey is usually substantially more difficult and costly than equivalent analysis of a cross-sectional survey. Longitudinal analysis of linked data from a series of surveys frequently involves extremely large data files.

The results of surveys are numerically coded and analyzed quantitatively, typically with the aid of computer statistical software. Quantitative data analysis techniques depend on whether the survey's purpose is descriptive or explanatory. Surveys (typically cross-sectional) that are primarily descriptive make use of simpler forms of analysis. Surveys (typically longitudinal) that sort out the relationships among the variables of interest require the use of more sophisticated data analysis techniques. Chapter 14 describes commonly used statistical methods for analyzing research, including survey data. The process of conducting survey research is explored in greater detail below.

PROCESS

Survey research consists of three major phases: planning, administration, and analysis. Each has a number of interrelated components.

Planning

Select a Topic

This first step in planning survey research is the same as in other types of research. Researchers decide on a topic of interest, select a problem to study within the identified topic, and formulate general hypotheses or research questions based on the selected problem. See Chapter 2 for conceptualizing health services research topics.

Review the Literature

Similar to other types of research, the next step is to review the relevant literature, including journal articles, books, and other published and unpublished materials, to determine what is known about the topic and what work remains to be done. During the course of this review, the investigator clearly states the research objectives, refines the problem, and specifies the research hypothesis or question in operational terms. A unique element in survey research is that investigators also search for and evaluate existing measures, scales, or instruments that may be incorporated in or adapted for the prospective survey.

Select the Unit of Analysis

The survey unit of analysis may be anything that can be counted, including either individuals or groups of individuals, such as households, organizations, cities, and the like. The choice of the unit of analysis is determined by the research objectives, specified hypothesis, or research question. If the population of interest as specified by the research objectives is individuals, then data need to be collected at the individual level. If the population of interest is groups of individuals, then data need to be collected from samples of groups. If the research objective is to examine causal relationships at the individual level, but the data are collected at the aggregate level, then the investigator commits the error of ecological fallacy. To avoid such an error, researchers need to collect data at the appropriate level.

Assemble the Survey Instrument

The next step is to assemble the instrument to be used for data collection. The survey instrument or questionnaire may be constructed by the researchers themselves or adapted from available instruments used by others. The particular variables selected depend on which characteristics should be studied in order to meet the research objectives. The advantage of using an established instrument is that reliability and validity measures of the instrument are likely to be available. The disadvantage is the possibly low degree of match between the researcher's interest and the available measures. Chapter 12 provides a detailed discussion of the preparation of research instruments.

Select the Survey Mode

Researchers need to also determine the appropriate survey mode or type to use for the study (Aquilino and Losciuto, 1990; Dillman, 2000). Two major survey modes are the self-administered questionnaire survey and interview survey.

Self-Administered Questionnaire Survey

In **self-administered questionnaire surveys,** respondents are asked to complete the questionnaires themselves by reading the questions and entering their own answers. There are many ways of conducting self-administered questionnaire surveys. They may be self-administered by mail, in person, or via the Internet.

The most common way is the use of a mail survey. The basic method is to send a copy of the questionnaire to respondents through the mail. This is accompanied by a cover letter explaining the purpose of the study and a self-addressed, stamped envelope for returning the completed questionnaire. If feasible, researchers may consider the use of a self-mailing questionnaire that eliminates the need to keep track of an envelope. The questionnaire may be folded so that the return address appears on the outside.

There are several postal options for mailing out the questionnaires and getting them returned. To mail out the questionnaire, the researcher can choose between first-class postage and bulk rate. First-class mail is faster and more certain, but bulk rate is cheaper. To get the questionnaires returned, the researcher can choose between business-reply permits and postage stamps. The advantage of using business-reply permits is that the researcher pays only for the questionnaires that are returned. This method is particularly appropriate for surveys that have a very low response rate per mailing. A disadvantage, however, is that for those returned questionnaires, the researcher pays for the mailing plus an additional surcharge. Another disadvantage, in terms of survey participants, is that the use of business-reply permits may seem less appealing to some respondents who consider them to be less personal. Since both business-reply permits and bulk rate mailings require establishing accounts at the post office, it is more appropriate if the survey is large in scale. The advantage of using stamps is that it may be more appealing to respondents and money may be saved if the response rate per mailing is high. The disadvantage is that the mailing of the questionnaires will have been paid for whether people return them or not. Before deciding on a particular option, the researcher needs to visit the local post office to find out the actual arrangements and rates.

Researchers may also consider administering the questionnaire simultaneously to a group of respondents gathered at one place. This approach is feasible when respondents can be assembled together. Its advantages include savings in terms of time and money (e.g., stamps), higher response rates, and the presence of researchers to provide introduction and assistance. Its disadvantages include potential time constraints and the inability of respondents to check for information. Of course, gathering respondents together for the survey is not always easy in the first place.

Questionnaires may be delivered by mail and picked up later by the research staff at a designated time. Using this strategy, the research staff has the opportunity to check for completeness. Conversely, questionnaires can be hand-delivered by the research staff, who explain the purpose of the study with a request that the respondents mail the completed questionnaires back to the investigators.

The Internet is an increasingly popular form of distributing self-administered questionnaires. Using the Internet to conduct surveys is emerging as a viable alternative to mail or telephone surveys, which experience declining response rates and rising costs. While mailed questionnaires remain essential for some surveys, the possibilities for electronic delivery of surveys are growing. A significant number of American households still lack Internet access. However, recent trends suggest this will not always be the case. According to the National Telecommunications & Information Administration (http://www.ntia.doc.gov), the percentage of U.S. homes with Internet access increased from 26 percent in 1998 to 54.6 percent in 2004. It is important to note that those households without Internet access are more likely to be low income, which has implications for survey research. Intuitively, Internet surveys are more likely to be successful when the targeted sample population has high rates of computer use (e.g., physicians or hospital administrators).

The practical advantages of using the Internet are clear: quick turnaround time, easy presentation of complex visual and audio materials to respondents, consistent delivery of questions and collection of responses, the flexibility to allow respondents to complete questionnaires whenever they like, lack of the pressure to move quickly (which is typical of telephone interviews), and the ability to track a respondent's answers across repeated waves of questioning. Furthermore, data entry is no longer a separate activity, and therefore the errors associated with data entry are reduced (Dillman, 2000). Postage and paper costs are eliminated. Barriers to reaching international respondents are lowered. Moreover, web graphics can make Internet surveys more attractive to respondents.

Conversely, barriers to Internet surveys also exist. The ability to read questions and navigate web pages is required, as is proficiency with a computer keyboard (and mouse when one is used). While increasing numbers of people are computer literate, there remains wide variation in people's familiarity with computer surveys (Dillman, 2000). With an Internet questionnaire, interviewers are removed from the equation and are therefore unable to demonstrate professionalism and commitment to the task, which can compromise respondent attentiveness and motivation. An Internet survey prevents the respondent and interviewer from having an interactive conversation that might clarify the meanings of ambiguous questions.

Also, obtaining e-mail addresses is a daunting task. Unlike telephone listings, there are limited e-mail listings except for captive populations (e.g., schools, companies, hospitals). Therefore, samples drawn may be of uncertain representativeness. Going through spam blockers is another challenge. With spam likely to make up a large portion of e-mail traffic, spam blockers or antispam tools have been built for most computers with Internet access, particularly in organizational environments. In theory, well-designed antispam filters won't challenge mail from known correspondents or mail that one actually asked to receive. Unfortunately, many current challenge-response systems are poorly designed, which could wreak havoc on mailing lists and other legitimate communications. Confidentiality of responses is another concern particular to potential Internet survey participants.

When considering whether to use web-based or e-mail surveys, one should take into account several factors (Dillman, 2000). First, e-mail is easier to compose and send. However, one needs the e-mail addresses of the respondents in order to use this method. Web-based surveys can be more visually stimulating and interactive but may appear differently depending on respondents' operating systems. Web survey designers need to design surveys than can be viewed on a variety of web browsers. Dillman (2000) suggested the development of user-friendly designs such as plain questionnaires without color and tables since questionnaires designed using extensive computer programming may not load properly on some web browsers. He recommended a series of principles for designing web surveys, including providing specific instructions on how to execute the computer action that is needed to flow through the form, using drop-down boxes sparingly, permitting respondents to answer one question before going on to another question, developing skip patterns that allow respondents to click on a link that takes them directly to where they need to be, and exercising restraint in using question formats that have known measurement problems (e.g., "check all that apply"). E-mail and web-based surveys can also be used in tandem. For example, respondents can be reached through e-mail and then sent via hyperlink to a web-based survey page. One can make a complex and appealing survey but leverage the personal touch of e-mail.

Another means of computer-based self-administered questionnaires is CAPI, or Computer-Assisted Personal Interviewing. The CAPI system requires researchers to bring computers to respondents' homes, schools, or work sites. Respondents record their responses on the computer while reading questions on the screen or while listening to a recording of an interviewer. Dillman (2000) expects CAPI will be largely replaced by Internet-based survey techniques.

Interview Survey

In **interview surveys**, respondents do not complete the questionnaire by themselves. Rather, researchers or interviewers ask the questions and answer categories (if applicable) orally, and then record the respondents' choices or answers. Interview surveys may be conducted face-to-face—either in person or via web camera—or by phone. Face-to-face interviews tend to obtain the most valid information because it is easier to build rapport with respondents in a face-to-face interview. The use of web cameras in conducting face-to-face interviews at a distance reduces the cost of traveling. Non-face-to-face interviews are more convenient to both interviewers and respondents. With the wide availability of telephones and cell phones, phone interviews are becoming more and more common. However, phone interviews are more likely to reach a nonrepresentative sample. On the one hand, many families and individuals have more than one phone (e.g., a landline, a cell phone, and in some cases a car phone as well), thus creating a problem of multiple counting. On the other hand, certain groups are still underrepresented in phone ownership, such as rural residents and the poor. Furthermore, the use of mobile phones, as compared with traditional landlines, not only makes it harder to reach someone but also realigns the telephone number concept from a household to a single individual. This complicates attempts to collect household data while creating opportunities for collecting individual data.

Computers play an increasingly significant role in phone interviews. A computer-assisted telephone interviewing, or CATI, system can greatly facilitate data collection, particularly for large-scale surveys (Baker and Lefes, 2001). The interviewer can sit in front of a computer terminal wearing a telephone-operator headset. The interviewer dials the number or the central computer randomly selects a telephone number and dials it. When the respondent answers the phone, the interviewer reads the instructions and interview schedule displayed on the computer screen. When the respondent answers the question, the interviewer types that answer into the computer terminal—either the code category for the appropriate answer to a closed-ended question or the verbatim response to an open-ended question (even text-based chats). All answers are immediately stored in the computer so that researchers can begin analyzing the data before the survey is complete, gaining a preliminary view of how the results will look.

Computer-Assisted Self-Interviewing (CASI) makes use of the video (Video-CASI) and audio (Audio-CASI) capabilities of personal and portable computers to present the questions on the computer monitors or over headphones to respondents, who then enter the answers on the computer keyboard (Aday and Cornelius, 2006).

The recent emergence of computer-based voice-over Internet protocol (VoIP) has had a great impact on telephone surveys. This new technology allows phone calls to be made by using a broadband Internet connection instead of using a standard phone line. Calls are made over the Internet by converting analog audio signals to digital data. The advantage of VoIP is the ability to place local and long-distance phone calls without paying extra phone charges.

Regardless of how interview surveys are conducted, the following are critical components: selecting the interviewers, training the interviewers, and conducting the interview (Fowler and Mangione, 1990; Suchman and Jordan, 1990).

Select the Interviewers

If the interview method is chosen and the respondents are too numerous for the researchers to interview alone, the field administration of the survey instrument begins with the recruitment of interviewers. The desirable qualities of interviewers include a high sense of responsibility, a pleasant personality that gains respondents' trust and cooperation, an interest in the research topic and in talking with people, an absence of prejudices toward the respondents, an ability to listen carefully and be articulate in conversation, and the skill to legibly and accurately record responses.

Train the Interviewers

In training interviewers, researchers first provide information about the study's general purpose, specific objectives, significance, sponsor, sampling method, planned uses, general guidelines, and procedures. Even though the interviewers may be involved only in the data collection phase of the project, it is useful for them to understand what will be done with the interviews they conduct and what purpose the interviews will serve. Motivation will be higher when interviewers know the purpose of the study and can identify with it (Babbie, 2006; Billiet and Loosveldt, 1988). However, to avoid or reduce interviewer bias, they should be blind to any type of outcome that is being tested.

Interviewers are then acquainted with the interview schedule or questionnaire item by item. The interview schedule consists of instructions to the interviewer, the questions to be asked, and the response categories. Each question and answer category is read out loud and the purpose of each question is explained. Questions or comments from the interviewers are then addressed. Interviewers must be able to read the questionnaire items fluently, without stumbling over words and phrases. They must be taught to follow question wording exactly.

The interviewers must be familiar with the instructions and specifications prepared in conjunction with the questionnaire, which are explanatory and clarifying comments about how to handle various situations that may arise with specific questions. They must be able to follow the instructions and determine when some questions will need to be tailored to fit a given respondent's situation.

Interviewers should learn how to record responses, especially when the questionnaire contains open-ended questions. Since open-ended questions aim at soliciting respondents' own answers, it is important that interviewers record the answers exactly as told without attempting to summarize or paraphrase. Interviewers need not worry about how the responses are to be coded. Researchers will decide on coding open-ended questions after the survey has been completed.

Basic interview techniques and rules are taught in terms of how to establish rapport with respondents and gain their cooperation, ask questions and probe in a manner that will not bias the response, record observations, and deal with interruptions and digressions. When respondents reply to a question with an inappropriate answer, probing is required. For example, the question may present an attitudinal statement and ask the respondent whether he or she strongly agrees, somewhat agrees, somewhat disagrees, or strongly disagrees with the statement. The respondent may reply that he or she agrees with the statement. The interviewer follows this reply with: "Would you say you strongly agree or agree somewhat?" If necessary, interviewers can explain that they must check one or the other of the categories provided.

To decrease the number of missing answers or "don't knows," interviewers can be instructed to probe for answers. For example, interviewers may ask, "If you have to choose an answer, which one do you consider the most appropriate choice?" Interviewers can also help to explain potentially confusing question-naire items. If respondents clearly misunderstand the intent of a question or in-dicate that they do not understand, interviewers can clarify the question so that responses are relevant.

Probes are more frequently required in eliciting responses to open-ended ques-tions. It is imperative that probes be completely neutral and that they not affect subsequent responses. Probes should be written in the questionnaire whenever a given question is suspected of requiring exploration for appropriate responses so that all interviewers will use the same probes whenever they are needed. This practice reduces the effect of interviewer bias.

Demonstrations are set up to show interviewers exactly how to conduct the interview. It is preferable that researchers interview a representative cross-section of true respondents. After the demonstrations, researchers should address any questions or concerns the interviewers might have. Then, interviewers are paired off to complete mock interviews themselves. Once the practice is completed, in-terviewers should discuss their experiences and ask any additional questions they might have. Next, interviewers are provided opportunities for real interviews un-der close supervision. When researchers are truly satisfied with the performance of a given interviewer, that person is then allowed to conduct independent inter-views. Continual supervision of the work of interviewers is necessary over the course of a study. Researchers should read the completed surveys and resolve any problems in a timely fashion.

Conduct the Interview

During the interview, interviewers should dress properly and remain courteous, tactful, and nonjudgmental throughout. Dress and appearance may send sig-nals as to a person's attitudes and orientations. Generally, interviewers should dress cleanly, neatly, and in a fashion not too different from that of the people they are interviewing. In demeanor, interviewers should be pleasant, friendly, interested, and relaxed without being too casual or clinging. They should try to communicate a genuine interest in getting to know the respondents but not engage in any debate or argument about anything that is reported. Information gathered in the course of the interview should not be revealed to anyone except the supervisor. To this end, the interviewer may be required to sign a nondisclo-sure agreement.

Interviewers can observe as well as ask questions. For example, observations can be made, in the case of a home visit, regarding the quality of the dwelling and the presence of various possessions, and note can be taken of the respondents' general reactions to the study and anything else that seems important. Interviewers can record these observations at the margins of the survey instrument.

It is the researchers' job to regularly check completed instruments to ensure that the survey questionnaire is properly filled out. At the initial stage of the study, they should sit in on interviews to make sure that respondents are interviewed properly. Throughout the study, investigators should remain available to interviewers to answer questions and provide assistance. Regular meetings with interviewers may be arranged to provide opportunities for interviewers to raise questions and receive solutions.

Choices

The choice of survey mode depends on a number of factors, including the research topic, type of respondents, sample size, and resources available to the researchers. Certain research topics are more amenable to interviews than questionnaires and vice versa. For example, if the purpose is to assess the knowledge level of the respondents, interview or in-person administration of a questionnaire is more appropriate than mail or Internet questionnaire surveys, because the latter cannot control for the possibility of respondents seeking outside help. In terms of respondents, the questionnaire is more appropriate for better-educated respondents and the interview for less-educated respondents.

The geographic distribution of respondents is also an important consideration. A well-dispersed survey population is better reached by mail or Internet questionnaire, or by telephone interview. Face-to-face interviews are not feasible in this situation. Survey sample size also dictates the mode chosen. The self-administered questionnaire survey is more likely to be used for larger samples and the interview for smaller samples. Among the resources important to survey research are funding and personnel. The most expensive and time-consuming mode of survey research is the face-to-face interview, the major costs being incurred from direct interviewing time and travel to reach respondents. The least expensive mode is the questionnaire survey. Chapter 13 provides more detailed comparisons of the pros and cons of data collection methods.

Survey Sampling Design

Survey sampling design depends on the characteristics and distribution of the population of interest, the availability of a sampling frame, and the survey mode chosen, as well as the overriding factor of cost (Kalton, 1983). For example, if population subgroups are disproportionately represented, a stratified sample may be chosen. If respondents are widely dispersed geographically, the most efficient sampling procedure for locating them is the use of the cluster sampling method. If mail survey or telephone interview is used, simple random or systematic sampling may be chosen, provided an adequate sampling frame that contains the list of addresses or phone numbers can be obtained. Decisions about the survey mode and sampling are closely related and made concurrently. Telephone interviews require access to a telephone directory comprising the target population. Similarly, e-mail questionnaires require access to respondents' e-mail addresses. And mail survey is only feasible where a mailing list is available. Finally, the sampling decision is influenced by cost and the resources available. Face-to-face interviews are the most costly, followed by telephone interviews and mail surveys. Chapter 11 examines various sampling methods.

Another potential selection bias, caused by unlisted numbers (typically, wealthier people request that their numbers not be published), had been reduced for some time in the 1990s through the **random digit dialing (RDD)** procedure. In RDD, known residential prefixes are sampled and the last four digits of the telephone number are selected by means of a table of random numbers. However, RDD is becoming less effective because of the omnipresence of answering machines, call-blocking devices, and caller ID (Dillman, 2000). The widespread use of mobile phones also constitutes a barrier to reaching potential respondents.

To overcome these barriers, researchers may blend RDD with targeted listed directories. Since sampling in the mobile phone era is becoming increasingly technical, researchers may consider using a professional contractor to help with sampling and/or data collection. A good contractor will have an excellent track record: he or she will be flexible in response to the client's demands, demonstrate knowledge of the targeted study populations and the broad subject matter of surveys, complete the tasks within the scheduled time frame, and offer a reasonable price.

Seek IRB Approval

Prior to data collection, investigators need to submit their study proposal for IRB review and approval. The Health Insurance Portability and Accountability Act (HIPAA) provisions have addressed the security and privacy of health data, establishing minimum federal standards for protecting the privacy of individually identifiable health information (National Institutes of Health, 2004; U.S. Department of Health and Human Services, 2005). These include the individual right to access and the right to amend one's personal health information and to obtain a record of when and why this information has been shared with others. Informed consent for survey studies is now a requirement. This statement of consent includes extensive detail on the benefits versus harm to study participants, information about the rights of anonymity and confidentiality, and an explanation as to how the participants' protected health information will be kept private.

Administration

Pretest the Survey Instrument

Whether the survey mode is an interview or questionnaire, the instrument should be pretested prior to actual use. A pretest consists of selecting a small but representative group of people and administering the survey instrument to them.

Probability sampling is not required in selecting the group for pretesting. The key is to choose those who share the major characteristics of the target population. A pretest is especially necessary if the instrument is newly designed for the purpose of the current study. Respondents are typically followed up and asked their views of the instrument in terms of clarity, choice of words, missing items, and length. A pretest is conducted to help determine whether further revision is needed, new items or categories should be added, and the clarity of the wording needs improving.

Obtain Access to Respondents

The next step is to obtain access to respondents. If respondents are from particular organizations, permission from the appropriate organizational administrators is needed. Endorsement from those who have an appeal to the respondents is also useful. A cover letter introducing the purpose and significance of the study may also facilitate access. In interviews, the cover letter is usually read to the respondent. In mail questionnaires, the cover letter is sent with the questionnaire either as a separate sheet or attached to the questionnaire. Internet-based questionnaires should also include an electronic version of a traditional cover letter. The major requirements of a general survey cover letter are to:

- indicate the general purpose and significance of the research
- specify the researchers and sponsors
- explain how respondents are selected for the study
- summarize the benefits of the study to the respondents and others
- list the incentives, if any, for participating in the study
- assure complete confidentiality
- estimate the time needed to finish the survey
- provide a telephone number for possible questions by respondents
- give directions as to how and when to return the completed survey

Administer the Survey

Surveys may be administered by mail, in person, or via telephone or Internet. Sometimes a combination of these methods can be used. For example, questionnaires may be mailed to respondents. Nonrespondents may be followed up with telephone interviews. See the earlier section "Select the Survey Mode" for a discussion of these methods.

Follow-up on Nonrespondents

The final step of field administration involves following up on nonrespondents to encourage their participation and increase the response rate (Cox and Cohen, 1985; James and Bolstein, 1990). Response rate is one important guide to the representativeness of the sample, because nonparticipants may differ in some important ways from respondents. A high response rate indicates less chance of significant response bias than a low response rate. Although no agreement exists as to what constitutes an adequate response rate, some researchers believe that in social science surveys, response rates of approximately 80 percent for face-to-face interviews, 70 percent for telephone interviews, and 50 percent for mailed questionnaires are generally considered acceptable. Internet-based surveys are still considered too new to determine what constitutes an adequate response rate. Response rates are generally higher for interviews than mail questionnaires. Reasons for the higher response rates include the intrinsic attractiveness of being interviewed (having someone's attention, being asked to talk about oneself, and the novelty of the experience), the difficulty of saying "no" to someone asking for something in person (respondents are more reluctant to turn down an interviewer than they are to throw away a mail questionnaire), and the fact that the importance and credibility of the research are conveyed best by a face-to-face interviewer who can show identification and credentials.

There are many ways to enhance the response rate for a given survey. Examples include shortening the questionnaire, obtaining sponsorship by a relevant authority, using a novel and appealing format, and paying respondents. Regardless of which alternatives have been used, a follow-up mailing is a required sequence for increasing return rates, particularly in large-scale mail surveys. In general, the longer a potential respondent delays replying, the less likely that person will do so at all. Properly timed follow-up mailings, then, provide additional stimuli for achieving responses.

Follow-up methods vary by survey modes. Since response rates are typically lower for mailed questionnaires, follow-up efforts are especially important with this mode. Usually, questionnaires are coded so that researchers know who has not responded. Researchers should closely monitor the returns of the questionnaires to look for clues for sending out the second follow-up mailing. A return-rate graph can be drawn that records the number of questionnaires returned for each day after the mailing. This information will enable researchers to know how long it takes for the first batch of questionnaires to be returned, when the peak is reached, when it trails off, and what the cumulative number and percentage of returns are. The dates of subsequent follow-up mailings should also be noted on the return-rate graph so that the effects of follow-up mailings can be monitored.

The first follow-up mailing is typically sent out to all nonrespondents about four weeks after the original mailing, to allow time for completion and for mailing in both directions. The return-rate graph will indicate that the return has stopped or significantly dropped off. A new questionnaire is included with each follow-up mailing along with a cover letter that contains a thorough explanation of why each respondent's cooperation is important to the validity of the findings, and all the basic information in the original cover letter. If the questionnaire is truly anonymous, follow-up questionnaires are sent to all persons in the initial sample. The cover letter includes a statement that expresses appreciation for those who have already sent in their completed questionnaire and encourages those who have not to do so immediately. In practice, three follow-up mailings (an original and two follow-ups) seems to be the most efficient approach.

In telephone interviews, follow-up procedures include calling back at different times of the day and/or different days of the week. In face-to-face interviews, neighbors or those knowledgeable about the whereabouts of the respondents may be asked as to when people are usually at home or how they might be contacted. In Internet surveys, e-mails may be sent repeatedly until responses are returned. The field administration phase concludes when follow-up efforts have been completed with the initially unresponsive persons in the sample.

Dillman (2000) identifies several strategies to improve survey response. These strategies rely on what he calls the "theory of social exchange," which postulates that "actions of individuals are motivated by the return these actions are expected to bring . . . from others" (p. 14). Improving survey response requires reducing the costs and increasing the rewards of responding. For instance, avoiding condescending language, inconvenience, and embarrassing questions lowers respondents' perceived costs of completing the survey. Showing positive regard, ensuring confidentiality, maintaining polite interactions, making the questionnaire interesting, and informing respondents of the importance of the research increase respondents' perceived rewards associated with responding.

Analysis

Process the Data

Before data can be analyzed, they have to be processed. Data processing entails correcting data-inputting errors, dealing with missing values, assigning weights, and recoding variables into conceptual categories to facilitate analysis. The handling of missing values and sample weights is discussed below. Chapter 13 details other listed procedures in data processing.

When surveys have large missing values, imputation is often used to minimize the effect on data analysis. Commonly used methods include deductive, cold-deck, hot-deck, statistical, and multiple (Aday and Cornelius, 2006; Rubin, 2004). **Deductive imputation** uses information from other parts of the questionnaire to fill in the missing pieces. For example, one can use the respondent's name to fill in missing information on gender. **Cold-deck imputation** applies group estimates (e.g., means) to individuals with missing values. The group estimate applied to individuals with missing values can be an overall group estimate or a subgroup estimate that more closely resembles the subgroup to which the individual with the missing value belongs. **Hot-deck imputation** uses the actual responses of individuals with similar characteristics and assigns those responses to individuals with missing values.

Statistical imputation uses statistical procedures for the assignment of missing values. For example, multiple regression may be used for data imputation by using nonmissing data to predict the values of missing data. Note that this may "overcorrect," introducing unrealistically low levels of error in the data. Consequently, the preferred method is stochastic substitution. Stochastic substitution uses the regression technique but adds a random value, such as the regression residual, from a randomly selected case from the set of cases with no missing values.

Multiple imputation generates multiple simulated values for each incomplete datum, then iteratively analyzes data sets with each simulated value substituted in turn. Multiple imputation methods yield multiple imputed replicate data sets, each of which is analyzed in turn. The results are combined and the average is reported as the estimate.

Before analysis is conducted, the sample data must also be weighted if subgroups of the sample were selected at different rates than others. Weighting is a process of statistically assigning more or less weight to some groups than others so that the distribution in the sample mirrors that of the population. To adjust for disproportional sampling, one computes the weight for each observation based on the inverse of the sampling fraction. For example, a study population has 10,000 whites and 1,000 blacks (totaling 11,000 people). The sample of 200 whites has a sampling fraction of $\frac{1}{50}$ ($\frac{200}{10,000}$). The sample of 100 blacks has a sampling fraction of $\frac{1}{10}$ ($\frac{100}{1,000}$). The inverse of the sampling fraction is 50 for whites and 10 for blacks. Multiplying the number of cases in the sample for each group by the inverse of its sampling fraction would yield the number of each group in the population, thus getting back to the actual distribution of each group in the population.

Analyze the Data

Data analysis applies appropriate statistical methods to survey data to test research hypotheses or answer research questions. Chapter 14 provides coverage of commonly used statistical methods for analyzing survey data.

STRENGTHS AND WEAKNESSES

Survey research is probably the best method to describe the characteristics of a population too large to observe directly. Probability sampling yields a group of respondents whose characteristics may be taken to reflect those of the larger population. Carefully constructed standardized measurements provide data consistent across all respondents so that the responses of different groups can be analyzed on a comparable basis.

Survey research has a high degree of transparency, or accountability. Methods and procedures used can be made visible and accessible to other parties (be they professional colleagues, clients, or the public audience for the study report), allowing the implementation, as well as the overall research design, to be assessed.

With surveys, a standardized language has been developed to describe most of the procedures involved, including introductory letters, the survey questionnaire, the codebook, analysis of nonresponse, and so on. The transparency of surveys facilitates systematic refinement of survey methods and techniques and the development of theoretical work.

Survey research covers a wide range of topics. Ethical and practical considerations make it difficult to study some topics experimentally, for example, the effect of high insurance premiums and deductibles on access to care or the experimental manipulation of patients and organizations. Survey research is often used instead.

Survey research can be an efficient data-gathering technique. While an experiment usually addresses only one research hypothesis, numerous research questions can be included in a single questionnaire instrument. The wealth of data collected through the survey method may help identify new hypotheses. Surveys may be reanalyzed as secondary data or with different theoretical perspectives, thus facilitating the cumulative development of scientific knowledge and methods.

Survey research has a number of difficulties and weaknesses. First, in many instances, the identification of an existing, suitable sampling frame poses problems, particularly if the group of interest is small or widely scattered. Second, the requirement for standardization makes certain questions appear artificial or superficial, particularly in the coverage of complex topics.

Third, certain topics may not be amenable to measurement through questionnaires. A survey cannot measure actual behavior and action; it relies almost exclusively on self-reports of recalled past behavior and action or of prospective or hypothetical behavior and action. As a result, data accuracy may be limited because of respondents' misinterpretation of questions, inaccurate recall, or purposeful misrepresentation of facts. A survey is also susceptible to reactivity, the tendency of respondents to give socially desirable answers to sensitive questions. Thus, survey results are generally weak on validity.

Fourth, survey research does not deal with the context of research setting. Although questionnaires can provide information in this area, a brief encounter for the purpose of administering a survey does not afford survey researchers the opportunity to develop a feel for the total situation and background in which respondents are thinking and acting. Neither does such a brief encounter give researchers a sense of the context within which behavior may be interpreted over an extended period of time.

Finally, survey research has severe limitations in explanatory analysis. Causal inferences from survey research generally are made with less confidence than inferences from experimental research. The three criteria for inferring causality include substantiating an association between the dependent and independent variables, establishing the time sequence so that the independent variable (cause) occurs before the dependent variable (effect), and ruling out alternative explanations. Experiments can satisfy these criteria by design, but surveys can meet only one of the criteria with complete confidence: establishing the association between variables. Since most surveys (longitudinal surveys excluded) collect data at a single point in time, it is difficult to establish the time sequence of variables. Whereas experiments control alternative explanations through randomization and direct control during the experiment, survey research uses statistical and modeling procedures to control these variables during data analysis.

SUMMARY

Survey research uses systematic methods to collect data from respondents. Its characteristics include large and randomly chosen samples, systematic instruments, and quantitative analysis. Its major elements consist of topic selection, literature review, unit of analysis, survey instrument design, choice of survey mode, sampling, pretesting, gaining access, survey administration, follow-up on non-respondents, data processing, and data analysis. Surveys may be self-administered, administered by others, cross-sectional, or longitudinal. The major strengths of survey research are related to its transparency or accountability, its efficiency, and its flexibility in terms of topics covered. However, survey research has a severe limitation in explanatory analysis.

REVIEW QUESTIONS

1. What purposes does survey research serve?
2. What are the essential elements of survey research?
3. What are the major types/modes of survey research? Describe situations that most appropriately fit each of these types.
4. Describe the process of conducting survey research.

REFERENCES

Aday, L. A., and Cornelius, L. J. (2006). *Designing and Conducting Health Surveys: A Comprehensive Guide* (3rd ed.). San Francisco: Jossey-Bass.

Aquilino, W. S., and Losciuto, L. A. (1990). Effects of mode of interview on self-reported drug use. *Public Opinion Quarterly, 54*(3), 362–391.

Babbie, E. (2006). *The Practice of Social Research* (11th ed.). Belmont, CA: Thomson/Wadsworth.

Bailer, B., and Lanphier, C. (1978). *Development of Survey Research Methods to Assess Survey Practices*. Washington, DC: American Statistical Association.

Baker, R. P., and Lefes, W. L. (2001). The design of CATI systems: A review of current practice. In R. M. Groves, P. N. Biemer, L. E. Lyberg, J. T. Massey, W. L. Nichols II, and J. Waksberg (Eds.), *Telephone Survey Methodology*. New York: Wiley.

Billiet, J., and Loosveldt, G. (1988). Interviewer training and quality of responses. *Public Opinion Quarterly, 52*(2), 190–211.

Converse, J. (1987). *Survey Research in the United States*. Berkeley: University of California Press.

Cox, B. G., and Cohen, S. B. (1985). *Methodological Issues for Health Care Surveys.* New York and Basel: Marcel Dekker.

Dillman, D. A. (2000). *Mail and Internet Surveys: The Tailored Design Method* (2nd ed.). New York: Wiley.

Fowler, F. J. (2002). *Survey Research Methods* (3rd ed.). Thousand Oaks, CA: Sage.

Fowler, F. J. and Mangione, T. W. (1990). *Standardized Survey Interviewing.* Newbury Park, CA: Sage.

James, J., and Bolstein, R. (1990). The effect of monetary incentives and follow-up mailings on the response rate and the response quality in mail surveys. *Public Opinion Quarterly,* 54(3), 346–361.

Kalton, G. (1983). *Introduction to Survey Sampling.* Beverly Hills, CA: Sage.

Miller, D. C., and Salkind, N. J. (2002). *Handbook of Research Design and Social Measurement* (6th ed.). Thousand Oaks, CA: Sage.

National Institutes of Health. (2004). Protecting personal health information in research: Understanding the HIPAA privacy rule. Retrieved July 10, 2007, from http://privacyruleandresearch.nih.gov/pr_02.asp

Singleton, R. A., and Straits, B. C. (2005). *Approaches to Social Research* (4th ed.). New York: Oxford University Press.

Suchman, L., and Jordan, B. (1990). Interactional troubles in face-to-face survey interviews. *Journal of the American Statistical Association,* 85, 232–241.

Rubin, D. B. (2004). *Multiple Imputation for Nonresponse in Surveys.* Hoboken, NJ: Wiley.

U.S. Department of Health and Human Services. (2005). Office for Civil Rights—HIPAA: Medical privacy: National standards to protect the privacy of personal health information. Retrieved July 26, 2007, from http://www.hhs.gov/ocr/hipaa

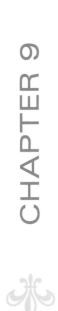

CHAPTER 9

Evaluation Research

KEY TERMS

cost–benefit analysis (CBA)
cost-effectiveness
   analysis (CEA)
discounting
evaluation research

process evaluation
quality-adjusted life
   year (QALY)

LEARNING OBJECTIVES

■ To understand the different types of evaluation research.

■ To become familiar with the process of
   evaluation research.

■ To be able to apply cost–benefit analysis
   and cost-effectiveness analysis.

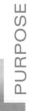

PURPOSE

Evaluation research serves two major purposes: program monitoring and improvement or policy application and expansion (Herman, Morris, and Fitz-

Gibbon, 1987; Stecher and Davis, 1987). The first purpose is concerned with the program itself. It examines the operations of a program, assesses whether and to what extent the stated objectives have been fulfilled, summarizes the strengths and weaknesses in its implementation, and identifies areas of improvement that can be made in program operations. Specifically, evaluators are interested in addressing the following questions: How has the program been implemented compared to the plans? What are the essential components? What are the characteristics of the participants? To what extent has the program served its intended purposes? Are there any impacts that are unintended or unplanned? How satisfied are the participants with the program? What is the attrition or dropout rate? How cost-effective and cost-efficient is the program? How can the program be improved in the future?

The second purpose extends beyond the program itself and is concerned with policy application as a result of program implementation. It focuses on the policy implications of the program and assesses whether it can be adapted in a different setting. Specifically, evaluators are interested in addressing the following questions: What policy implications can be derived from the program? How generalizable are the findings? How likely could the program be adopted in other settings? What are the conditions or prerequisites for such an adoption? What adaptations, if any, have to be made before the program can be introduced to other settings? What will be the likely costs and benefits of the program in other settings?

The major difference between these two purposes is that the first purpose is limited to assessing and/or improving the effectiveness of a specific program within a particular setting and usually satisfies the needs of the management or administration within that setting. The second purpose serves to enlighten policy makers (at the federal, state, or local level) and funders by providing pertinent information regarding how to solve particular health and social problems and how to modify and expand the program to other settings.

Both efficacy and resource scarcity provide the impetus for conducting evaluations. Not all new programs are beneficial and conducive to solving the problems encountered. The usefulness of a program needs to be tested and confirmed before the program is expanded or promulgated. Program efficacy is all the more critical in the face of resource constraints. Both human and financial resources are limited at the business and governmental levels. Resource constraints make it necessary to prioritize problem areas on which to concentrate and to choose the programs that can most effectively and efficiently address these areas. Evaluation research is thus conducted to establish the validity of programs and to dismiss those programs that are ineffective and/or inefficient.

Evaluation of programs and policies is often required to receive funding (Centers for Disease Control and Prevention [CDC], 1999). The Government Performance and Results Act of 1993 mandates that federal agencies set performance goals and measure annual results. In addition, independent grant makers and foundations routinely call on grant recipients to perform evaluations.

DEFINITION

In health services research, **evaluation research** is the use of one or more research methods in assessing various aspects of a program or policy, including components, operation, impact, and generalizability. The evaluation target may be a particular product (e.g., drug), service (e.g., family planning), or problem (e.g., lack of access). Since evaluation usually focuses on particular programs, evaluation research is sometimes called program evaluation. It can be conducted at the individual, group, institution, community, county, state, or national level.

Evaluation research has a number of characteristics (Rossi, Lipsey, and Freeman, 2004). First, evaluation research is technical. Using established research methods, evaluators design, implement, and examine a program in ways replicable by other investigators. Rigorous application of scientific research methods is necessary for the evaluation results to be valid and legitimate. Thus, for evaluation to be successful, evaluators must be knowledgeable about commonly used evaluation methods and be capable of applying them.

Evaluation research is applied. In contrast to basic research, evaluation research is undertaken to solve practical organizational and social problems. The growth of evaluation research reflects the increasing desire by health services researchers to actually make a difference in the delivery of health care services. The applied nature of evaluation research is typically reflected in the sponsors and funders of a project, who may be managers or administrators in a business, government, service, or private funding agency. The influence of increased evaluation requirements, particularly at the federal level, that must accompany new programs, and the set-aside of evaluation funds to fulfill those requirements, cannot be neglected. The value of evaluation often depends on its utilization by sponsors and funders. To maximize the use of evaluation research, evaluators should be knowledgeable about the social dynamics of the setting in which they perform the evaluation, as well as the subject matter related to the evaluation.

Evaluation research should maintain objectivity. Results obtained objectively are more valid and useful in the long run for both organizations and society. Funders, sponsors, administrators, and evaluators all have the responsibility of making the evaluation objective. On the part of program funders and administrators, the results of evaluation should not be tied to the current or future reward of the evaluator. If evaluators are personally or financially tied to the project they evaluate, they may be hesitant to report negative findings and could become "hired guns" of their sponsors. On the part of evaluators, they should not let the process of gaining trust and rapport affect their perspectives. Regardless of the sponsor's intent, changing policy expectations, resources, or other constraints, evaluators should strive to maintain ethical integrity and scientific objectivity.

Examples of important evaluations related to health services abound in the literature. One of the most notable is the Women's Health Initiative, which evaluated the health risks and benefits of hormone replacement therapy (HRT) for postmenopausal women (Writing Group for the Women's Health Initiative, 2002). For decades, HRT was routinely prescribed to help prevent coronary heart disease, despite the lack of evidence of HRT's long-term effects. Beginning in 1993, the Women's Health Initiative conducted a rigorous randomized controlled trial, enrolling more than 16,000 women, to assess the associations between HRT and coronary heart disease, breast cancer, stroke, pulmonary embolism, endometrial cancer, colorectal cancer, and hip fracture. After a mean 5.2 years of follow-up, the trial was stopped due to the finding that women using HRT experienced unacceptably high rates of invasive breast cancer.

This trial of a women's health intervention illustrates the tenets of evaluation described above. First, the HRT evaluation was technical: it was designed and implemented using established research methods that other researchers could replicate. Second, the HRT evaluation was applied: the study's findings had a direct impact on clinical practice. Finally, the HRT evaluation maintained objectivity: despite many years of HRT popularity, the Women's Health Initiative study proved scientifically that this practice posed greater risks than benefits.

TYPES

The field of evaluation is marked by diversity in disciplinary training, perspectives on appropriate method, and evaluation activities and arrangements. Evaluation itself may be classified into various types according to different purposes. The major types include needs assessment, process evaluation, outcome evaluation, and policy analysis (Brownson, Baker, Leet, and Gillespie, 2003; Herman et al., 1987; Neutens and Rubinson, 1997; Patton, 2002; Rossi et al., 2004; Stokey and Zeckhauser, 1978).

Needs Assessment

The purpose of **needs assessment** is to identify weaknesses or deficiency areas (i.e., needs) in the current situation that can be remedied, or to project future conditions to which the program will need to adjust (Herman et al., 1987). The results of a needs assessment can be used to allocate resources and efforts to meet identified unfulfilled needs.

Needs assessment can be performed at the organization or the community level (Barker et al., 1994; Brownson et al., 2003; Dignan and Carr, 1987; Farley, 1993; Green and Kreuter, 1991; Herman et al., 1987; Kark, 1981; Young,

1994). In either case, data are identified and collected from a variety of sources and stakeholders, including available databases, provider and patient/client focus groups, interviews, surveys, and meetings. The objectives are to identify and diagnose organizational or community-wide problems, prioritize them based on their critical nature and complications, and determine desired outcomes to be sought.

In an organizational needs assessment, the following questions may be asked: What are the key components of the current services and programs, including medical, social, and health services? What are the problems of each service or program? What are the possible causes of the identified problems? Examples of problems include services that are absent; inadequate; insufficient; poorly managed, coordinated, or delivered; inefficient; ineffective; incompatible with service objectives; or either overextended or underutilized. What are the possible solutions to identified problems for each service or program? Examples of solutions include adding new services or redesigning and improving current ones in terms of management, coordination, or delivery. For each solution identified, what are the organizational consequences with respect to service objectives, management, staff, clients, finance, and service delivery? What optimal course of action can be chosen based on needs assessment? An optimal course of action is one that takes into account all the consequences of all alternatives, both positive and negative, and has the greatest net benefit among all alternatives.

In a community needs assessment, the following questions may be asked: What are the populations at risk or in need within the community? Populations at risk or in need typically include the uninsured, underinsured, minority groups, unemployed, and single mothers and their children. What are the most frequently encountered health problems? What are the most costly health problems? What are the current services and programs, including primary, secondary, and tertiary, that target the population at risk or in need? Examples of services and programs include prenatal care, primary care, vision and hearing screening, dental services, and mental health services, which may include drug and alcohol abuse programs, counseling, long-term transitional housing for chemically dependent women with children, and low-income housing for displaced mothers.

What are the problems and deficiencies of current community services and programs? Examples of problems include lack of effectiveness, gaps between current community services/programs and needs, lack of knowledge of services and programs on the part of providers and patients, lack of coordination, inadequate referral transfer patterns, duplication, misinformation, poor information management, poor patient education, and maldistribution of current services and providers. What strategies can be tried to improve current community services and programs? Examples of viable strategies include developing an integrated service system that is consumer-focused and addresses the consumer's social, medical, and health needs; involving providers, funders, and clients in the planning, development, and implementation of services and programs; coordinating funding sources; regularly evaluating services and programs and their impact; improving awareness of services and programs; and improving accessibility to services (e.g., relocating services, extending hours, providing transportation services, standardizing service eligibility requirements).

How can a course of action be implemented to solve the most pressing community-wide problems? A recent community-level needs assessment conducted in Louisiana illustrates how this question can be answered. It is an important form of evaluation that can inform public health planning. Researchers examined tobacco use among ninth-grade students in south central Louisiana by surveying more than 4,800 students about their tobacco habits (Johnson, Myers, Webber, and Boris, 2004). The study team confirmed the self-reported survey results by collecting saliva samples from a subset of students. About 58 percent of the ninth graders reported they had smoked a cigarette at some point, with 25 percent reporting they had smoked within the previous 30 days, and 17 percent reporting they had smoked within the past 7 days. The study identified which racial and ethnic groups were most likely to be smokers, and what types of social relationships and attitudes were associated with smoking. The results from this needs assessment provided the state of Louisiana with data to guide health promotion and tobacco control efforts among young people.

Process Evaluation

Process evaluation is concerned with how a particular program actually operates. It focuses on the staffing, budget, activities, services, materials, and administration of the program. Process evaluation serves a monitoring function, assessing whether the program has been implemented as planned, whether it is in compliance with legal and regulatory requirements, and whether any problems have been encountered in the implementation stage. Based on process evaluation, changes may be made in certain aspects of the program to address unintended consequences or to resolve unexpected problems.

There are many reasons for monitoring the process of implementing a program. Rossi et al. (2004), in their comprehensive discussion of evaluation research, have summarized the following. First, program monitoring ascertains that program administrators conduct their day-to-day activities efficiently and, if they do not, identifies ways to enhance efficiency. Second, program monitoring provides evidence to funders, sponsors, or stakeholders that the program is being implemented as planned and according to the purpose for which it was funded. Third, process evaluation identifies unexpected problems that need to be corrected immediately rather than held for the end of the normal duration of the program. Fourth, process evaluation is often a prelude to outcome evaluation. There is no point in assessing the impact or outcome of a program unless it has indeed taken place in the way intended. Finally, monitoring program costs and resource expenditures provides essential information for estimating whether the benefits of a program justify the costs.

Important questions to be addressed in process evaluation include: What are the critical activities and services of the program and what are their schedules?

How are they operated? How are resources—including staff, budget, and time—allocated and managed? What is the relationship between program activities and program outcomes or objectives? To what extent has the program been implemented as planned? Is the program implemented efficiently? What problems, both anticipated and unforeseen, have been encountered in the implementation stage? What adjustments in program operation and management are necessary to address the problems?

Many of the data elements required for process evaluation are either available or can be incorporated into an organization- or a program-wide management information system that routinely collects information on a client-by-client basis. Relevant data elements include sociodemographic data, services provided, service providers, diagnosis or reasons for program participation, costs, outcome measures, and satisfaction. The information is essential for program monitoring as well as assessment at a later stage.

Vidaro, Earp, and Altpeter (1997) provide a detailed account of their efforts to design and conduct an ongoing eight-year process evaluation for a comprehensive breast cancer screening intervention for African-American women in five rural North Carolina counties. Vidaro and her colleagues describe how the study team created process evaluation objectives to mirror the objectives of the program being evaluated. For instance, the breast cancer screening program's objectives centered on reducing barriers to screening and encouraging women to seek screening. Therefore, the process evaluation objectives included exploring local health care providers' knowledge and practice of breast cancer screening as well as factors shaping patients' attitudes, knowledge, beliefs, and practices regarding screening. The study team developed a number of data collection instruments to pursue these process evaluation objectives, including patient interviews, provider surveys, service statistics, and project documents.

Over the course of the process evaluation, Vidaro et al. (1997) encountered several challenges, including: (1) coping with funding constraints (the value of process evaluation is not always readily apparent to funders, who tend to be more interested in final health outcomes); (2) finding ways to reallocate staff time so that the process evaluation could take place without disruption of other activities; (3) striking a balance between breadth and depth of the process evaluation (in a complex, multifaceted program, one must choose whether to evaluate all program components with little depth, or focus on fewer components with greater depth); and (4) determining how best to use process evaluation findings to improve the breast cancer screening program. Vidaro and her colleagues' frank discussion of their experiences provides great insight into the real-world challenges associated with process evaluation. This example also highlights the fact that every evaluation is different, because each program and policy under evaluation is unique. While this chapter provides an overview of theory and techniques for evaluation, there is great variation in the application of these skills.

Outcome Evaluation

Outcome evaluation, also called impact assessment, focuses on the accomplishments and impact of the service, program, or policy and its effectiveness in attaining the intended results that were set prior to program or policy implementation (Herman et al., 1987). Program results may be compared with the status quo or some competing alternative program or policy with the same goals. The results of outcome evaluation enable sponsors and stakeholders to decide whether to continue or discontinue a program, or whether to expand or reduce it. Examples of outcome measures include health status (e.g., recovery from an illness), behaviors (e.g., primary care visits), performance (e.g., smoking cessation), cognitive (e.g., knowledge or skill gained), and affective (e.g., satisfaction level). While evaluation is primarily concerned with explicitly defined goals and objectives, evaluators should also watch for unintended or unanticipated outcomes, both positive and negative.

Due to resource constraints, knowledge of program accomplishments alone is insufficient; the results produced by a program or policy must be compared with the costs incurred in implementing the program. Cost–benefit analysis is conducted and the program's net benefit is compared with some objective standard or that of a competing program with the same goals. Programs that are continued and promulgated are likely to be cost-effective.

Important questions to be addressed in outcome evaluation include: What are the goals and objectives of the program or policy? How are they measured and assessed? What programs are available as alternatives to this program? How are the program's essential components (e.g., activities, services, staffing, budget, and administration) related to achieving program goals and objectives? How successful isthe program in accomplishing its intended results? How effective is the program in comparison with alternative programs or by some objective standards? How costly is this program in comparison with alternative programs? What are the effects of the program and its components? Which program components best accomplish each of the program goals and objectives? What gaps exist in meeting the program goals and objectives? What changes should be made that might lead to better attainment of the goals and objectives? What are the unanticipated outcomes, both positive and negative, associated with the program? What decisions can be made regarding program continuation, expansion, modification, and promulgation?

Outcomes research conducted at the patient level is called medical outcomes or effectiveness research. Typically, research focuses on the most prevalent, costly medical conditions, for which there are alternative clinical strategies or pathways. Outcomes research involves linking the type of care received by a variety of patients with a particular condition to positive and negative outcomes in order to identify what works best for which patients (Guadagnoli and McNeil, 1994). Type of care refers not only to medical or surgical interventions, such as the use of a particular drug or surgical procedure, but also to diagnostic, preventive, and rehabilitative care.

Generally, outcome measures refer to the health status of patients (Greenfield and Nelson, 1992). They include the traditional outcome measures of mortality and morbidity, as well as assessments of physical functioning, mental well-being, and other aspects of health-related quality of life (Bergner, 1985; Greenfield and Nelson, 1992; Steinwachs, 1989; Ware, 1986).

The following are examples of the structured instruments that exist for most dimensions of health status:

- general health measures: Nottingham Health Profile, the Sickness Impact Profile, and the Medical Outcomes Study Instrument/SF-36, which provide global profiles of health including well-being, function, and social and emotional health (Bergner et al., 1976; Bergner et al., 1981; Hunt and McEven, 1980, 1985; Riesenberg and Glass, 1989; Tarlov, Ware, Greenfield, Nelson, and Perrin, 1989)

- physical functioning measures: Lambeth Disability Screening Questionnaire, which determines levels of disability, impairment, and physical function within general populations (Patrick et al., 1981)

- pain measures: McGill Pain Questionnaire and the visual analogue scale (Dixon and Bird, 1981; Melzack, 1983; Scott and Huuskisson, 1979)

- social health measures: Social Health Battery (Williams, Ware, and Donald, 1981)

- psychological measures: General Health Questionnaire, which identifies people with psychological or psychiatric morbidity (Goldberg and Hillier, 1979)

- quality of life measures: Four Single Items of Well-being and the Quality of Life Index, which seek to measure the overall satisfaction and well-being of individuals (Andrews and Grandall, 1976; Spitzer, Dobson, and Hall, 1981)

- specific disease measures: Arthritis Impact Measurement Scale and the Oswestry Low Back Pain Disability Questionnaire (Fairbank, Couper, Davies, and O'Brien, 1980; Meenan, Gertman, and Mason, 1980)

Another important aspect of outcomes research is concerned with the costs of medical care. By associating costs with alternative clinical pathways or strategies, outcomes research contributes to a clear understanding of the financial implications associated with alternative clinical strategies for the treatment of the most prevalent and costly conditions. Such information benefits health services managers and medical directors in their efforts to operate efficiently in the managed care environment. Two interrelated trends of immediate and critical importance to health services organizations are the movement to managed care and the organization of previously independent health care providers into integrated networks (Bureau of Primary Health Care, 1994a, 1994b, 1995; Ginzberg, 1994). Managed care organizations combine the organization, financing, and delivery of health care in ways that respond to the demographics and economics that prevail in different regions of the country (Shortell, Gillies, and Anderson, 1994). In a managed care setting, health services organizations will be placed at risk by way of capitation and will be expected to cope with externally imposed controls on utilization.

The interest in the measurement of health-related outcomes and their predictors has escalated in recent years because of the increasing number of therapeutic options available to patients, the concomitant increase in health care costs, and the resultant need for health care reform to control these costs (Parkerson, Broadhead, and Tse, 1995). Both the public (e.g., federal and state government) and private sectors are under considerable pressure to control the rapid increases in expenditures for Medicaid, Medicare, and private insurance programs and at the same time improve the quality of care (Bailit, Federico, and McGivney, 1995). In part, these objectives can be achieved by allocating their limited resources to treatments of established effectiveness (Kitzhaber, 1993).

The emergence of using evidence-based medicine (EBM) in clinical service delivery systems has resulted in increased research support in this area. In the 1990s, the Agency for Healthcare Research and Quality (AHRQ), then called the Agency for Health Care Policy and Research, launched the Medical Treatment Effectiveness Research Program, which provided research funding for comparative analyses of disease prevention, diagnosis, treatment, and/or management. In fall 2005, the AHRQ announced a $15 million Effective Health Care Program that supports the development of new research on the outcomes of various health services and treatments, including pharmaceuticals. This initiative is described in depth at the AHRQ website (http://www.effectivehealthcare.ahrq.gov).

A salient example of the importance of outcome evaluation can be found in the area of community health center services for people who are low-income and/or uninsured. In 2001, President Bush identified the expansion of community health centers, which are located in medically underserved urban and rural areas in every state and territory, as a priority of his administration (Address of the President to the Joint Session of Congress, 2001). Because community health centers receive a significant portion of their operating budgets from federal grants and from Medicaid reimbursement, outcome evaluations of their performance are critically important to Congress and the executive branch, who determine funding allocations. Numerous outcome evaluations of community health center performance report that the centers provide high-quality, cost-efficient primary and preventive health care services (e.g., Falik et al., 2006; O'Malley, Forrest, Politzer, Wulu, and Shi, 2005; Shin, Markus, and Rosenbaum, 2006). In addition, there is growing evidence from outcome evaluations that expansion of community health centers is a promising strategy for reducing racial and ethnic disparities in health and health care (e.g., General Accounting Office, 2003; Shi, Stevens, Wulu, Politzer, and Xu, 2004; Shin, Jones, and Rosenbaum, 2003).

Policy Analysis

Policy analysis lays out goals, identifies alternatives for meeting the goals, uses logical and rational processes to evaluate identified alternatives, and chooses the best or optimal way to reach the prescribed end. Policy analysis is typically performed with constraints on time, information, and resources. Its purpose is to inform policy and decision makers of available options, provide a framework for valuing them, predict their consequences, and assist in rational and informed problem solving. Policy analysts rely heavily on the techniques developed in economics, mathematics, operations research, and systems analysis.

The five-step framework (Stokey and Zeckhauser, 1978) for policy analysis includes: (1) establishing the context, (2) identifying the alternatives, (3) predicting the consequences, (4) valuing the outcomes, and (5) making a choice. Each of these steps contains important questions and issues to be addressed by the policy analysts. For example, to establish the context of analysis, policy analysts must find the underlying problem and outline the goals to be pursued in confronting it.

To lay out the alternative courses of action, analysts need to be knowledgeable about the particular policy and program in question and about how to obtain further information for analysis. Also, the alternatives should be designed to take advantage of additional information as it becomes available. This enables policy and decision makers to change the course of action as they learn more about the real world.

In predicting the consequences or estimating the likelihood of the alternatives, researchers rely heavily on the analytic techniques of the management sciences, in particular economics and operational research (e.g., forecasting and simulation, cost–benefit analysis, discounting, decision analysis, linear programming, critical path method, and Markov models).

To value the predicted outcomes, analysts try to choose objective (often quantitative) standards or criteria against which policy choices can be evaluated. Since some alternatives will be superior with respect to certain goals and inferior with respect to others, analysts may have to address the goals separately and descriptively.

In selecting the alternative, analysts draw all aspects of the analysis together to identify the preferred course of action. Sometimes, the analysis is straightforward and the best alternative will emerge and be selected. At other times, the analysis may be so complex that researchers have to rely on a computer program to keep track of all the options and their possible outcomes. In most situations, the choice among competing policy alternatives is difficult, for the future is uncertain and the trade-offs among viable options are both inevitable and painful.

Health policy analysis is performed by a wide range of people and organizations, including academics, government officials, think tanks, and consulting firms. These different types of analysts produce different types of policy analysis products. For instance, academics tend to produce policy analysis articles or books for publication, government officials tend to produce policy memos or issue briefs to inform policy makers, and think tanks and consulting firms tend to produce reports tailored to particular clients in the health care industry or in government. The Rand Corporation, a nonprofit research and analysis organization, routinely produces this third type of health policy analysis, an example of which is a recent report on the diffusion of health information technology (HIT)

(Fonkych and Taylor, 2005). In this report, Rand follows the classic strategies of policy analysis. First, the company establishes the context for HIT by summarizing the current state of HIT adoption by the U.S. health care system and identifying factors predicting its adoption. Rand proceeds to identify policy alternatives to improve HIT diffusion, discusses the consequences of each alternative, and makes policy recommendations based on the empirical findings.

PROCESS

Before conducting an evaluation, the investigator is first designated as an evaluator. The selection of an evaluator often hinges on many considerations including credibility, level of competence, availability, cost, and time, among others. Perhaps the most important consideration is credibility. Evaluation has to be credible to be useful. For evaluation to be credible, the evaluator has to be trustworthy. An evaluator's credibility is enhanced when that person is competent, knowledgeable, personable, and reliable.

Competence can be indicated by credentials (degrees, certificates, and licenses), reputation, relevant experience (past projects in similar areas or using similar skills), perceived technical skills that are critical to the project, and the validity and reliability of the evaluation design and the data-gathering and analysis methods adopted. Competence also means that evaluators are articulate about their chosen evaluation methods. Since most users or sponsors are not sophisticated in terms of research methodology and people are usually more skeptical of methods and arguments they do not comprehend, evaluators should try to keep the design and the data-gathering and analysis methods sufficiently simple and straightforward, yet valid.

Knowledge of the subject matter is another way to gain credibility. Both research and work experience can enhance knowledge level. Personality is important because conducting an evaluation often requires gaining trust and building a rapport with administrators, participants, and users or audiences. Strong interpersonal skills have to be nurtured. At the same time, evaluators should remain objective in their work, taking care not to be constrained by friendships, professional relations, or the desire to land future evaluation jobs. Finally, a good track record on relevant research projects is helpful for establishing an evaluator's credibility.

There are many ways to conduct evaluation research. The following is a description of a representative six-step process: (1) determine the scope of evaluation, (2) get acquainted with the program, (3) choose the methodology for evaluation, (4) collect the data, (5) analyze the data, and (6) report the findings. While evaluators may use this as a framework, they should be aware that adaptations may be necessary for their unique projects.

Determine the Scope of the Evaluation

To determine the scope of an evaluation, the evaluator first reviews all pertinent information. Then some background investigation is conducted to find out more about the nature of the assignment. Finally, the evaluator negotiates and reaches agreements with the sponsor about their mutual expectations.

Review Information About the Evaluation

Once selected, in most situations the evaluator is likely to be presented with a lot of information about the program or project to be evaluated, as well as about the scope of work. In other cases, the evaluator may have to help locate any pertinent information related to the program or project. Regardless of how information is collected, the evaluator should review these materials carefully and have a clear sense of the scope or boundaries of the assignment. After the review, the evaluator should find answers to the following questions: What is the ultimate objective of this assignment? What is to be evaluated? What issues or questions will the evaluation address? What is the nature of this evaluation? Is it a needs assessment (e.g., planning for the future), a process evaluation (e.g., improving an ongoing program or project), an outcome evaluation (e.g., making judgments about program results and impact), a policy analysis (e.g., evaluating alternatives and making a choice), or a combination of these? What specific tasks must be accomplished? How are these tasks related to the objective of the evaluation? What resources (e.g., budget, data sources, staff, informants) are made available to the evaluator? What is the duration of the evaluation? What deliverables are expected from the evaluator in the course and at the end of the project? What is the time schedule for these deliverables? How will the evaluation results be utilized? What additional information will be provided to the evaluator? If some of these questions cannot be answered from the materials provided, the evaluator may contact the host to obtain additional information.

After obtaining answers to these questions, the evaluator then critically assesses the assignment. Does the sponsor require more than someone can possibly deliver both in terms of scope of work and time frame? Does the evaluator fill the role of a researcher or analyst, or is he or she required or expected to be an advocate? Many researchers find it inappropriate to mix research with advocacy. An advocacy role could also have a potentially negative impact on the credibility of the evaluation. The evaluator should let the sponsor know this concern. Are resources (e.g., budget, data sources, staff, informants) sufficient for carrying out the necessary tasks? What additional resources are required? The evaluator should record all the concerns along with elements missing from the previous sets of questions. He or she also needs to consider potential designs to be used for data collection and analysis and must develop a preliminary evaluation plan. Such advance preparation will enable the evaluator to be both knowledgeable and sensitive in the first meeting with the sponsor and enable him or her to use that meeting productively to probe and clarify the intended scope of the assignment.

Conduct Background Investigation

Next, the evaluator conducts some background investigation to find out more about the program and evaluation. Also, he or she reviews related literature about the subject area and the evaluation methods relevant for this type of assignment. If the evaluator is not already familiar with this type of program or project, he or she should contact someone who is. Consulting with such a person can help the evaluator know more about the program, its context and setting, the political nature of the evaluation, the problems in the program, and potential pitfalls in evaluating the program. Such information is valuable in conducting the evaluation work effectively.

Background investigation should help the evaluator assess the extent to which important stakeholders are likely to be affected by either the program or the evaluation. Possible stakeholders include policy and decision makers, program sponsors, evaluation sponsors, the program target population, participants, managers and staff, and competitors. The evaluator should understand the relationships among the various stakeholders.

Meanwhile, the evaluator will find it beneficial to examine the literature of the subject to see what has been written about this type of program or about specific components of the program. Access to earlier evaluations of this or similar programs will also be valuable. The review of evaluation methods will be helpful in refining the approach and improving the plan.

Negotiate the Contract

Having become familiarized with the scope of work and identified areas of missing information or concerns, the evaluator meets with the project sponsor. The sponsor may be the funder or primary user of the evaluation. The purpose of this meeting is to reach a common understanding about the exact scope and nature of the evaluation. Failure to do so could lead to wasted money and effort, frustration, and acrimony if sponsors or evaluators feel they do not get what they expected. The evaluator and sponsor should go over the scope of work and reach an agreement about all stipulations. If any areas are unsatisfactorily addressed in the scope of work, the evaluator should make sure they are clarified. At the end of the session, after negotiation, both sides should agree on the following:

- The general purpose of the evaluation assignment.
- The users and audiences for the evaluation.
- The program or project components to be evaluated.
- A description of the questions or issues to be addressed.
- The respective roles, tasks, or responsibilities of the evaluator and sponsor or staff in the evaluation process. For example, for the evaluator, the specific tasks to be performed, the assignments to be turned in, and the time frame for accomplishing these. For the sponsor or staff, the kinds of access (e.g., data, informants, assistants, a coordinator, program records, files, computers, copy machine, fax machine, telephone), the required resources (e.g., persons as-

signed to the project, staff time to administer instruments), and the types of cooperation, collaboration, and assistance (e.g., random assignment possibility, pilot test feasibility) to be provided.

- A set of criteria to be used to judge the successful completion of the evaluation.

- The methodology or general approach to be used, including evaluation design (e.g., experiment, time series, case control, case study), data collection methods (e.g., tests, observations, interviews, questionnaires), instrument types (readily available or to be designed), measurements (particularly those related to outcome), criteria for success or failure, and data analysis methods. The administrative requirements underlying the proposed methodology should also be considered and laid out. If certain methods are not feasible, the potential trade-offs between administrative feasibility and technical quality should be made clear and must be well understood by both sides.

- The style of report to be produced. This may include the major sections of the report, the extent to which quantitative or qualitative information is reported, whether the evaluator will write technical reports, brief notes, or confer with the staff, and whether revisions will be necessary and under what conditions.

- The evaluation budget. The budget is prepared based on the tasks and schedules specified for conducting the evaluation. It includes both fixed- and variable-cost items. Examples include personnel (the evaluator and assistants, including the time spent reviewing the project; outside consultants; statisticians), travel and transportation, subcontracting (e.g., the collection of both primary and secondary data), postage (for questionnaires, draft reports, and so on), photocopying, printing, computer hardware and software (and/or computing time, when access is to a mainframe computer), and phone calls (including long-distance). If in-kind support is provided for certain items, this should be so indicated.

- A schedule of all the major project activities, meetings, and assignment due dates.

- A plan for utilizing the evaluation results.

- A contingency plan that specifies the conditions under which the evaluation plan may be changed, who will make decisions about changes, and who will implement them. Examples of such conditions include unexpected illness, delay in data collection, change of policy, and so forth.

The agreement reached as a result of this meeting should be documented, reviewed, and signed by both parties. The meeting between the evaluator and sponsor will result in a formal contract on terms agreeable to both parties. The final contract will include the following: a description of the evaluation questions to be addressed by the evaluator; the methodology to be used, including design and data collection and analysis methods; a timeline for these activities; a list of the tasks and responsibilities of program staff or others in support of the evaluation; a schedule of reports and meetings, including tentative agendas where possible; and a budget estimating anticipated costs.

Get Acquainted with the Program

Once the contract has been signed, the evaluator officially proceeds with the evaluation. The first task is to get fully acquainted with the program or project to be evaluated. Specifically, the evaluator should find out about the program's goals and objectives; its principal activities, organizational arrangements, staffing, and roles and responsibilities; the relationships between program operations and outcomes; the profiles of clients served and services provided; financial performance; and primary problems. The level of understanding at this phase should be more specific than during the background investigation phase. In addition, some contextual information about the organization that administers the program will be useful. Such information includes the organization's mission, history, services, staff and client characteristics, and so on.

Often, the evaluator's organizational collaborators or coordinators are the best sources of such information. They can at least suggest where to find the information. Some common sources include the following:

- funding proposal written for the program and the request for proposals (RFPs) written by the sponsor or funding agency

- program brochures and other materials, program implementation directives and requirements, administrative manuals, and annual reports

- the organizational chart and descriptions of administrative and service positions and responsibilities, patient or client records, and daily schedules of services and activities

- the program budget and actual spending reports, memos, meeting minutes, and newspaper articles

- documents describing the history of the program or the social context in which it has been designed to fit

- legislation, administrative regulations, completed evaluation studies, and perspectives and descriptions from program managers, participants, sponsors, or users

If feasible, the evaluator may want to personally experience some or all of the program components and activities. At a minimum, he or she should conduct one site visit to obtain firsthand impressions of how the program actually operates. The evaluator then directs his or her attention to the goals, objectives, and outcomes of the program and their measurements. The goals and objectives specified for the program will be used as a benchmark. Program staff and planners will be consulted to make sure these are indeed the goals and objectives of the program. The evaluator may ask them to write a clear rationale describing how the particular activities, processes, materials, and administrative arrangements of the program will satisfy the goals and objectives specified. The evaluator may also look for additional sources of program goals and objectives. For example, are there written federal, state, or local guidelines for program processes and goals to which this program must conform? What are the needs of the community or constituency that the program is intended to meet? Utilizing this information, the evaluator can recreate a detailed description of the program, including statements identifying program goals and objectives, cross-classifying them with program components, and comparing how the program is supposed to operate with how it actually does.

Information about the outcomes of the program may be obtained from published documents, performance records, productivity indicators, patient or client databases, and cost data, such as financial records, insurance claims, and workers' compensation claims. Often it may be necessary to conduct additional studies to find out more about the program and its performance. For example, participant and/or staff surveys or interviews may be conducted to obtain additional or supporting data to back up the description of program events, operations, and outcomes. Past evaluations of this or a similar program, if available, will provide insight into how measurements can be constructed. Books and articles in the evaluation literature that describe the effects of similar programs are also valuable. If feasible, the evaluator should personally observe or monitor the program outcomes.

At this stage, creation of a logic model is often useful (Brownson et al., 2003). A logic model is a diagram or table that connects the program's goals to specific objectives or activities and to the desired outcomes. The logic model incorporates measures to determine whether program activities are achieving these outcomes. Creation of this model serves several purposes. First, it allows the evaluator to become intimately familiar with the program in question. Second, it fosters collaboration among the evaluator, the program staff, and other stakeholders. Often, people involved in different aspects of a program disagree about its goals, objectives, and desired outcomes. The creation of the logic model forces discussion and consensus on these issues. Finally, the completed logic model acts as a blueprint of sorts for the rest of the evaluation. It can help guide the evaluation design, instrument, and measures, as well as the data collection and analysis methods. In addition, the logic model may serve as the outline for the final evaluation report.

Finalize the Methodology for the Evaluation

Although the evaluation plan must be thought about at the start, now that the evaluator has become acquainted with the program, it is time to finalize the methodology. Specifically, the evaluation design, data instruments and measures, data collection methods, and data analysis techniques should be decided upon. The evaluator is encouraged to involve the primary potential users in the planning of the evaluation to facilitate their ownership of the study and enhance trust and cooperation. A detailed schedule should also be drawn up indicating when and for how long each activity will be performed, by whom, and using what resources. The schedule will be used to monitor progress so that the evaluation can be completed in a timely fashion.

Evaluation Design

Evaluation design is concerned with choosing the appropriate research methods, both quantitative and qualitative, and selecting the unit of analysis and sampling techniques (Alkin, Kosecoff, Fitz-Gibbon, and Seligman, 1974; Brownson et al., 2003; Campbell and Stanley, 1966; Cook and Campbell, 1976; Fitz-Gibbon and Morris, 1987; Rossi et al., 2004).

Many research methods can be used in evaluation research including surveys, experiments, case studies, and so on. The choice depends mainly on the objectives of the evaluation and the constraints of the situation. The evaluator should choose the best possible design from a methodological and practical standpoint, taking into account the potential importance of the program, the practicality and feasibility of each design, the resource constraints, and the validity and generalizability of the results.

In choosing evaluation methods, the evaluator may incorporate both quantitative and qualitative approaches. Quantitative approaches (such as surveys, experiments, longitudinal research, and secondary analysis) are necessary to measure, summarize, aggregate, and compare program outcomes and effects; attribute their causes; and generalize program results to the population as a whole.

Qualitative approaches (such as focused group interviews, observation, case studies, and fieldwork) are important to understand the meaning of a program and its outcomes from the participants' perspectives. The emphasis is on detailed descriptions and on in-depth understanding as it emerges from direct contact and experience with the program and its participants. Qualitative approaches are appropriate when the evaluator is interested in detailed descriptive information, the dynamics of processes and implementation, specifics of problem areas, and unanticipated outcomes and side effects. Qualitative approaches add depth, detail, and meaning to empirical findings.

The combination of both quantitative and qualitative methods may be needed for the purpose of evaluation. If the program components, operations, and outcomes are well defined, a quantitative approach can easily be used to determine program effectiveness. If these elements are poorly defined, a qualitative approach may be used first to identify critical program features and potential outcomes before employing a quantitative approach to assess their attainment. A quantitative approach can be used to assess whether program objectives have been reached. A qualitative approach can be used to understand how and why program objectives have or have not been reached. A quantitative approach can show the breadth of information about the program. A qualitative approach can add depth and sensitivity to program information.

The design of an evaluation also considers the unit of analysis and sampling procedures. The choice of the unit of analysis depends on the program objectives and is related to the target the program or intervention is designed to affect. If the objective is to see progress made at the individual level, then individuals are the unit of analysis. If the objective is to see progress at the organizational level, then the organization is the unit of analysis. Other examples include groups, communities, associations, neighborhoods, hospitals, companies, districts, counties, states, and nations. Sometimes, multiple units of analysis are necessary.

A sampling plan specifies how the unit of analysis will be selected for study. Sampling is used when it is too expensive and time consuming to study every unit. This is a good way to increase the kinds of information to be collected given limited budget and time. If interviews or surveys are to be conducted, a random sampling method should be used to select subjects. If a focus group is to be employed, participants should be selected based on their representativeness with respect to different organizational units and responsibilities as well as personal demographic characteristics. Chapter 11 provides a detailed discussion of the frequently used sampling methods.

Evaluation Instrument and Measures

Once the evaluation method has been chosen, the evaluator then selects or designs instruments containing measures of the variables to be studied. The principal advantage of using an existing instrument is that the validity and reliability of the measures may be available. However, if no relevant instrument is available or accessible, or only portions of the measures are available, a new instrument has to be developed.

The instrument, whether available or newly constructed, should include all important measures related to the evaluation objectives and, if possible, to advancing the development of associated scientific theories. The program sponsor and staff should be invited to participate in the selection and/or design of the research instrument. At minimum, the draft instrument should be circulated to them for inputs and changes. The involvement of potential users is important to gain their trust and cooperation. The completed instrument should be pilot-tested and revised, and the validity and reliability of the measure documented. In general, the following measures are usually examined as part of an evaluation:

- participant characteristics (e.g., age, sex, race and ethnicity, education, income, occupation, attitudes and beliefs, experience, and baseline data on performance to be affected by the intervention)

- characteristics of the program structure or context that might affect the intervention (e.g., staff characteristics, organizational setting, and environmental impact)

- characteristics of program implementation or processes (e.g., types of intervention; activities; services including materials, staffing, and administration)

- characteristics of program outcomes, both long-term and short-term (e.g., measures of program goals and objectives, including health status, condition, knowledge, attitude, satisfaction level, behavior changes, and unanticipated outcomes—both positive and negative)

- costs associated with the program (personnel, materials, equipment, facilities, and indirect opportunity costs) and benefits associated with program outcomes (e.g., improved health status, reduced use of costly services, and savings on opportunity costs)

Data Collection Methods

Data for evaluation research may be obtained through surveys, interviews, administrative records, observations, or content analysis. The evaluator should first try to find useful information that has been or is being collected routinely in the setting. Some data elements may already exist in the agency's files, reports, journals, logs, service records, provider records, participant records, and information systems, which can be copied and processed to provide information for the evaluation. Computer-based management information systems are becoming more popular and sometimes indispensable for health and other human services programs. They produce periodic tables and reports containing information regularly used by staff and management. Service records can be narrative reports or highly structured data forms on which project staff check which services were given, how they were received, and what results were observed. Provider data may cross-list services delivered to clients as well as provider's characteristics. Participant data may record services received as well as participants' characteristics.

Other data elements may be developed and incorporated into the system or collected firsthand. When there is no record-keeping system, the evaluator may suggest its establishment to collect needed information. He or she might persuade program staff to establish record-developing systems that will benefit both the evaluation and the program. A good way to increase the amount of information collected is by involving assistants and program staff in data collection. Not only should the evaluator specify which data collection methods to use, and when to use them, the evaluator must also understand whose responsibility it is to collect or provide different data elements.

Data Analysis

The types of data analyses conducted are related to the evaluation design (Fitz-Gibbon and Morris, 1987; Patton, 1987, 2002). When designs consist of control groups or nonbiased comparison groups, the analysis is quite straightforward. Comparisons can be made between the outcomes of the experimental and control groups, together with statistical procedures for determining whether observed differences are likely to be due to chance variations. For programs with nonuniform coverage, evaluators may take advantage of variations in intervention in order to approximate quasi-experimental designs, and program effect can be assessed in the same way as with experimental designs. However, variables measuring program intensity should be included in the analysis.

When no control groups are built into the design, as in the case of full-coverage programs, the impact of intervention is difficult to assess with confidence. Designs without control groups generally are evaluated by using before-and-after time-series designs in which there are multiple measurements before and after the program is introduced. Specifically, preprogram and post-program outcome measurements are compared to see if the differences are significant.

More sophisticated multivariate statistical procedures are available for causal analyses and for providing statistical controls. For example, a regression analysis that includes both the program and other competing measures can be conducted to test whether the program is a significant predictor of outcome. A number of procedures can be performed, including modeling all but the program variable against the outcome measure. Then the program measure can be added to the regression equation to assess its impact on the overall variance explained, over and above the variance explained by the other measures included in the analysis. Chapter 14 examines the statistical methods that can be used in data analysis.

Collect the Data

Once the evaluation methodology has been finalized, the evaluator then proceeds with the tasks as scheduled. Much of the initial research will involve implementing the planned methodology, including design, sampling, and data collection and processing. Usually, there will be different kinds of data and different ways of collecting them. Data may be collected cross-sectionally or longitudinally. They may be collected from program staff and/or participants themselves. Staff surveys might indicate that services have been delivered. Participants' surveys are valuable for a number of reasons. First, they provide evidence to corroborate the staff's response. If the response is not corroborated, then different perspectives can be obtained. Second, securing participant data enables providers and program planners to measure recipients' comprehension of and satisfaction with the program, as well as their perception of which program elements are important. Finally, participant surveys are a valuable way to find out not only whether services were delivered, but what services were actually delivered and whether they were utilized as intended. Collecting a variety of information enables the evaluator to gain a broad and thorough perspective on the program and to obtain additional indicators of program effects.

The evaluator should make sure that the instruments are administered, interviews and observations conducted and coded, secondary data gathered and processed, and scheduled deadlines met. If necessary, the investigator should see to it that proper training has been given to those responsible for data collection (sending out questionnaires and monitoring their return, or conducting telephone or face-to-face interviews, observations, fieldwork, and so on).

Analyze the Data

Data analyses are conducted according to the techniques specified in the methodology section. The major objective is to determine the net outcome of the program, that is, whether or not a program produces desired levels of effects, reflected by the outcome measures, over and above what would have occurred either without the program or with an alternative program. Net outcome may be expressed as gross outcome subtracting the effects from non-program-related extraneous confounding factors and design effects. The net outcome may then be compared with that from other programs or some objective standards. In this section, we review the literature concerning some commonly used approaches to analyzing evaluation data: program coverage measurement, cost–benefit analysis, cost-effectiveness analysis, decision analysis, and modeling. Chapter 14 presents statistical techniques useful for evaluation analysis.

Measuring Program Coverage

Often, one of the program goals is related to program coverage or exposure. The program sponsor and administrators are interested in the extent of program coverage because they need to be accountable for spending. Program coverage is also a precondition for achieving program effect. After all, how can the intervention be expected to work without first being implemented?

Rossi et al. (2004) have discussed a number of measures of program coverage based on program participants' characteristics. The overcoverage rate may be expressed as the number of program participants who are not in need, compared with the total number of participants in the program or with the total number not in need in a designated population, if this number is available:

$$\text{Overcoverage rate} = 100 \times \frac{\text{number of program participants not in need}}{\text{total number of program participants} \atop \text{or those not in need in a designated population}}$$

The program coverage rate refers to the proportion of the target population in need of the program who actually participate in it. This may be expressed as:

$$\text{Program coverage rate} = 100 \times \frac{\text{number of program participants who are in need}}{\text{total target population who are in need}}$$

The undercoverage rate refers to the proportion of the target population in need of the program who have not participated in it. This may be expressed as:

$$\text{Undercoverage rate} = 100 \times \frac{\text{number of nonparticipants who are in need}}{\text{total target population who are in need}}$$

or

$$\text{Undercoverage rate} = 100 - \text{program coverage rate}$$

The efficiency of a program depends on both maximizing the number served who are in need and minimizing the number served who are not in need. This may be expressed as:

$$\text{Coverage efficiency rate} = 100 \times \left(\frac{\text{number of program participants who are in need}}{\text{total target population who are in need}} - \frac{\text{number of program participants not in need}}{\text{total number of program participants or those not in need in a population}} \right)$$

The coverage efficiency rate ranges from +100 to −100 with +100 indicating total coverage of people in need of the program and −100 indicating total coverage of those not in need.

Cost-Benefit Analysis and Cost-Effectiveness Analysis

Purpose

Both cost-benefit analysis (CBA) and cost-effectiveness analysis (CEA) are means of analyzing or judging the efficiency of programs (Blaney, 1988; Department of Veterans Affairs, 1989; Drummond, Sculpher, Torrance, O'Brien, and Stoddard, 2005; Patrick, 1993; Pearce, 1981; Rossi et al., 2004; Rowland, 1995; Stokey and Zeckhauser, 1978; Veney and Kaluzny, 2005). Efficiency analyses provide a framework for relating program costs to program results.

Significance

Efficiency analysis, as provided by CBA and CEA, is crucial for decisions related to the planning, implementation, continuation, and expansion of health services programs. Since programs are usually conducted under resource constraints, only those that are effective in achieving the intended goals and/or are efficient in terms of resource consumption deserve to be continued or expanded. Funders and decision makers often make decisions regarding continuing program support based on a consideration of the bottom line (the goal being financial benefits, or the equivalent, that outweigh costs). CBA and CEA help identify and compare the actual or anticipated program costs with the known or expected program benefits and provide valuable information for efficiency analysis. Recent examples of health services research using CBA include a study of the economics of vaccinating restaurant food handlers against hepatitis A (Meltzer, Shapiro, Mast, and Arcari, 2001) and an evaluation comparing the costs and benefits of using whole-cell pertussis vaccine versus acellular vaccine for childhood immunizations in the United States (Ekwueme et al., 2000). Cost-effectiveness analysis has recently been used to explore such salient health services issues as the value of breast magnetic resonance imaging to screen BRCA1/2 mutation carriers (Plevritis et al., 2006) and lung cancer screening with helical computed tomography in older adult smokers (Mahadevia et al., 2003).

Definitions

Cost-benefit analysis (CBA) compares the benefits of a program with its costs. Both direct and indirect benefits and costs are identified and included in the analysis. Both benefits and costs are quantified and translated into a common monetary unit. Both benefits and costs may be projected into the future to reflect the lifetime of a program, or the future benefits and costs may be discounted to reflect their present values. Certain assumptions can be made in order to translate particular program elements (both inputs and outputs) into monetary figures. The basis for the assumptions underlying the translation and analysis must be specified and discussed. Different analyses may be undertaken based on different sets of assumptions. The net benefits are typically used to judge the efficiency level of the program, or they may be compared with those of other competing programs.

Cost-effectiveness analysis (CEA) also compares the benefits of a program with its costs, but it requires monetizing only the costs of programs and not the benefits. Program benefits in CEA are expressed in outcome units, such as the **quality-adjusted life year (QALY)**, which integrate a measure of quality or desirability of a health state with the duration of survival (Haddix, Teutsch, and Corso, 2003). The efficacy of a program in attaining its goals or in achieving certain outcomes is assessed in relation to the monetary value of the resources or costs spent in implementing the program. Cost-effectiveness analysis is more appropriate than cost–benefit analysis when there are controversies about converting outcomes into monetary values (e.g., human lives saved).

Differences

The difference between CBA and CEA is related to how program outcomes or effects are expressed. Program outcomes are expressed in monetary terms in CBA, but in nonmonetary or substantive terms in CEA. For example, a cost–benefit analysis of a health promotion program to reduce cigarette smoking would focus on the difference between the dollars spent on the antismoking program and the dollars saved from reduced medical care for smoking-related diseases, decreased sick leave, and so on. A cost-effectiveness analysis of the same program would estimate the dollars spent to convert each smoker to a nonsmoker, or a heavy smoker to a moderate smoker. Whereas CBA compares benefits to costs in monetary terms, CEA compares costs expressed in monetary terms to units of substantive goals achieved. Cost–benefit is mainly concerned with cost relative to output. Cost-effectiveness first assesses the degree to which a program achieves its goals and then examines the efficiency level in goal attainment.

Use

Cost–benefit or cost-effectiveness analysis can be used during all phases of a program including planning, implementation, and evaluation. In the planning phase, CBA may be undertaken to estimate a program's anticipated costs and benefits. Assumptions must be made about the magnitude of a program's potential positive net impact and its costs. Cost–benefit conducted before program implementation is particularly appropriate for programs that are expensive, time consuming, resource intensive, or difficult to abandon once they have been put into place. In the implementation phase, CBA and CEA can be used to monitor the progress of a program toward anticipated benefits and costs. Program adjustments may be needed if great variations between anticipated and actual benefits or costs are noted. These kinds of analysis are most commonly undertaken after program completion as part of the evaluation strategy to assess the net impact of a program. The efficiency of a program may be assessed in either absolute or comparative terms. Cost–benefit and cost-effectiveness analyses are particularly valuable when decision makers are considering alternative programs as opposed to merely deciding whether to continue an existing one.

Method of Cost-Benefit Analysis

Specify the Accounting Perspectives

In CBA, the costs and benefits may be considered from different perspectives, such as from the viewpoint of program participants, the program sponsor, or society as a whole (Rossi et al., 2004). Program participants are individuals, groups, or organizations that receive the program or services. The program sponsor is the funding source of the program intervention or services and may be a private, for-profit firm; a community nonprofit agency; a foundation; or a government agency. Society's perspective takes the point of view of the community affected either directly or indirectly by the program intervention or services.

A cost-benefit analysis based on the program participants' perspective often produces higher net benefits than one that uses other perspectives, because much of the program costs may be borne or subsidized by the program sponsor or society. A CBA based on the program sponsor's perspective resembles a profitability analysis conducted by private firms. It may be used by private firms sponsoring a program for its employees or constituents, or by sponsors who must make choices between alternative programs in the face of limited financial resources. The social perspective is the most comprehensive one, taking into account all identifiable costs and benefits. However, it is usually the most complex, largely because of how difficult it is to obtain all relevant information for analysis. Different accounting perspectives may not only cause differences in the choice of cost and benefit items, but they may also value those items in varying ways. For example, the social perspective differs from the individuals' or the sponsor's perspective in valuing or monetizing costs and benefits (Stokey and Zeckhauser, 1978).

Deciding which accounting perspective to use is generally the task of the evaluation sponsor. The evaluator has the responsibility to make clear to the sponsor the choices available and their implications. It may also be possible to conduct the analysis based on different or all perspectives. As a minimum, the evaluator needs to specify which perspective has been chosen and the rationale for such a choice.

Identify Costs and Benefits

After the accounting perspective has been selected, the next step is to identify all costs and benefits of the program. Those whose accounting perspectives were chosen may be surveyed to identify their costs and benefits related to the program. Other useful sources include program documents and previous literature. All relevant cost and benefit components must be included to ensure CBA results are valid. Identifying program costs and benefits is typically more difficult before rather than after the program because the anticipated program costs and benefits are merely speculations and may over- or underestimate the true effects of the program. Also, information is more limited before the program. However, if a CBA is planned, it is important from the very beginning to keep accurate and complete accounts of all the costs and benefits associated with the program. In addition, depending on the complexity of the study, the research team should include a researcher whose specialty is CBA, to ensure, for the sake of future analysis, that the costs and benefits are properly collected from the outset.

Measure Costs and Benefits

After program costs and benefits are identified, the next step is to measure them in terms of a common monetary unit. There are various ways of measuring program costs and benefits. The most straightforward approach is to use the actual monetary costs and benefits. Another approach is to value program costs and benefits at their fair market prices, that is, based on how much the current market would charge for certain program inputs or outputs. When market prices are not readily available, program or service providers or recipients may be asked to assign a value to them for providing or receiving a particular service.

In measuring cost, the evaluator should not neglect opportunity costs. **Opportunity costs** reflect alternative ways resources can be utilized. For example, if the resources were not spent on a particular program, they might be used for alternative choices. Therefore, the costs of a program may be estimated by the worth of the forgone options for which these resources might be used. Sick leave is another example of opportunity cost in that the time spent in receiving treatment and recuperating cannot be used for earning income. Even when sick leave is part of the employment benefit, it represents an opportunity cost for the employer, who may have to hire a replacement, pay overtime to existing employees to perform the additional work, or reschedule program activities.

In measuring benefits, the evaluator should not forget to factor in program externalities, or the unintended spillover consequences, of the program. Program externalities may be beneficial or harmful. The beneficial externalities should be added to the total program benefits and the harmful externalities to the total costs. Because such effects are not the intended outcomes, they may be inappropriately omitted from cost–benefit calculations if special efforts are not made to include them.

The evaluator should try to measure or monetize all identified cost and benefit components and specify the measurement methods. When cost items are omitted, the program will seem more efficient than it really is. When benefit items are omitted, the program will seem less efficient than is the reality. Either situation will likely produce biased results. However, sometimes it may be impossible or unethical to measure certain elements or there may be considerable disagreement as to the monetary values applied to a particular element (such as the value of a human life). The general approach for the evaluator is to produce elements that can be valued and then list those that cannot. If essential elements or too many elements cannot be valued, CBA may not be the appropriate evaluation method to use. Cost-effectiveness analysis might be a preferred alternative.

Value Costs and Benefits

After costs and benefits have been measured in the monetary unit, the evaluator then conducts the actual valuation. Often, a computer spreadsheet program is used to facilitate the valuation. In setting up the spreadsheet, the evaluator may need to choose the relevant time periods and associated discounting factors for noncurrent time periods. The inclusion of different time periods may be required because: (1) the program is long and overlaps different time periods; (2) there are several programs to be compared and they take place in different time periods with each period reflecting a particular monetary value; or (3) the program produces benefits that may also be derived in the future, sometimes long after the intervention has taken place. Indeed, holding everything else equal, the longer the time horizon chosen, the more likely the program will appear beneficial.

To facilitate analysis, costs and benefits occurring at different time periods are brought into the same time period. If the chosen common time period is the present, then present values must be calculated for all costs and benefits that are expected in the future. If the chosen common time period is some future time period, then future values must be calculated for all costs and benefits that are expected for that future time period. **Discounting** is the technique to reduce costs and benefits that are spread out over time to their present values or to their common future values.

The results of discounting, and the whole cost-benefit analysis, are particularly sensitive to the discount rates applied. Why particular discounting rates are selected needs to be explained. Often, to resolve the controversies surrounding the choice of discount rates, evaluators conduct cost-benefit analysis using several different rates. One of the discount rates chosen might be the internal rate of return of the program, that is, the discount rate the program would have to obtain for its benefits to equal its costs. Another rate might be the prevailing lending rate at a local bank. Not only may different discounting rates be used but different assumptions may be applied. Indeed, such sensitivity analyses using varying discounting rates and assumptions to estimate their consequences for program results are often considered signs of a well-conducted cost-benefit analysis.

Another factor that needs to be taken into account when comparing costs and benefits at different time periods is inflation (or deflation, which is much less common). Inflation factors are often published for different years, and adjustments can accordingly be made to reflect the true value of money for different periods of time.

The final step in valuing costs and benefits is to compare total program costs to total program benefits by subtracting costs from benefits. If the result is positive, then the program has a net benefit. If the result is negative, then the program has a net loss. The net result of one program may be compared with that of another program or some objective standard to get a sense of the relative success of a particular program.

Method of Cost-Effectiveness Analysis

The identification, measurement, and valuation of costs, including assumptions and discounting factors, are similar between CBA and CEA (Guttentag and Struening, 1975; Rossi et al., 2004; Stokey and Zeckhauser, 1978). Cost-effectiveness analysis, however, does not require program benefits to be reduced to a monetary unit. Instead, program benefits are measured in terms of whether the program has reached its substantive goals or at least significant portions of these goals. If the goals have been reached, or substantially reached, then the program is considered effective. Cost-effectiveness analysis is often used to compare the efficiency (i.e., the monetary value of program costs) of programs that share the same or similar goals and outcome measures. The key is to determine which program components are more efficient. Programs may be ranked in terms of their costs for reaching given goals. If different programs have different degrees of goal achievement, CEA can be used to describe the various inputs required for achieving different degrees of the goals. Cost-effectiveness analysis may be used both before and after the program.

In 1996, the U.S. Panel on Cost-Effectiveness in Health and Medicine, a nongovernmental panel of experts in CEA, clinical medicine, ethics, and health outcomes measurement, was convened by the U.S. Public Health Service to establish recommendations for conducting and reporting CEA. In light of wide variations in the methods used, the panel attempted to create standards for CEA that would allow for comparisons across studies. The panel's most important recommendations pertained to how to measure health outcomes associated with the various interventions investigated in the course of CEA. The panel concluded health effectiveness should be measured in terms of the QALY (quality-adjusted life year), which incorporates changes in survival and changes in health-related quality of life by weighting years of life to reflect the value of health-related quality of life during each year (Weinstein, Siegel, Gold, Kamlet, and Russell, 1996). The QALY is calculated using scoring systems, such as the EuroQOL, the Quality of Well-Being instrument, the Health Utility Index, and the SF-6D, that measure people's perceptions of quality of life in different states of health. These instruments essentially measure what trade-offs people are willing to make to achieve a certain health state. The use of standardized QALY in CEA facilitates comparisons of different health interventions.

Limitations

In spite of their value, there are also limitations in the use of CBA and CEA. First, the identification of costs and benefits may be incomplete or subject to controversy. Even though efficiency analyses are largely quantitative and rigorous, there is no single right analysis. Different costs and outcomes may be taken into account, depending on the perspectives and values of sponsors, stakeholders, targets, and evaluators themselves. Second, the valuation of costs and benefits may be problematic. Controversies may result from placing economic values on particular input or outcome measures. Different ways of valuing costs and outcomes may be used, depending on the perspectives and values of sponsors, stakeholders, targets, and evaluators themselves. Third, complete use of CBA or CEA may not be feasible, practical, or wise in many evaluation projects. The required data elements for undertaking cost-benefit calculations may not be fully available.

Cost-benefit and cost-effectiveness analyses may be appropriately performed when the program has independent funding, but not when program costs or benefits cannot be separated from those related to other nonprogram activities. It may be too expensive or time-consuming to collect all the data needed. Some measures of inputs or outcomes cannot be meaningfully converted into monetary terms. Neither form of analysis can be performed when program impact and magnitude of impact are not known or cannot be validly estimated.

Decision Analysis

Decision analysis allows the evaluator to visually and conceptually map out uncertain events and different policy or programmatic alternatives in order to determine which alternative is most likely to produce the best outcomes (Owens, 2002). Decision analysis is comprised of three main steps: (1) identify the decision maker and the alternatives, (2) anticipate the uncertain events that lead to different outcomes, and (3) assign values to the different outcomes. This process can be displayed visually as a decision tree.

Figure 9.1 is a simple example of a decision tree for an evaluation of a breast cancer screening program. In this diagram, the square represents the decision to be made, and the circles represent chance events. The question the evaluator ultimately hopes to answer is whether the screening program in question results in earlier treatment for women who have breast cancer.

The first step in decision analysis is to identify the decision maker and the alternatives. In this case, the decision maker could be the funder of the program, the agency or organization running the program, or society as a whole. Choosing society as the decision maker, as is often done in decision analysis, entails the evaluator's assessment of the breast cancer screening program must account for a broad range of perspectives (e.g., government recommendations, clinical guidelines, and patients' perceived quality of life). It is the evaluator's responsibility to research all of the perspectives accordingly.

The second step of decision analysis is identifying the uncertain events that lead to different outcomes. In this case, the uncertain event is whether a person

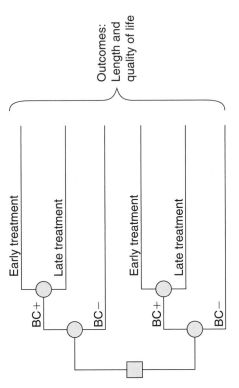

Figure 9.1. Decision tree example: Breast cancer screening

with breast cancer receives early treatment or not. The evaluator must search the epidemiologic, clinical, and policy literature in order to assign probabilities to each of the uncertain event branches of the decision tree.

Assigning values to these outcomes of interest is step three of the process. This step is also called "averaging out and folding back" and involves taking a weighted average of the outcomes based on the probability of occurrence (Owens, 2002). The outcomes of interest in this decision analysis could be length and quality of life. Depending on whether a woman with breast cancer was screened or not, and depending on the timing of her treatment, her length and quality of life will differ. Determining the magnitude of this difference through decision analysis may be of great interest and use in the evaluation of the breast cancer screening program.

Modeling

Models are constructed to reduce the complexity of the problem to be solved by eliminating trivial and noncritical elements so that attention can be focused on the essential features of the program. They are an abstraction of the real world designed to capture the essential elements of the problem. One major advantage of modeling is that it helps a person think rationally before acting. Consider, for example, the common notion that we should improve access to physicians in medically underserved areas. However, providing rural people with access to doctors and other health care providers is merely a means to an end. The goal, frequently overlooked, is to improve people's health. It is possible for a decision maker to be so involved with access that the health of the population becomes a side issue.

Another advantage of modeling is that it forces us to focus on fundamental principles rather than nonessential elements. Models convert a complex situation into one that clearly lays out the critical elements. The process of constructing a model forces us to fully understand the situation and the types of information needed to construct an accurate model. The difficulty experienced in constructing a model may indicate how little we know about the problem and how much more we need to understand about the system to be modeled. Understanding the system is not simply a matter of establishing the relationships among variables; it is also a matter of obtaining accurate information. The effective analyst should not only talk to those knowledgeable about the system, but look for independent corroboration before relying on the information obtained.

Also, modeling is less expensive and more feasible than is experimenting with the system itself. For example, in designing the construction of a hospital, planners need to find out the impact of many variables on design, including patient load, intensive-care load, and emergency rate, to name a few. To experiment with an actual hospital would be prohibitively expensive in terms of time and money, and dangerous to patients' health. Modeling, on the other hand, allows us to gain insights into the potential impact of various combinations of the essential variables of interest.

We have already discussed many examples of models. Graphs and charts are a type of model. Flow charts and logic models, which show connections between different programmatic elements, are types of diagrammatic models. Decision trees that identify uncertain events and outcomes are yet another type of model.

Models may be classified as deterministic or probabilistic, and as descriptive or prescriptive (Stokey and Zeckhauser, 1978). Deterministic models describe or predict outcomes that are assumed to be certain. Probabilistic models refer to situations where the result following a particular action is not a unique outcome but consists of a range of possible outcomes with associated probabilities of happening. When confronted with uncertain consequences of a policy choice, and, in particular, if the possible consequences differ widely from one another, the analyst can construct a decision tree and estimate the probability of each outcome.

Descriptive models attempt to describe or explain how variables of interest operate, predict how they will respond to changes in other parts of a system, or show what outcomes will likely result from choices or actions. Prescriptive models encompass elements of descriptive models that delineate the choices available to decision makers and predict the outcome of each. They further include procedures that help decision makers choose among alternative actions, taking into account decision makers' preferences among alternative choices and outcomes. Prescriptive models are so named because they help prescribe courses of action. They may also be termed normative or optimizing models.

Report Findings

Evaluators have many ways to report their findings. Program results can be conveyed through informal meetings with program and evaluation sponsors as well as by way of memos, newsletters, formal presentations, formal written reports, and scholarly publications (Morris, Fitz-Gibbon, and Freeman, 1987). For program sponsors, a formal written report is perhaps the most important product of evaluation and is required from the evaluator. To enhance their utility, evaluation results should be presented in a way that nonresearchers can easily understand. The evaluator may share any draft reports with the clients for review before turning in the final product.

The formal evaluation report typically starts with an executive summary that presents the highlights of the major sections, with particular emphasis on the major findings of the evaluation. In the introduction, the purposes of the evaluation and the major evaluation questions to be discussed are briefly reviewed.

In the evaluation methods section, the design of the evaluation, sources of data, and techniques for data analysis are described. Their limitations, if any, should be discussed along with other constraints of the evaluation (e.g., limited budget and time, political and organizational constraints).

In the program implementation section, the evaluator summarizes the major features of the program, how the program is operating, whether it is being implemented as planned, major problems encountered during operation, and external and internal factors that have influenced the program. When a program includes more than one site, the evaluator should also compare similarities and differences in program staffing, administration, targets, implementation, and surrounding environments among the sites.

In the evaluation results section, the outcome of the analysis is presented with particular emphasis on the effects of the program, that is, the extent to which the goals and objectives of the program have been achieved. The presentation should be organized to address all the objectives of the evaluation. Both quantitative and qualitative results should be presented. Tables and graphs may be used to summarize major quantitative analysis results. Qualitative results may be presented as cases, anecdotes, or quotes. While quantitative analysis reveals the outcomes of the program, qualitative analysis explores how the outcomes have been achieved.

In the discussion and recommendations section, the evaluator first delineates the major findings (both statistical and substance significance should be taken into account), summarizes the primary strengths and weaknesses of the program, assesses to what extent program goals and objectives have been achieved, and discusses the generalizability of program effectiveness to other similar settings. Then, specific recommendations are made to indicate areas for further improvement related to the program, its staffing, activities, and administration.

STRENGTHS AND WEAKNESSES

The principal strength of evaluation research is its potential for making an impact on policy. Evaluation research can contribute to the improvement of the design and implementation of health programs and interventions aimed at improving the health status of the population. Compared with other types of research, evaluation has greater policy-making relevance and significance and has practical utility for policy and decision makers who are looking for research evidence. The evaluator's challenge is to get the best possible information to policy and decision makers and then to get those people to actually use the information for policy purposes.

There are many ways evaluation results may be utilized. Evaluation results may be directly used in program development and modification. Evaluation research may have an indirect impact on policy and decision makers whose future policy and program planning is influenced by evaluation results on a conceptual level.

Evaluation research frequently encounters some potentially limiting factors. For example, the internal validity of evaluation may be limited by the unfeasibility of random assignment as a result of resistance from subjects, sponsors, administrators, or staff. The resulting selection bias and the later differential attrition rates could enhance or mask the true impact of the program.

The external validity of evaluation may be threatened by other commonly encountered features of health programs. For example, the program may be effective in a particular geographic setting where external factors are crucial to its implementation. When the effectiveness of a program is dependent on the personal qualities and interests of the staff who administer it, program results might not be generalizable to widespread application of the program by staff who may be less capable, committed, or interested in program success. The knowledge that one is a participant in an experimental health program can generate enthusiasm and cooperation that might not be there when the program is no longer novel or being evaluated. These potential threats to external validity should be watched carefully, or the extension of a program or policy to other participants or beneficiaries could be hampered.

Time, financial limitations, and political climate are important constraints affecting the scope and depth of program evaluation. The amount of time the evaluator can devote to the project may determine the choice of evaluation methods and affect the ultimate breadth and quality of an evaluation. The amount of time and effort the evaluator will devote to the project is also dependent on available budget. The political climate could influence an evaluation in several ways. It might place constraints on evaluation design and data collection. The use of research results may be influenced by political considerations. When evaluation results contradict deeply held beliefs or vested interests, they may not be taken very seriously. After all, an evaluation is only one ingredient in a political process of balancing interests and making decisions.

SUMMARY

Evaluation research serves the purposes of both program monitoring and refinement and policy application and expansion. It is the systematic application of scientific research methods for assessing the conceptualization, design, implementation, impact, and/or generalizability of organizational or social (including health services) programs. Evaluation research is technical, applied, and should be objective. The major types of evaluation consist of needs assessment, process evaluation, outcome evaluation, and policy analysis. The six-step process of conducting evaluation research involves determining the scope of evaluation, getting acquainted with the program, choosing the methodology for evaluation, collecting the data, analyzing the data, and reporting the findings. The principal strength of evaluation research is its potential for having an impact on policy. However, the validity of evaluation is often limited due to the impracticality of applying strict scientific design.

REVIEW QUESTIONS

1. What is evaluation research? What are the different types of evaluation? What kinds of questions are usually asked for each type of evaluation?
2. How does a researcher conduct an evaluation? What are the elements to be considered in designing an evaluation?

3. Draw the distinctions between cost-benefit analysis and cost-effectiveness analysis. Use an example to illustrate their differences.

4. What are the potential limitations of an evaluation? How can researchers guard against them?

REFERENCES

Address of the President to the Joint Session of Congress. (2001, February 27). Washington, DC: Office of the Press Secretary.

Agency for Healthcare Research and Quality. (2005, September 29). AHRQ launches new "effective health care program" to compare medical treatments and help put proven treatments into practice [Press release]. Retrieved July 11, 2007, from www .ahrq.gov/news/press/pr2005/effectivepr.htm

Alkin, M. C., Kosecoff, J., Fitz-Gibbon, C. T., and Seligman, R. (1974). *Evaluation and Decision-Making: The Title VII Experience* (CSE Monograph Series in Evaluation No. 4). Los Angeles: Center for the Study of Evaluation.

Andrews, F., and Grandall, R. (1976). The validity of measures of self-reported well-being. *Social Indications Research, 3*, 1–19.

Bailit, H., Federico, J., and McGivney, W. (1995). Use of outcomes studies by a managed care organization: Valuing measured treatment effects. *Medical Care, 33*(4), AS216–AS225.

Barker, J. B., Bayne, T., Higgs, Z. R., Jenkin, S. A., Murphy, D., and Synoground, G. (1994). Community analysis: A collaborative community practice project. *Public Health Nursing, 11*, 113–118.

Bergner, M. (1985). Measurement of health status. *Medical Care, 23*, 696–704.

Bergner, M., Bobbitt, R., Carter, W. B., and Gilson, B. S. (1981). The sickness impact profile: A development and final revision of a health status measure. *Medical Care, 19*(8), 787–805.

Bergner, M., Bobbitt, R., Kressel, S., Pollard, W. E., Gilson, B. S., and Morris, J. R. (1976). The sickness impact profile: Conceptual formulation and methodology for the development of a health status measure. *International Journal of Health Services, 6*, 393–415.

Blaney, D. R. (1988). *Cost-Effective Nursing Practice: Guidelines for Nurse Managers.* Philadelphia: Lippincott.

Brownson, R. C., Baker, E. A., Leet, T. L., and Gillespie, K. N. (2003). *Evidence-Based Public Health.* Oxford: Oxford University Press.

Bureau of Primary Health Care. (1994a, October) *BPHC-Supported Primary Care Centers Directory.* Bethesda, MD: U.S. Department of Health and Human Services.

Bureau of Primary Health Care. (1994b, December). *Community Health Centers' Performance under Managed Care.* Bethesda, MD: U.S. Department of Health and Human Services.

Bureau of Primary Health Care. (1995, February) *Integrated Service Networks and Federally Qualified Health Centers.* Bethesda, MD: U.S. Department of Health and Human Services.

Campbell, D. T., and Stanley, J. C. (1966). *Experimental and Quasi-experimental Designs for Research.* Chicago: Rand McNally.

Centers for Disease Control and Prevention. (1999). Framework for program evaluation in public health. *Morbidity and Mortality Weekly Report, 48*(No. RR-11).

Cook, T. D., and Campbell, D. T. (1976). The design and conduct of quasi-experimental and true experiments in field settings. In M. Dunnette (Ed.), *Handbook of Industrial and Organizational Psychology*. Chicago: Rand McNally.

Department of Veterans Affairs. (1989). *Cost–Benefit Analysis Handbook*. Washington, DC: Office of Planning and Management Analysis.

Dignan, M., and Carr, P. (1987). *Program Planning for Health Education and Health Promotion*. Philadelphia: Lea and Febiger.

Dixon, J. S., and Bird, H. A. (1981). Reproducibility along a 10cm vertical visual analogue scale. *Annuals of Rheumatic Diseases, 40*, 87–89.

Drummond, M. F., Sculpher, M. J., Torrance, G. W., O'Brien, B. J., and Stoddard, G. L. (2005). *Methods for the Economic Evaluation of Health Care Programmes* (3rd ed.). New York: Oxford University Press.

Ekwueme, D. U., Strebel, P. M., Hadler, S. C., Meltzer, M. I., Allen, J. W., and Livengood, J. R. (2000). Economic evaluation of use of diphtheria, tetanus, and acellular pertussis vaccine (DTaP) or diphtheria, tetanus, and whole-cell pertussis vaccine (DTwP) in the United States. *Archives of Pediatrics & Adolescent Medicine, 154*, 797–803.

Fairbank, J. C. T., Couper, J., Davies, J. B., and O'Brien, J. (1980). The Oswestry low back pain disability questionnaire. *Physiotherapy, 66*, 271–273.

Falik, M., Needleman, J., Herbert, R., Wells, B., Politzer, R. M., and Benedict, M. B. (2006). Comparative effectiveness of health centers as regular source of care: Application of sentinel ACSC events as performance measures. *Journal of Ambulatory Care Management, 29*(1), 24–35.

Farley, S. (1993). The community as partner in primary health care. *Nursing and Health Care, 14*, 244–249.

Fitz-Gibbon, C. T., and Morris, L. L. (1987). *How to Design a Program Evaluation*. Newbury Park, CA: Sage.

Fonkych, K., and Taylor, R. (2005). *The State and Pattern of Health Information Technology Adoption*. Santa Monica, CA: Rand.

General Accounting Office (GAO). (2003). *Health Care: Approaches to Address Racial and Ethnic Disparities*. Washington, DC. GAO-03-862R.

Ginzberg, E. (1994). Improving health care for the poor. *Journal of the American Medical Association, 271*(6), 464–466.

Goldberg, D., and Hillier, V. (1979). A scaled version of the General Health questionnaire. *Psychology Medicine, 9*, 139–145.

Green, L., and Kreuter, M. (1991). *Health Promotion Planning: An Educational and Environmental Approach*. Mountain View, CA: Mayfield.

Greenfield, S., and Nelson, E. C. (1992). Recent developments and future issues in the use of health status assessment measures in clinical settings. *Medical Care, 30*(Suppl), MS23–MS41.

Guadagnoli, E., and McNeil, B. J. (1994). Outcomes research: Hope for the future or the latest rage? *Inquiry, 31*(1), 14–24.

Guttentag, M., and Struening, L. (Eds.). (1975). *Handbook of Evaluation Research* (Vol. 2). Beverly Hills, CA: Sage.

Haddix, A. C., Teutsch, S. M., and Corso, P. S. (2003). *Prevention Effectiveness: A Guide to Decision Analysis and Economic Evaluation* (2nd ed.). Oxford: Oxford University Press.

Herman, J. L., Morris, L. L., and Fitz-Gibbon, C. T. (1987). *Evaluator's Handbook*. Newbury Park, CA: Sage.

Hunt, S., and McEwen, J. (1980). The development of a subjective health indicator. *Social Health and Illness, 2*(3), 231–246.

Hunt, S., and McEwen, J. (1985). Measuring health status: A new tool for clinicians and epidemiologists. *Journal of Royal College General Practitioners, 35,* 185–188.

Johnson, C. C., Myers, L., Webber, L. S., and Boris, N. W. (2004). Profiles of the adolescent smoker: Models of tobacco use among 9th grade high school students. *Preventive Medicine, 39,* 551–558.

Kark, S. L. (1981). *The Practice of Community-Oriented Primary Health Care.* New York: Appleton-Century-Crofts.

Kitzhaber, J. A. (1993). Prioritizing health services in an era of limits: The Oregon experience. *BMJ (British Medical Journal), 307,* 373.

Mahadevia, P. J., Fleisher, L. A., Frick, K. D., Eng, J., Goodman, S. N., and Powe, N. R. (2003). Lung cancer screening with helical computed tomography in older adult smokers. *Journal of the American Medical Association, 289*(3), 313–322.

Meenan, R., Gertman, P., and Mason, J. (1980). Measuring health status in arthritis. *Arthritis and Rheumatism, 23*(2), 146–152.

Meltzer, M. I., Shapiro, C. N., Mast, E. E., and Arcari, C. (2001). The economics of vaccinating restaurant workers against hepatitis A. *Vaccine, 19,* 2138–2145.

Melzack, R. (Ed.). (1983). *Pain Measurement and Assessment.* New York: Raven Press.

Morris, L. L., Fitz-Gibbon, C. T., and Freeman, M. E. (1987). *How to Communicate Evaluation Findings.* Newbury Park, CA: Sage.

Neutens, J. J., and Rubinson, L. (1997). *Research Techniques for the Health Sciences.* Needham Heights, MA: Allyn & Bacon.

O'Malley, A. S., Forrest, C. B., Politzer, R. M., Wulu, J. T., and Shi, L. (2005). Health center trends, 1994–2001: What do they portend for the federal growth initiative? *Health Affairs, 24*(2), 465–472.

Owens, D. K. (2002). Analytic tools for public health decision making. *Medical Decision Making, 22*(Suppl.), S3–S9.

Parkerson, G. R., Broadhead, W. E., and Tse, C. J. (1995). Health status and severity of illness as predictors of outcomes in primary care. *Medical Care, 33*(1), 53–66.

Patrick, D. (1993). *Health Status and Health Policy: Quality of Life in Health Care Evaluation and Resource Allocation.* New York: Oxford University Press.

Patrick, D., Darby, S., Green, S., Horton, G., Locker, D., and Wiggins, R. (1981). Screening for disability in the inner city. *Journal of Epidemiology Community Health, 35,* 65–70.

Patton, M. Q. (1987). *How to Use Qualitative Methods in Evaluation.* Newbury Park, CA: Sage.

Patton, M. Q. (2002). *Qualitative Evaluation and Research Methods* (3rd ed.). Thousand Oaks, CA: Sage.

Pearce, D. W. (1981). *The Social Appraisal of Projects: A Text in Cost–Benefit Analysis.* London: Macmillan.

Plevritis, S. K., Kurian, A. W., Sigal, B. M., Daniel, B. L., Ikeda, D. M., Stockdale, F. E., and Garber, A. M. (2006). Cost-effectiveness of screening BRCA1/2 mutation carriers with breast magnetic resonance imaging. *Journal of the American Medical Association, 295*(20), 2374–2384.

Riesenberg, D., and Glass, R. M. (1989). The medical outcomes study. *Journal of the American Medical Association, 262*(7), 943.

Rossi, P. H., Lipsey, M. W., and Freeman, H. E. (2004). *Evaluation: A Systematic Approach* (7th ed.). Thousand Oaks, CA: Sage.

Rowland, N. (1995). *Evaluating the Cost-Effectiveness of Counseling in Health Care.* New York: Routledge.

Scott, J., and Huuskisson, E. C. (1979). Vertical or horizontal visual analogue scales. *Annuals of Rheumatic Diseases, 38,* 560.

Shi, L., Stevens, G. D., Wulu, J. T., Politzer, R. M., and Xu, J. (2004). America's health centers: Reducing racial and ethnic disparities in perinatal care and birth outcomes. *Health Services Research, 39*(6, Pt. 1), 1881–1901.

Shin, P., Jones, K., and Rosenbaum, S. (2003). *Reducing Racial and Ethnic Health Disparities: Estimating the Impact of High Health Center Penetration in Low-Income Communities.* Washington, DC: National Association of Community Health Centers.

Shin, P., Markus, A., and Rosenbaum, S. (2006). *Measuring Health Centers against Standard Indicators of High Quality Performance: Early Results from a Multi-Site Demonstration Project* [Interim report]. Minnetonka, MN: United Health Foundation.

Shortell, S. M., Gillies, R. R., and Anderson, D. A. (1994). The new world of managed care: Creating organized delivery systems. *Health Affairs, 13*(5), 46–64.

Spitzer, W. O., Dobson, A. J., and Hall, J. (1981). Measuring quality of life of cancer patients: A concise QL-Index for use by physicians. *Journal of Chronic Disease, 34,* 585–597.

Stecher, B. M., and Davis, W. A. (1987). *How to Focus an Evaluation.* Newbury Park, CA: Sage.

Steinwachs, D. M. (1989). Application of health status assessment measures in policy research. *Medical Care, 27*(Suppl.), S12–S26.

Stokey, E., and Zeckhauser, R. (1978). *A Primer for Policy Analysis.* New York: W. W. Norton.

Tarlov, B. R., Ware, J. E., Greenfield, S., Nelson, E. C., and Perrin, E. (1989). The medical outcomes study. *Journal of the American Medical Association, 262*(7), 925–930.

Veney, J. E., and Kaluzny, A. D. (2005). *Evaluation and Decision Making for Health Services* (3rd ed.). Chicago: Health Administration Press.

Vidaro, C. I., Earp, J. L., and Altpeter, M. (1997). Designing a process evaluation for a comprehensive breast cancer screening intervention: Challenges and opportunities. *Evaluation and Program Planning, 20*(3): 237–249.

Ware, J. E. (1986). The assessment of health status. In L. H. Aiken and D. Mechanic (Eds.), *Applications of Social Science to Clinical Medicine and Health Policy.* New Brunswick, NJ: Rutgers University Press.

Weinstein, M. C., Siegel, J. E., Gold, M. R., Kamlet, M. S., and Russell, L. B. (1996). Recommendations of the panel on cost-effectiveness in health and medicine. *Journal of the American Medical Association, 276*(15), 1253–1258.

Williams, A., Ware, I., and Donald, C. (1981). A model of mental health, life events and social supports applicable to general populations. *Journal of Health and Social Behavior, 22,* 324–336.

Writing Group for the Women's Health Initiative. (2002). Risks and benefits of estrogen plus progestin in healthy postmenopausal women: Principal results from the Women's Health Initiative randomized controlled trial. *Journal of the American Medical Association, 288*(3), 321–333.

Young, K. R. (1994). An evaluative study of a community health service development. *Journal of Advanced Nursing, 19,* 58–65.

Design in Health Services Research

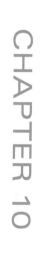

KEY TERMS

accuracy
complexity
efficiency
external validity
Institutional Review
   Board (IRB)

internal validity
measurement reliability
measurement validity
precision

research design
research method
research/study population

LEARNING OBJECTIVES

- To understand the major considerations in designing a study.
- To summarize the characteristics of commonly used research methods.

- To appreciate the general guidelines in choosing appropriate research methods.

PURPOSE

Research design is concerned with the planning of research and specifies the hypotheses or questions to be studied, the data to be collected, the methods of data collection, and the types of analysis to be used. It is the blueprint of research that lays out the strategy and framework, integrating different phases of the research activities and providing the basic direction (Creswell, 2002; Keppel and Wickens, 2004; Miller and Salkind, 2002). Even though research design is a distinctive stage in itself, it is built upon knowledge of many previous and subsequent stages of the research process. The conceptualization stage (Chapter 2) lays the foundation of research questions to be studied. If the research is based on available data, the groundwork stage identifies the sources of relevant available data (Chapter 3). If the research is based on a primary source of data, the sampling stage (Chapter 11) provides the appropriate sampling method, and the data collection stage (Chapter 13) indicates the best method of data collection. The data analysis stage (Chapter 14) targets the most appropriate and efficient methods of data analysis. These chapters cover many of the relevant issues involved in designing a study.

A particularly important aspect of HSR design, often considered simultaneously when choosing the specific design for a study, is the selection of an appropriate research method. **Research method**, or methodology, consists of a body of knowledge that reflects the general philosophy and purpose of the research process, the assumptions and values that serve as rationale for research, the general approach of data collection and analysis, and the standards used for interpreting data and reaching conclusions.

Chapters 4 through 9 have presented the major types of research methods useful for health services research. These include research review, meta-analysis (Chapter 4), secondary analysis, research analysis of administrative records (Chapter 5), qualitative research, case study (Chapter 6), experiment, quasi-experiment (Chapter 7), survey research, longitudinal research (Chapter 8), and evaluation research (Chapter 9). Each of these methods has its own unique characteristics, strengths, and weaknesses. In choosing a method, researchers need to compare the characteristics between the various approaches and their particular studies and select the methods that optimally match the study requirements and constraints.

In this chapter, the major considerations in designing a study will be summarized. Then, the characteristics of the key types of research methods will be discussed. Finally, an approach to choosing the methods most suitable for the investigator's intended study will be suggested.

CONSIDERATIONS IN DESIGNING A STUDY

When designing a study, health services researchers typically consider the following: (1) What is the research population and the most appropriate sampling strategy? (2) What is the most appropriate research method or combination of methods for this population? (3) Which data collection method or methods will best capture the characteristics of this study population? (4) How can the response rate be enhanced so that the sample adequately represents the study population? (5) Which design strategy will be used and what are the potential

Specify:

- the research population and sampling strategy
- the research methods
- the data collection methods
- the strategy to enhance response rate
- the design strategy and the potential threats to validity
- the measures to be used
- the statistical models and analyses to be conducted
- the concerns and tactics related to human subjects
- the administrative concerns
- the time frame and major milestones

Figure 10.1. Designing a research study: Practical considerations

threats to validity, both internal and external? (6) Which measures will be used to validly and reliably capture all elements of the conceptual framework, answer the research questions, and test the hypotheses? (7) What statistical models and analyses will be conducted to test the research hypotheses and answer the research questions? (8) What ethical issues related to human subjects need to be taken into account in the course of the study? (9) What administrative concerns need to be addressed to ensure the successful and timely completion of the study? and (10) What are the major milestones and the timeline of this study? Figure 10.1 summarizes these considerations and further elaboration follows.

Research Population and Sampling Strategy

Researchers need to be clear about their **research** or **study population**, the target group to which study results are generalized. While considering which sampling strategy best captures this study population, investigators may consider the following criteria: **precision**, which refers to the degree to which further measurements will produce the same or similar results, a function of random sampling error (sample size); **accuracy**, which indicates how close the estimates derived from a sample are to the true population value, a function of systematic sampling error (sampling frame and procedure); **complexity**, which means the amount of information to be gathered and the number of sampling stages; and **efficiency**, which involves obtaining the most accurate and precise estimates at the lowest possible cost. Often, trade-offs are necessary when selecting a sampling strategy that maximizes representation and minimizes costs. To be competent in designing a sampling strategy, researchers must become familiar not only with different sampling methods, but also with their logical trade-offs. See Chapter 11 for an in-depth description of sampling methods.

Research Method

Once the population and sampling strategy are in place, investigators then must decide which research method to use in carrying out the study. All research methods have their particular strengths and weaknesses, but some may be better suited to certain situations than to others. Often, a study can be conducted using a range of methods or approaches. Sometimes, a combination of methods is the optimal strategy. Deciding upon the right methods requires that researchers become acquainted with those that are commonly used, while also understanding how to make trade-offs among the multiple considerations of a study. Sometimes, investigators become too specialized in their own method (e.g., experimenter, evaluator, qualitative researcher, survey methodologist, or secondary data analyst) to recognize alternative approaches. The later sections of this chapter summarize the characteristics of the main research methods and suggest an approach to choosing the most suitable methods for a given study.

Data Collection Method

Data may be collected primarily by researchers themselves or secondarily by using existing sources. The key consideration is that data collection methods adequately represent the study population. Chapter 13 compares various data collection methods and their respective impact in terms of data quality, sample size, cost, time, and demands placed on the research project, research subjects, interviewers, and the instrument. Knowledge of these trade-offs is critical for selecting an optimal data collection strategy.

Strategy to Enhance the Response Rate

Once the data collection method is decided upon, researchers need to specify a strategy to achieve an adequate response rate. A high response rate is critical to ensure that the sample represents the study population. Chapter 13 describes commonly used methods to enhance survey response rates, such as follow-up efforts, sponsorship, length of questionnaires, introductory letters, types of questions, inducement, anonymity/confidentiality, time of contact, and method of return. Many of these approaches are also appropriate for other study types, such as experimental research. If the response rate is too low and the sample cannot adequately represent the study population, investigators may have to expand their data collection effort or revise the initial research population.

Design and Potential Threats

The design of the study needs to be considered in terms of frequency of data collection, unit of analysis, and the use of control or comparison groups. If data are collected only once, a cross-sectional method (e.g., survey) can be used. If data are collected multiple times, a longitudinal method (e.g., experiment or quasi-experiment) may be used. Data may be collected at the individual, aggregate, or mixed level. If the unit of analysis is at the individual level, then data may only be collected about the individuals. If the unit of analysis is at the aggregate (nonindividual) level, then data may only be collected about that aggregate (e.g., organization, community, social group). If the unit of analysis is at the mixed level, which includes both individual and nonindividual, then data may need to be collected at both individual and nonindividual levels.

To test the impact of an intervention, inclusion of a control (or comparison) group is critical. Chapter 7 describes various experimental and quasi-experimental designs and threats to internal and external validity. A study maintains **internal validity** to the extent that it rules out the possibility that extraneous variables, rather than the manipulated independent variable, are responsible for the observed outcome. **External validity** is related to the generalizability of results. A study is considered externally valid if its effect can be generalized to the population, setting, treatment, and measurement variables of interest. Knowledge of these design options, their pitfalls, and strategies to enhance validity is critical for designing and carrying out research.

Measures

The purpose of measurement is to operationalize the concepts portrayed in the study's conceptual framework, which encompasses the research hypotheses and questions. Measurements need to achieve both validity and reliability. **Measurement validity** refers to the extent to which important dimensions of a concept and their categories have been taken into account and appropriately operationalized. **Measurement reliability** refers to the extent to which consistent results are obtained when a particular measure is applied to similar elements. In finalizing their measurements, researchers need to know when to use existing measures and when to develop and validate new ones. Chapter 12 provides a detailed discussion of measurement-related concerns.

Statistical Models and Analysis Methods

The purpose of conducting statistical analyses is to test research hypotheses and answer research questions. During study design, the proper analytic models and statistics for each research hypothesis and question need to be specified. Approaches to data exploration, coding, and reduction need to be discussed. Chapter 14 provides an illustrative discussion of major descriptive, comparative, and multivariate statistics used in HSR.

Concerns and Tactics Related to Human Subjects

As Chapter 1 points out, respecting human subjects is a fundamental ethical principle of scientific inquiry that governs health services research. Research institutions have an **Institutional Review Board (IRB)**, or office for research subjects, to provide guidance and oversight. Researchers need to be familiar with the process of seeking approval and carrying out ethical research as established through their IRB. Typically, the process is as follows: (1) the Principal Investigator (PI) and Study Team prepare and submit an application to the IRB; (2) a research specialist assigned to the project completes an administrative review and schedules and manages the committee review of the project; (3) the IRB conducts a committee review and expresses any concerns and/or provides approval to the PI; and (4) the PI and Study Team conduct research, report adverse events, and submit requests for amendments and for continuing reviews until study completion. Figure 10.2 presents the Johns Hopkins University template for IRB submission as an example.

Administrative Concerns

When designing a study, investigators should also consider the practical aspects of conducting the study, including forming a research team and assigning roles, locating space, gaining access to research subjects, establishing quality control measures, and developing strategies to handle unexpected events. Chapter 3 discusses these administrative concerns as part of the groundwork preparation for carrying out a study.

Timeline and Milestones

Finally, researchers need to specify the timetable for performing the study and identify associated milestones. Typical milestones include the following: finalizing study design; developing study measures; piloting, validating, and finalizing study measures; collecting data; inputting data; "cleaning" and exploring data; analyzing data; writing the draft report; and writing the final report. A detailed timeline and milestones will not only force the investigator to consider the whole project prospectively, but will provide a measure of the study's progress. Should the study be delayed due to extraordinary circumstances, the timeline should be adjusted accordingly.

CHARACTERISTICS OF RESEARCH METHODS

There are various ways to consider the characteristics of research methods (Creswell, 2002). Research methods may be classified as primary or secondary, quantitative or qualitative, and cross-sectional or longitudinal. The purposes of research methods may be exploratory, descriptive, or causal. Research methods may be considered in terms of their cost, time, sample, depth of information provided, design, and analysis. This section examines how the research methods differ in terms of these characteristics. Table 10.1 summarizes the results

Research Question

Rationale
Problem, background, aim

Methods
Study design and rationale

Population
Sample size, power calculations, inclusion/exclusion criteria, gender, age, and locale

Procedures
Recruitment process, study procedures in sequential order, methods of intervention, methods for dealing with adverse events, methods for dealing with illegal reportable activities, methods for storing samples beyond the end of the study

Risks/Benefits
Description of risks, description of measures to minimize risks, description of potential benefits, description of level of research burden

Compensation
Type of compensation, amount of compensation, schedule of compensation

Disclosure/Consent Process
Description of the consent process, including who, when, and where consent will be obtained

Safety Monitoring
Description of who will perform safety monitoring, their affiliation and expertise; safety endpoints (i.e., AEs or SAEs) to be monitored; frequency of review by the safety monitor or DSMB of aggregate summaries of expected AEs or SAEs; plan for promptly providing to CHR the reports of all safety monitoring reviews of AES or SAEs; and plan for reporting to CHR expected AEs or SAEs that occur more frequently or more severely than described in the research plan or on the consent form

Confidentiality Assurances
Certificate of confidentiality (if applicable), data security, plan for record keeping, person responsible and telephone number, plan for disposition of identifiers at end of study, plan for secure storage of data, person who will have access to data

Collaborative Agreements
Description of the collaboration, letters of collaboration, name of institution/person, role of collaborative organization, role of institutional investigator

Figure 10.2. Institutional Review Board (IRB) submission template
Source: Adapted from Johns Hopkins University Office of Research Subject IRB Template.

Table 10.1. **Characteristics of major types of health services research methods**

Characteristics	Research Methods									
	Research Review	Meta-analysis	Secondary Analysis	Administrative Records	Qualitative Research	Case Study	Experiment Quasi-experiment	Survey Research	Longitudinal Research	Evaluation Research
DATA										
Primary					X	X	X	X	X	X
Secondary	X	X	X	X	X	X			X	X
ANALYSIS										
Quantitative		X	X	X		X	X	X	X	X
Qualitative	X		X		X	X				X
TIME										
Cross-sectional			X	X	X	X		X		
Longitudinal	X	X	X	X	X	X	X	X	X	X
PURPOSE										
Exploratory					X	X				
Descriptive	X	X	X	X		X		X	X	X
Causal		X	X	X	X	X	X	X	X	X
COST										
expensive						X	X		X	X
moderate					X	X	X	X	X	X
cheap	X	X	X	X	X	X		X		X

	C1	C2	C3	C4	C5	C6	C7	C8	C9	C10
TIME										
lengthy							X	X	X	
moderate					X	X	X	X		
short	X	X	X	X						X
SAMPLE SIZE										
large	X		X	X				X		
moderate		X					X		X	X
small					X	X				
DEPTH										
great					X	X				X
moderate	X		X	X			X	X	X	
low	X	X	X	X			X	X	X	
DESIGN										
complex							X		X	X
moderate					X	X		X		X
easy	X	X	X	X						
STATISTICS										
sophisticated		X	X	X				X	X	X
moderate			X			X	X			X
simple	X				X	X				

of the comparisons. It is important to consider these summaries as suggestive rather than definitive since there are many variations with each research method.

Primary versus Secondary Research

Research is considered primary when the data originate with the study. Research is considered secondary when the data were collected for some other purpose(s). In general, compared with secondary research, primary research tends to produce data more relevant for the study. However, it is also more costly and time consuming to collect primary rather than secondary data.

Among the research methods discussed, experiment, quasi-experiment, and survey are primary research methods. Research review, meta-analysis, secondary analysis, and research analysis of administrative records are secondary research methods. Qualitative research, case study, and longitudinal research are mainly primary methods, although they may also include elements of secondary analysis. Evaluation research can be either primary or secondary.

Quantitative versus Qualitative Research

Quantitative research focuses on using numbers in the analysis. Qualitative research focuses on using statements in the analysis. Compared with qualitative research, quantitative research is able to cover more people and hence presents broader and more generalizable findings. By contrast, qualitative research tends to produce more in-depth and detailed information, and hence its findings tend to be more valid.

Among the research methods discussed, meta-analysis, research analysis of administrative records, experiment, quasi-experiment, survey, and longitudinal research are quantitative research methods. Research review, participant observation, and focused interview are qualitative research methods. Evaluation research, case study, and secondary analysis can be either quantitative or qualitative.

Cross-Sectional versus Longitudinal Research

Cross-sectional research refers to using data collected at one point in time. Longitudinal research refers to using data collected at two or more points in time. Collecting cross-sectional data is cheaper and less time consuming than collecting longitudinal data. Longitudinal data tend to be more extensive and better suited for causal research than cross-sectional data. However, attrition is a potential problem when designing longitudinal studies.

Among the research methods discussed, research review, meta-analysis, experiment, quasi-experiment, and evaluation research tend to be longitudinal. Secondary analysis, research analysis of administrative records, qualitative research, case study, and survey research can be either cross-sectional or longitudinal.

Exploratory and Descriptive versus Causal Research

Exploratory research is conducted when little is known about the subject matter. The purpose is to gain an initial insight into the topic, finding out its critical issues and concepts. Descriptive research provides a more detailed account of the distributions of the major characteristics of the subject matter. Causal research explains subject matter, testing hypotheses and examining relationships, including cause and effect, among variables. Generally, the design of causal research is most rigorous, followed by descriptive and exploratory research. There is often a time sequence among the three research purposes. Exploratory research is conducted first to provide categories and concepts of characteristics important to a subject. Descriptive research is performed next in an effort to understand the distributions of these characteristics. Causal research then is carried out to assess the relationships among these characteristics.

Among the research methods discussed, research review tends to be descriptive. Experiment and quasi-experiment tend to be causal. Secondary analysis, research analysis of administrative records, and survey research are mostly descriptive, although they can be causal if proper statistical methods are used. Meta-analysis, evaluation, and longitudinal research tend to be causal, although they can also be descriptive. Qualitative research can be exploratory or causal, and case study can be exploratory, descriptive, or causal.

Cost

The cost of research is primarily concerned with the cost of data collection and analysis. It usually costs more to conduct: (1) primary research compared with secondary research, because data have to be collected firsthand; (2) longitudinal research compared with cross-sectional research, because data have to be collected at multiple points in time; and (3) causal research compared with exploratory or descriptive research, because the design is typically more difficult to implement.

Among the research methods discussed, longitudinal research, experiment, and quasi-experiment generally tend to be most expensive, followed by survey research. Methods of relatively low-cost inquiry include research review, meta-analysis, secondary analysis, and research analysis of administrative records, primarily due to savings in data collection. Qualitative research and evaluation research can vary in cost depending on the scope of the investigation, the methods used, and the time permitted. Case study is typically of moderate to low cost because of the limited samples chosen for investigation.

Time

The time spent in conducting research derives primarily from data collection and analysis. As with cost, more time is usually spent in primary research than secondary research, longitudinal research than cross-sectional research, and causal research than exploratory or descriptive research. Indeed, there is a close correlation between research time and cost.

Among the research methods discussed, longitudinal research, experiment, and quasi-experiment tend to be lengthier than other methods, followed by survey research. Research review, meta-analysis, secondary analysis, and research analysis of administrative records usually require less time. The time spent for case study tends to be moderate. Qualitative research and evaluation research have the greatest variations in terms of time spent, depending on the scope and urgency of the study.

Sample

The sample is drawn from the population of interest and, if well chosen, its characteristics may be used to generalize results to that population. The size of the sample depends on many factors. Research purpose is related to sample size in that exploratory research typically requires a smaller sample than causal or descriptive research. The homogeneity of population characteristics is also associated with sample size. A smaller sample size is adequate for a more homogeneous population. Budget and time also influence sample size. A larger sample requires more time and money than a smaller one. Chapter 11 provides a more systematic review of how to determine the sample size for a study.

Among the research methods discussed, the less costly quantitative methods, such as survey research, secondary analysis, and research analysis of administrative records, generally use large sample sizes. More costly quantitative methods, such as experiment, quasi-experiment, and longitudinal and evaluation research, generally use moderate sample sizes. Qualitative methods such as case study tend to use small sample sizes. While research review tries to use maximal samples, meta-analysis uses moderate samples because of the difficulty of locating relevant research articles for secondary analysis.

The type and quality of the sample will affect the study's external validity. External validity, as discussed in Chapter 7, is defined as a study's generalizability to the population, setting, treatment, and measurement variables of interest. National survey research has high external validity because the selection of participants is random and the population in the study is representative of the population of the nation as a whole. In contrast, convenience sampling within a small town yields low external validity because the sample is not randomly chosen and the population is not representative.

Depth

The depth of research has to do with how much detailed information can be collected from the subjects. Given the same research budget, there is a trade-off between the scope of coverage (i.e., how many respondents can be surveyed as reflected by the sample size) and the depth of coverage. Generally, qualitative research sacrifices scope in favor of depth, and quantitative research sacrifices depth in favor of scope. Exploratory research emphasizes depth whereas descriptive and causal research emphasize scope. The depth of coverage is also more limited for longitudinal than for cross-sectional studies because of the greater amount of missing data.

Among the research methods discussed, qualitative research and case study provide great depth of coverage. Quantitative methods such as survey research, secondary analysis, experiment, quasi-experiment, research analysis of administrative records, and longitudinal research provide moderate to low depth of coverage. Meta-analysis usually has low depth because of the lack of common variables in all relevant studies. Research review has moderate to low depth depending on how much research has been conducted on a particular subject. The depth of evaluation research varies based on the method used and the extent of evaluation.

Design

As stated at the beginning of this chapter, design is the planning phase of research. Design involves specifying research questions and data sources and determining the methods for data collection and analysis. Research design is usually more complex for causal research than exploratory or descriptive research, for longitudinal than cross-sectional studies, and for quantitative than qualitative research. The complexity of design is also positively correlated with time and cost.

Among the research methods discussed, experiment, quasi-experiment, and longitudinal research generally have the most complex design, since much of the research effort goes into improving and implementing the design. Specific tasks include refining the number of conditions, measuring key variables, providing instructions to subjects, pretesting, introducing intervention, and collecting data. The design for survey research, qualitative research, and case study is of moderate difficulty. Research review and meta-analysis have relatively easy designs. The design for secondary analysis and research analysis of administrative records depends on the availability of designs and is therefore easy for today's investigators given the prevalence of designs. The design of evaluation research relies on the method chosen for the evaluation. Many health services are intended to achieve certain outcomes, for example, by improving health status, increasing utilization, and so forth. Evaluation research that aims to determine whether health services (or other interventions) actually accomplish their purposes is typically related to experiment or quasi-experiment.

The research design has implications for the study's internal validity. For instance, randomized experimental designs have fewer threats to internal validity than many quasi-experimental designs. Through randomization, the researcher is better able to control for factors influencing internal validity, such as equivalence of groups and the potential influence of extraneous variables on study outcomes.

Analysis

Data analysis involves applying statistical methods to the collected data and generating results to answer the research hypotheses and questions. Data analysis is generally more difficult for quantitative than qualitative research, longitudinal than cross-sectional studies, and causal than exploratory or descriptive research. The difficulty of analysis positively influences the time and cost of research.

Among the research methods discussed, longitudinal research, secondary analysis, research analysis of administrative records, meta-analysis, and survey research generally require more complex data analysis. In contrast, the analysis of experimental and quasi-experimental data is relatively easy and straightforward. The statistical analysis requirement of research review is low. The difficulty of analyzing data from case studies and evaluation research depends on the type and number of methods chosen for the investigation. Since qualitative analysis is more narrative than quantitative, the use of statistics is kept to a minimum.

CHOOSING APPROPRIATE RESEARCH METHODS

Each of the major research methods offers particular strengths and weaknesses and serves, in its own way, a desired end. For example, research review, meta-analysis, secondary analysis, and research analysis of administrative records all have the principal advantages of speed and relatively low cost compared with other study methods. Their principal disadvantage is that the scope and depth of the investigation is constrained by available studies or data. Further, for research in which the data were collected for another purpose, gaining familiarity with the data elements and evaluation of the data quality become difficult and may be time consuming. Experimental and longitudinal research have the principal advantage of validity in study design. However, these methods are usually very costly and sometimes not appropriate. Survey research is the most widely used method because it is the most efficient for obtaining a larger sample size per dollar spent than any other method. However, data analysis requires great effort and skill, especially when causal relationships are studied.

Because research methods involve differing strengths and weaknesses, they constitute alternative, rather than mutually exclusive, strategies for research. In many situations, a combination of methods can be used in the same study. The first task in choosing a research method should be to sort out the various methods and their relative merits, deciding whether one approach makes sense or two or more methods should be combined. In this section, some guidelines are suggested for choosing the appropriate methods for investigation. These guidelines are not prescriptive and should be evaluated based on the investigator's particular research situation.

Research Purpose

The choice of research methods is closely related to the purpose of the investigation. If researchers are conducting exploratory research on a topic about which they have little prior knowledge, a qualitative method—such as a case study, fieldwork, or observation—is generally more appropriate. If they are conducting a descriptive study in order to provide a detailed description of the major characteristics of the topic, then survey research is preferred. On the other hand, if they are conducting causal or explanatory research to determine the relationships among various factors, experimental, quasi-experimental, or longitudinal research may be considered. Secondary analysis and research analysis of administrative records may be selected for both descriptive and causal research if available data are relevant to the research purpose. When investigators are asked to perform an evaluation of a program or project, evaluation research comes into play. If there are large numbers of prior studies on a subject, researchers may want to conduct a research review or meta-analysis (when study results are published quantitatively) before undertaking their own study.

Available Resources

The choice of research method is also related to the availability of resources. Valuable resources include knowledge, money, time, support, and analytic skills. The investigator's knowledge and familiarity with various research methods play a significant role in the method chosen. Some researchers are limited in their research training and experience. The options available to them are correspondingly limited to those with which they are most familiar and comfortable. An interdisciplinary research team can overcome this problem by including people from different scientific disciplines and research backgrounds.

The available budget is critical for decisions about the type of method to be used and the scope of study. Limited case study is generally cheaper than large-scale investigation. Survey research is cheaper than experimental research. Cross-sectional study is cheaper than longitudinal study. Research population, data sources, sample size, data collection, and analysis methods are all tied to monetary considerations. Like money, time plays an essential role in the choice of the research method. For example, the time allowed for evaluation often dictates which and how many methods can be chosen.

Staff support is important because, for any given amount of time, more staff support usually means more data collected. The interview survey is perhaps the best example. After subjects have been identified and located, the number of qualified interviewers that researchers have available to them dictates how soon the interviews can take place. Finally, analytic skills are crucial for data analysis. After all, data have to be analyzed to address important research questions. Analytic skills often involve statistical and computer skills. They are especially important for large-scale studies or studies using data from multiple sources. Indeed, the absence of these skills may limit the investigator to generally descriptive analysis, which does not make full use of the data collected.

Access

Access to research subjects or available data is an important determinant in selecting research methods. The willingness of research subjects may dictate whether experimental techniques can be used or a quasi-experiment must be employed. Subject attrition is a critical concern for longitudinal research designs. The data collection methods chosen for survey research—whether mail questionnaires or telephone or face-to-face interviews—may depend on the characteristics of the subjects. Qualitative research relies heavily on the subjects' compliance and willingness to be studied, observed, or interviewed. The availability of, and accessibility to, relevant data sources may determine whether secondary research can be conducted in lieu of primary research. Access to available data and subjects also determines the types of methods chosen for evaluation research.

Combining Research Methods

In choosing methods for study, investigators need not be confined to a single method. Often, a combination of methods can more effectively fulfill the research purpose (Creswell, 2002; Greene, Caracelli, and Graham, 1989). For example, research review is typically conducted before any study is conceptualized and often included in the final research report. Meta-analysis can be performed as an independent study as well as an integral, preliminary part of primary research. Secondary data may be used in combination with primary sources to compensate for missing data elements. Qualitative research can be used in combination with quantitative research, with the former laying the groundwork as well as providing interpretations for data drawn from large-scale examples of the latter. Many more possible configurations of combined research methods may be cited. Figure 10.3 summarizes those combinations.

Specifying the Limitations

Finally, investigators should explicitly specify the limitations or constraints facing their study, as well as be clear about what can, and cannot, be achieved by the study. Frequently, investigators have to scale down the design, modify the research question, or select alternative methods because of uncontrollable factors. The specification of study constraints is important for the reader or other researchers who may not be limited by the identified constraints. When faced with budgetary or other constraints, researchers should sacrifice the scope of the study to maintain the validity and reliability of the findings. For example, costs

Primary Types	Possible Additional Types
Research review (Chapter 4)	Meta-analysis
Secondary analysis (Chapter 5)	Research review, survey research
Qualitative research (Chapter 6)	Research review, case study, observation, focused interview
Experiment, quasi-experiment (Chapter 7)	Research review
Survey research (Chapter 8)	Research review, qualitative research
Evaluation research (Chapter 9)	Research review, experiment, quasi-experiment, survey research, secondary analysis, longitudinal research, qualitative research

Figure 10.3. Combining the different types of health services research methods

can typically be reduced by having smaller sample sizes, more clustered or narrowly defined samples, and shorter questionnaires.

SUMMARY

In designing a study, researchers specify the research population and sampling strategy, the research methods, the data collection methods, the strategy to enhance the response rate, the design strategy, the measures, the statistical models and analyses, the concerns and tactics related to human subjects, the administrative concerns, and the timeline and major milestones. Research methods may be classified as primary or secondary, quantitative or qualitative, cross-sectional or longitudinal. Their purposes may be exploratory, descriptive, or causal. They may be considered in terms of their cost, time, sample, depth of information provided, design, and analysis. In choosing appropriate research methods for a study, investigators should consider such factors as the purpose of the research, the available resources, access to research subjects or available data, and the possibility of using a combination of methods. The limitations or constraints of the design should also be specified.

REVIEW QUESTIONS

1. Please specify the major considerations in designing a study.

2. What are the commonly used types of research methods? Differentiate their major characteristics.

3. What factors need to be considered in choosing the appropriate research methods?

REFERENCES

Creswell, J. W. (2002). *Research Design: Qualitative, Quantitative, and Mixed Methods Approaches* (2nd ed.). Thousand Oaks, CA: Sage.

Greene, J. C., Caracelli, V. J., and Graham, W. E. (1989). Toward a conceptual framework for mixed-method evaluation designs. *Educational Evaluation and Policy Analysis, 11*(3), 255–274.

Keppel, G., and Wickens, T. D. (2004). *Design and Analysis: A Researcher's Handbook* (4th ed.). Englewood Cliffs, NJ: Prentice Hall.

Miller, D. C., and Salkind, N. J. (2002). *Handbook of Research Design and Social Measurement* (6th ed.). Thousand Oaks, CA: Sage.

CHAPTER 11

Sampling in Health Services Research

KEY TERMS

cluster sampling
convenience sampling
nonprobability sampling
observation unit
parameters
population
power
probability sampling
purposive sampling
quota sampling

random error
random number
   generator (RNG)
sample size
sampling
sampling bias
sampling design
sampling element
sampling error
sampling fraction

sampling frame
sampling unit
simple random sampling
snowball sampling
statistics
stratified sampling
systematic error
systematic sampling
unit of analysis
variable

LEARNING OBJECTIVES

- To understand the logic of sampling and commonly used sampling terms.

- To describe the major types of probability and nonprobability sampling.

- To identify factors considered in determining sample size.

DEFINITION

Sampling is the process of selecting a subset of observations from an entire population of interest so that characteristics from the subset can be used to draw conclusions or make inferences about the population (Babbie, 2006; Henry, 1990).

Logic of Sampling

The logic of sampling is that a large population of interest can be studied efficiently and accurately through examination of a carefully selected subset or sample of the population. Efficiency has to do with obtaining information at an acceptable cost. Accuracy is concerned with minimizing sampling error or the differences between sample estimates and population parameters.

Sampling is a familiar activity to most people. Few would consume the whole pot of soup just to determine whether it was properly seasoned. Often, a sample of a spoonful of soup would be sufficient. Likewise, sampling is an efficient way to study a population. Rather than observing every individual unit within the population, sampling selects a subset of the units, thus saving money and time that would have been incurred if all units within the population were observed.

Since the purpose of sampling is to make generalizations about the whole population of interest—that is, make estimates and test hypotheses about population characteristics based on data from the sample—a sample must be carefully selected to adequately represent population variability and make statistically valid inferences. In the physical and medical sciences, because sampling elements often share a high degree of homogeneity, not many units would be needed to adequately represent the properties of the elements. One test tube of blood, for example, will be quite similar to another. In the social sciences, including health services, sampling elements often involve humans and are far less homogeneous than physical or chemical elements. Thus, the sample must be carefully selected to make sure that all major population variations are adequately represented. When the population of interest is large, a well-selected sample can generate more accurate and informative results about the population than information from the entire population. This is because the quality of data collection can be improved and there are less opportunities for introducing clerical and measurement errors that may arise from collecting, processing, and analyzing data for a large population.

The central limit theorem provides the theoretical foundation for sampling. It states that sample means are normally distributed (i.e., in a bell-shaped curve) around the population mean, and that the sample distribution will approximate population distribution as the sample size increases. Therefore, when carefully used, sampling will enable us to generate information about the population. Specifically, given sufficient sample size, 68 percent of the sample observations will fall within one standard deviation of the population mean, 95 percent within two standard deviations of the population mean, and 99 percent within three standard deviations of the population mean.

In addition to efficiency and accuracy considerations, sampling is sometimes necessary due to access problems. Not all sampling elements are known, or if identified, accessible. When there is no **sampling frame**, or a list of the study population, it may be too time consuming, let alone costly, to enumerate all the population elements. A stratified sampling plan that enumerates elements within selected strata might be more reasonable and preferred. Sometimes, even when investigators intend to study every member of the population, some members may refuse to be studied. Research ethics dictate that informed consent is a prerequisite of research participation. Some individuals are considered ethically at risk, including minors (those under 18), prisoners, the mentally disabled, and institutionalized or hospitalized people. When these people are included in the population being considered, special efforts should be made to ensure informed consent. These efforts include seeking permission from parents or guardians, and conducting reviews through institutional review boards (IRBs).

Sampling Terms

Before describing the different types of sampling methods commonly used in health services research, we must first define some terms frequently used in sampling (Babbie, 2006; Fowler, 2002; Henry, 1990; Rubin, 1983). These include unit of analysis, sampling element, sampling unit, observation unit, population, sampling frame, sampling design, sampling error, sampling bias, variable, statistics, and parameters.

Unit of Analysis

Unit of analysis refers to the object about which the researcher wishes to draw conclusions based on the study. The purpose of the study typically dictates what or who is to be studied and hence what the appropriate unit of analysis is. A variety of units may be studied, including individuals (e.g., patients or doctors), groups (e.g., families, couples, census blocks, cities, or geographic regions), institutions (e.g., hospitals, nursing homes, or group practices), or events (traffic accidents or diseases). Units of analysis in a study are typically also the sampling elements and the units of observation. When aggregate data are used, the conclusions may be drawn only at the aggregate level, not at the individual level, to avoid committing an ecological fallacy.

Sampling Element

Sampling element refers to the unit of sample to be surveyed, and provides the information base for analysis. The sampling element must be specified before sampling can be undertaken. The choice of a particular sampling element depends on the unit of analysis to be used for a study. The unit of analysis, in turn, depends on the purpose of the study and the target population about whom study results are to be generalized. In applied research, practical policy-related considerations, such as the level at which legislation becomes operative, often determine the relevant unit of analysis. It is important to understand the concept of ecological fallacy: information collected at the aggregate level, from organizations, counties, or states, may not be generalized to the level of individuals.

In health services research, typically, sampling units are individuals, households, or organizations. Social groups, industries, or nation states can also be used as sampling elements. When individuals are used in sampling, they can be further specified in terms of individual characteristics to be included or excluded from a study, such as age, sex, race, occupation, income, and education, as well as other characteristics pertinent to the study, including those with a particular disease or receiving a particular service. When households are used as the sampling element, they may be further defined in terms of family characteristics, such as presence of children or elderly members, number of parents and generations, and the like. When organizations are used as the sampling element, they can be further described in terms of organizational characteristics, such as profit status, services provided, size, and so forth.

Sampling Unit

Sampling unit is the actual unit that is considered for selection. The sampling unit and sampling element are the same in single-stage sampling but different in multistage sampling. An example of multistage sampling would be when one wants to select a sample of counties, then a sample of hospitals within the selected counties, and finally, a sample of patients within the selected hospitals. In this example, the sampling units are county, hospital, and patient, but only the last (patient) is the sampling element, because individual patients will be the unit of analysis.

Observation Unit

Observation unit is the unit from which data are actually collected. The observation unit and sampling element may be different when, for example, heads of households (observation unit) are surveyed about all household members (sampling element), or administrators (observation unit) are questioned about characteristics of organizations or their clients (sampling element).

Population

Population refers to the target for which investigators generate the study results. A population may be defined as universe or study relevant. A universe population consists of a theoretically specified aggregation of sampling units. A study population includes only the aggregation of sampling units from which the sample is to be selected. A study population is usually smaller than a universe population, because some sampling units may be omitted from the sampling frame available. Investigators should find out which types of sampling units are likely to be omitted or inadequately represented in the study population so that generalization about the universe population can be adjusted accordingly.

Sampling Frame

Sampling frame is a list of sampling units from which the sample is actually selected. Examples include telephone directories, membership lists, student rosters, patient records, and the like. Although researchers hope that the sampling frame represents the entire universe population, this is seldom the case, because the sampling frame is typically incomplete and not up to date. The sampling frame determines the scope of the study population.

Sampling Design

Sampling design refers to the method used to select the sampling units and may be classified into probability and nonprobability sampling methods. In **probability sampling**, all sampling units in the study population have a known, nonzero probability of being selected in the sample, typically through a random selection process. Random does not mean haphazard or arbitrary; rather, an unbiased probability method is used to select the sample. Specifically, all sampling units have an equal or known chance of being selected in the sample, and the selection of one unit will not affect the chance of selecting another unit. Random selection produces an unbiased sample whose results may be validly generalized to the population of interest.

In **nonprobability sampling**, the probability of selecting any sampling unit is not known because units are selected through a nonrandom process. A nonprobability sample may be biased because certain units may be more or less likely to be included in the sample. A biased sample will produce results that cannot be validly generalized to the population of interest.

Sampling Error

Although a sample is expected to reflect the population from which it comes, there is no guarantee that any sample will be precisely representative of the population. Chance may dictate that a disproportionate number of untypical observations will be made. When a sample does not represent the population well because of chance, **sampling error** occurs. Sampling error comprises the differences between the sample and the population that are due solely to the particular units that happen to have been selected. Sampling error is also known as **random error**. Sources of random error include sampling variability, subject-to-subject differences, and measurement errors. It can be controlled and reduced to acceptably low levels by using average measures, increasing the sample size, and repeating the experiment.

Sampling Bias

Sampling bias is a tendency to favor the selection of units that have particular characteristics. It describes deviations that are not a consequence of chance alone. Sampling bias is also known as **systematic error**. Sampling bias can yield an estimate very far from the true value, even in the wrong direction. An example of selection bias is when the subjects studied are not representative of the target population from which conclusions are to be drawn.

For example, a researcher may try to estimate the prevalence of smoking in residents of a county by selecting a random sample from all the patients registered with local primary care physicians, and sending them a questionnaire about their smoking habits. With this design, one source of error would be the exclusion from the study sample of residents not registered with a primary care doctor. These excluded subjects might have different rates of smoking from those included in the study. Also, not all of the subjects selected for study will necessarily complete and return questionnaires. Nonresponders may have different smoking habits from responders. In addition, certain kinds of patients (e.g., older and more educated) are more likely to be selected into studies presumably due to a higher level of participation (i.e., a high response rate) among the older and better-educated group. In contrast, lower-socioeconomic-status groups are less likely to participate (i.e., a low response rate), resulting in inadequate representation of these groups in many of the national population-based surveys. To reduce sampling bias, disproportionate stratified sampling may be used to oversample the less represented groups.

Variable

A **variable** is a set of mutually exclusive attributes. Variables are collected with an instrument (e.g., questionnaire or interview guide) from observation units to gain information about sampling elements. For example, hospital administrators (observation unit) may be asked about the age, sex, race, and insurance characteristics (variables) of their patients (sampling element).

Statistics and Parameters

Statistics refers to the summary numerical description of variables about the sample. **Parameters** refers to the summary numerical description of variables about the population of interest. Statistics are combined from information collected from the sample and used to provide estimates of the population parameters. The accuracy of the estimation may be assessed by the confidence intervals of the sample statistics.

PROBABILITY SAMPLING

Probability sampling requires the specification of the probability that each sample element will be included in the sample. The process of probability sampling consists of using a sampling frame and some random procedure of selection that makes probability estimation and the use of inferential statistics possible. Random sampling, however, does not guarantee that any single sample will be representative of the population. The extent that a sample represents the population depends on the variability within the population and the sample size. If the investigator is certain that a random sample produces unusual and nonrepresentative cases, based on previous experience of the population, he or she should not replace the atypical cases with more typical ones. Rather, the entire sample may be discarded and a new sample drawn instead. Sometimes, it may be necessary to increase the sample size.

Probability sampling methods are generally used at later rather than exploratory phases of research, when accuracy of samples is critical so that sample finding may be validly generalized to the population. Commonly used probability sampling methods include simple random sampling, systematic sampling, cluster sampling, and stratified sampling. The choices among these methods are typically based on the nature of the population under study, the purpose of the study, and the available resources. If the population is homogeneous, simple random and systematic sampling methods are more likely to be used. If the population is heterogeneous, stratified sampling is more likely to be used. If the population is scattered, cluster sampling would be the method of choice. The purpose of the study will determine how accurate the data collected need to be and the types of strata that need to be sampled and analyzed. Resource constraints in terms of time and money will favor cluster over simple random or systematic sampling when face-to-face interviews are planned. The availability of a sampling frame will also affect the choice of a particular method. Figure 11.1 summarizes the trade-offs among the probability sampling methods.

Simple Random Sampling

Simple random sampling means that every unit in a population has an equal probability of being included in the sample. The procedure for conducting simple random sampling is:

1. Define the population of interest that constitutes the complete set of units or elements of the universe under study.

2. Establish the sampling frame that lists all units or elements in the population of interest. The sampling frame represents the study population. Whether the simple random sampling method is feasible or preferred depends largely on whether or not there exist accurate and complete lists of the population elements from which the sample is to be drawn. It would be prohibitively expensive and time consuming to compose such a sampling frame.

3. Assign a number to each element in the sampling frame from 1 to N.

4. Decide upon the desired sample size (n).

5. Select n different random numbers between 1 and N using a table of random numbers. The sample elements corresponding to the selected n random numbers become the sample.

Appendix 5 contains a table of random numbers. Suppose researchers want to sample 400 (n) patients from one year of patient records that

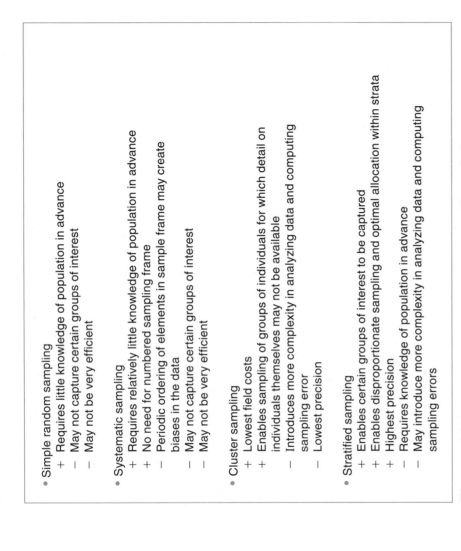

- Simple random sampling
  + Requires little knowledge of population in advance
  − May not capture certain groups of interest
  − May not be very efficient

- Systematic sampling
  + Requires relatively little knowledge of population in advance
  + No need for numbered sampling frame
  − Periodic ordering of elements in sample frame may create biases in the data
  − May not capture certain groups of interest
  − May not be very efficient

- Cluster sampling
  + Lowest field costs
  + Enables sampling of groups of individuals for which detail on individuals themselves may not be available
  − Introduces more complexity in analyzing data and computing sampling error
  − Lowest precision

- Stratified sampling
  + Enables certain groups of interest to be captured
  + Enables disproportionate sampling and optimal allocation within strata
  + Highest precision
  − Requires knowledge of population in advance
  − May introduce more complexity in analyzing data and computing sampling errors

Figure 11.1. Trade-offs among probability sampling methods

includes 5000 patients (N). The patient records system may already have assigned codes to patients, say, from 0001 to 5000. Since the numbers in Appendix 5 are completely random, it makes no difference where one starts or whether one chooses numbers by moving down columns or across rows. However, in order to remain random, researchers need to decide how to begin. Once researchers start using the numbers, they should not use the same numbers again. Say a researcher closes his or her eyes and points a finger at the sixth number down in the second column: 74717. Since the population of patients totals 5000, or four digits, only four digits of numbers will be needed and the researcher may choose to use either the first four or the next four numbers. Say the researcher chooses to use the next four digits; the first sampled patient is number 4717. Moving down the column, the second patient becomes 0805. The next number, 7602, is beyond the total population size (5000) and hence should be ignored. The next patient selected is 2135. This procedure is used until all 400 sample elements or patients are selected. When researchers come across a number they have already selected, they should simply ignore it and move on. When the numbers on one page are used up, the investigators go to the next page.

Instead of using random number tables, researchers may opt to use an Internet-based **random number generator (RNG)** to obtain desired random numbers. An RNG is a computational device designed to generate a sequence of numbers that lacks any pattern, that is, that appear randomly. Wikipedia, the free online encyclopedia, recommends the following Internet-based RNGs (http://en.wikipedia.org/wiki/Random_number_ generator): Blum-Blum-Shub pseudorandom number generator, ISAAC, Lagged Fibonacci generator, Linear congruential generator, Linear feedback shift register, and Mersenne twister.

6. Collect information from the selected sampling elements. See Chapter 13 for data collection methods.

Systematic Sampling

Systematic sampling selects every *k*th element from the sampling frame after a random start. The procedure for conducting systematic sampling is:

1. Define the population of interest.

2. Establish the sampling frame that contains a complete list of the population.

3. Decide upon the desired sample size (n).

4. Calculate the sampling interval, which is the distance between elements to be selected for the sample. The sampling interval may be calculated by dividing the population size N (total elements in the sampling frame) by the sample size n, or N/n. For instance, if there are 5000 patients and the researcher wishes to select 400, then the sampling interval is 12.5 (5000/400).

5. For a random start, randomly choose a number from 1 to k, with k being the sampling interval. In our example, a number from 1 to 13 will be selected. This can be accomplished by drawing a number from a hat containing 13 pieces of paper numbered 1 to 13.

6. Select every *k*th number until the total sample is selected. In our example, since a patient cannot be divided by half, researchers may alternately sample every 12th and then every 13th patient until a total of 400 patients are selected. Supposing the randomly selected number is 10, the sample then would include patients numbered 10, 22, 35, 47, 60, . . . , 4998.

Systematic sampling is easier to draw than simple random sampling because the investigator does not have to read from the random numbers all the time to draw the sample or have to number all the list of elements if they are not prenumbered. Therefore, it is often used in lieu of simple random sampling, particularly if the sampling list is long or the desired sample size is large. Systematic sampling is commonly used when choosing a sample from city or telephone directories or other preexisting but unnumbered lists.

However, researchers should be cautious about the existence of periodicity or cyclical patterns that may correspond to the sampling interval. For example, if a household survey decides to select every 10th housing unit from the block and the 10th unit happens to be at the corner of the block, then all corner houses would be selected. If there are systematic differences between corner houses and other houses (for example, in terms of size, expensiveness, and so on), then the sample would be biased. In sampling months from a large number of years, if the sampling interval happens to be 12, the investigator will end up selecting the same month within each year, a month that might coincide with a peak patient volume or the worst bad debt ratios. To guard against periodicity, the investigator should carefully examine the sampling frame. If periodicity is detected, systematic sampling can still be used simply by having a random start on every page of the sampling list.

Cluster Sampling

Cluster sampling first breaks the population into groups or clusters, and then randomly selects a sample of clusters. In single-stage cluster sampling, all elements of selected clusters are studied. In multistage cluster sampling, two or more stages of sampling are performed and elements from the selected clusters of the last stage sampling may be randomly selected. The sampling units in the first stage of sampling are called primary sampling units (PSUs); those in the second stage of sampling are called secondary sampling units; and so on. Clusters are usually natural groupings, such as organizations or associations, or geographic units, such as regions, states, counties, census tracts, cities, towns, neighborhoods, and blocks. The procedure for conducting cluster sampling is:

1. Define the population of interest.
2. Identify the clusters within the population. For example, if researchers are interested in studying the individual households within a state (i.e., population of interest) in terms of their use of medical services, they may use such clusters as counties (i.e., primary sampling units), residential areas (i.e., secondary sampling units), and street blocks (i.e., tertiary sampling units).
3. Decide upon the desired sample size (n). Knowledge of the total population size and population elements in different clusters will be useful to determine how many units are to be selected for each stage of cluster sampling. In our example, the numbers of households within a state and county are readily available from the census data, but those within residential areas and street blocks may have to be estimated with the help of staff from the Census Bureau.
4. Establish the sampling frame that contains a complete list of the population elements within the clusters selected at the last stage of sampling. In our example, researchers need only compile lists of households for all the selected blocks, not lists for all households in the state.

5. Either choose all the elements within the clusters selected at the last stage of sampling or randomly select a sample of these elements. In our example, researchers may either interview one owner or adult resident from each of the households from the blocks selected, or randomly select the households from the block and then interview one owner or adult resident.

Deciding whether to study all the elements within the cluster or to randomly select the elements for study usually depends on the heterogeneity (or variations) of the elements within the clusters. The more heterogeneous (or various) the elements, the greater the proportion of them that should be studied. Since usually there are more variations between clusters than within clusters, researchers sample more clusters and select fewer elements within clusters to generate more representative samples. The downside of this practice, however, is that it is more expensive both in terms of sample frame preparation and data collection. Population lists have to be compiled for more clusters and, if interviewing is the method of data collection, people have to be sent to more places to conduct the interviews. When natural clusters are not of the same size, researchers may sample clusters with probabilities proportional to the population size so that the equal probability requirement is not violated.

An example of cluster sampling is the National Health Interview Survey, a cross-sectional national household interview survey using a multistage cluster area probability design. The first stage consists of a sample of 358 primary sampling units (PSUs) drawn from approximately 1,900 geographically defined PSUs (i.e., clusters) that cover the 50 states and the District of Columbia. A PSU consists of a county, a small group of contiguous counties, or a metropolitan statistical area. Within a PSU, two types of second-stage units are used: area segments and permit area segments. Area segments are defined geographically and contain between eight and twelve addresses. Permit area segments cover geographical areas containing housing units built after the 1990 census. The permit area segments are defined using updated lists of building permits issued in the PSU since 1990 and contain an expected four addresses. Within each segment, all occupied households at the sample addresses are targeted for interview.

The principal advantage of cluster sampling lies in its efficiency, particularly when the populations of interest are unlisted or widely dispersed. Considerable amounts of money and time can be saved because cluster sampling does not require that complete lists of each and every population unit be constructed. Only the population elements in the last-stage clusters need to be listed so that a sample of elements can be drawn from these lists. Data-gathering costs may be reduced significantly, particularly when face-to-face interviews is the method of choice. Individuals within clusters are obviously much less dispersed than individuals within the entire population. Therefore, travel-related time and costs for the purpose of conducting interviews are greatly reduced.

The potential drawback of cluster sampling is its representativeness. If significant differences exist among clusters in terms of the important variables being studied, then cluster sampling may be biased if particular clusters are not sampled. Increasing the sample size of clusters will improve the probability that different clusters are sampled, but this will increase sampling costs, therefore defeating the major benefit of cluster sampling.

Stratified Sampling

In **stratified sampling** the population is divided into nonoverlapping groups or categories, called strata, and then independent simple random samples are drawn for each stratum. It may be used either for the purpose of making comparisons among subgroups of the population or for making estimates of the entire population. Stratified sampling may be proportional or disproportional, depending on the probability of each sampling element to be selected. In proportional stratified sampling, all population strata are sampled proportional to their composition in the population, so that all sampling elements will have an equal probability of being selected. Proportional stratified sampling allows direct generalization from sample to population without any statistical adjustments.

In disproportional stratified sampling, different probabilities are used to sample different population strata so that sampling elements will have an unequal probability of being selected. Typically, more units are sampled from the strata with a smaller proportion of the population. Disproportional stratified sampling is used when one or more strata within the population are underrepresented and would not otherwise appear in sufficient numbers in simple random sampling. In general, disproportional sampling is used whenever a simple random sample would not produce enough cases of a certain type to support the intended analysis.

Disproportional stratified sampling does not affect analysis within each stratum. However, if researchers want to combine different strata, disproportional stratified sampling does not allow direct generalization from sample to population because the probability of selection varies from stratum to stratum. In generalizing from sample to population, estimates must be weighted by the inverse of the **sampling fraction** to compensate for over-sampling in some strata and reflect the proportion that each stratum represents in the population. The sampling fraction reflects the proportion of subjects to be sampled for the study. For example, if 10 percent of black patients were selected versus 5 percent of white patients, then to generate population estimates, the proper weighting for black patients would be 10, or the inverse of the sampling fraction 10/100, and for white patients 20, or the inverse of the sampling fraction 5/100. The weighting procedure may be simplified by giving every white patient a weight of 2 (20/10) and no weighting for black patients, or by giving every black patient a weight of 0.5 (10/20) and no weighting for white patients. Statistics software (e.g., SPSS and SAS) usually has detailed descriptions of how weighting can be performed and analyzed. The procedure for conducting stratified sampling is:

1. Define the population of interest.
2. Identify the strata within the population. Strata could be demographic characteristics, such as sex, age, and race; socioeconomic status, such as

income, education, and occupation; or any variables that have significant bearing on the dependent variables. One or more strata may be used at the same time.

For example, if researchers want to find out the relationship between certain patient characteristics such as race, sex, and insurance status and medical treatment procedures for one particular illness, the strata of interest will be race (white, black, other), sex (male, female), and insurance (private insurance, Medicare only, Medicaid only, no insurance).

3. Decide upon the desired sample size (n). Knowledge of the total population size and population elements at different strata will be useful to determine how many units to be selected for each strata. In our example, total population size refers to all patients admitted for the particular illness of interest. Population elements at different strata refer to patient distributions according to race, sex, and insurance status, that is, the number of patients who are white, male, and have private insurance; white males with Medicare only; white males with Medicaid only; white males with no insurance; the number of patients who are black, male, and have private insurance; and so on.

4. Establish the sampling frame that contains a complete list of the population elements within the strata selected. In our example, each patient is classified into groups or strata based on race, sex, and insurance. Therefore, researchers will have a list of white male patients with private insurance, a list of white male patients with Medicare insurance only, and so on. Preparing sampling frames that classify elements into strata may be difficult if the information needed is not readily available or too costly to obtain.

5. Apply a simple random sampling method to select elements from each stratum using the sampling frame prepared for this purpose. Either a proportional or a disproportional sampling method may be used. In proportional sampling, patients from all strata have the same probability of being selected. In disproportional sampling, they have different probabilities of being selected. Disproportional sampling is used when certain strata have relatively few patients so that an insufficient number of them will be selected if proportional sampling is used. Indeed, the principal advantage of stratified sampling is to increase representation particularly for strata with small proportions of elements in the population.

Many national surveys incorporate stratified sampling in overall sampling design. For example, since 1995, the National Health Interview Survey has included race/ethnicity as a stratum and over-sampled (i.e., disproportionately sampled) both black and Hispanic persons. The Medical Expenditure Panel Survey also includes stratified sampling by over-sampling policy-relevant population subgroups, beginning with the 1997 panel. Initially, these subgroups included: (1) adults with functional impairments, (2) children with limitations, (3) individuals between the ages of 18 and 64 predicted to have high levels of medical expenditures, and (4) individuals with family incomes less than 200 percent of the poverty level.

NONPROBABILITY SAMPLING

Nonprobability sampling does not require the specification of the probability that each sample element will be included in the sample (Babbie, 2006; Henry, 1990; Patton, 2002). Typically, nonrandom procedures are used to select sampling elements. Nonprobability sampling may not be representative of the population of interest and hence may not be generalizable to the population. Sampling error cannot be calculated and selection biases are not controlled. However, it is much more convenient, less expensive, and less time consuming than probability sampling and may be useful when probability sampling methods cannot be used. For example, when there are very few population elements (e.g., cities or hospitals in the region), random sampling may not generate a representative sample, and sampling based on expert judgment may be more reliable.

Nonprobability sampling methods are frequently used in the early or exploratory stage of a study where the purpose is to find out more information about the topic, discover interesting patterns, and generate hypotheses for later, more formal investigation. It is also used when data accuracy is not very important, when resources such as time and money are very limited, or when certain subjects are difficult to locate or access. Commonly used nonprobability sampling methods include convenience sampling, quota sampling, purposive sampling, and snowball sampling.

Convenience Sampling

Convenience sampling relies on available subjects for inclusion in a sample. Available subjects may be people encountered in the street, volunteers who answered an advertisement, or a captive audience, such as students in classrooms, patients in hospitals, employees in organizations, and the like. Convenience sampling is quick and easy but generally does not represent the population of interest. It may be used at an early stage of research when a mere feel for the subject matter is needed.

Quota Sampling

Quota sampling specifies desired characteristics in the population elements and selects for the sample-appropriate ratios of population elements that fit the characteristics. The desired characteristics may be age, sex, race, income level, education, occupation, or geographic region. Quota sampling is similar to stratified random sampling in that both methods divide the population into relevant strata. However, the two methods are fundamentally different because unlike stratified random sampling, quota sampling does not provide all population elements an equal or known probability for being selected. Investigators may use any method to select population elements to fulfill their assigned quota. Quota sampling is cheap, easy, convenient, and saves time in terms of data collection. Its representativeness is often questionable, particularly when investigators select subjects who are most conveniently available.

Purposive Sampling

Purposive sampling selects sampling elements based on expert judgment in terms of the representativeness or typical nature of population elements and the purposes of the study. Purposive sampling may be used when sample size is small and simple random sampling may not select the most representative elements. It is an economical way of generating a representative or typical sample using few elements. However, considerable prior knowledge of the population is required before the sample is selected.

Snowball Sampling

Snowball sampling relies on informants to identify other relevant subjects for study inclusion. Those other subjects may in turn provide leads to additional relevant subjects. The term *snowball* is used because, like a snowball that starts small but becomes bigger and bigger as it rolls downhill, sampling based on chain referrals starts with a small number of subjects but expands as subjects refer additional people for inclusion. Snowball sampling is particularly useful for studying populations who are difficult to identify or access, for example, persons with HIV/AIDS or drug abusers. Since the sample depends heavily on referrals by the investigators' informants, its representativeness is limited to the investigators' network of informants.

SAMPLE SIZE DETERMINATION

Sample size is determined by a number of factors including the characteristics of the population, the nature of the analysis to be conducted, the desired precision of the estimates, the resources available, the study design, and the anticipated response rate. Often these factors have to be considered simultaneously and trade-offs made before the final sample size is decided upon.

Population Characteristics

Since the sample is drawn to represent a population, certain population characteristics, such as heterogeneity and size, have a significant impact on the size of a representative sample. In general, the more heterogeneous a population, the larger the sample size required. On the other hand, the less heterogeneous a population, the smaller the sample size required. In the extreme case, where all population elements are different, a census of every element is required. When there is no heterogeneity or variability among population elements, a sample of one is sufficient. In health services research, as in other social sciences research, the populations of interest are generally much more heterogeneous than they are in most other disciplines.

The accuracy of a sample estimate may be indicated by its standard error, calculated with the standard deviation divided by the square root of the sample size ($\sigma/\sqrt{N}$). The standard error reflects the magnitude of differences in the measured variable among study subjects. The formula indicates that the standard error of the sample estimate is directly related to the standard deviation or heterogeneity of the population and is indirectly related to the sample size. In other words, the more heterogeneous the population, the larger the sample size required to minimize the standard error. Specifically, because of the square root function, in order to reduce the standard error by one half, researchers must increase the sample size by four times. It can be seen that at a certain point, for example, after 2,000, there is a diminishing return in the reduction of standard error by sample size increases. As a rule of thumb, a minimum sample of 100 is preferred for the purpose of statistical analysis.

In addition to heterogeneity, the size of the population also affects the sample size. Given the same heterogeneity, a larger population requires a larger sample size than a smaller population. However, contrary to intuition, sample size does not need to increase in proportion to population size. An examination of the complete formula for the standard error makes this clear. According to Kish (1965), the complete formula for the standard error for finite populations is $SE = (\sigma/\sqrt{N})(\sqrt{1-f})$, where f is the sampling fraction. For a large population, the sample fraction is generally so small that the correction factor $\sqrt{1-f}$ is very close to $\sqrt{1}$ or 1, having negligible impact on the standard error. Only when the population is small does the sampling fraction have a significant impact on standard error.

Analysis

The sample size is also determined by the nature of the analysis to be performed. Specifically, the number of comparisons that will be made and the number of variables that have to be examined simultaneously have a significant influence on the sample size. In general, the more comparisons or subgroup analyses to be performed, the larger the sample size should be. For example, before surveying the patient population, researchers need to decide how many levels of analyses or breakdowns they will have. Possible breakdowns include age (under 65 and 65 and above), sex (male and female), race (white, black, and other), insurance status (Medicare, Medicaid, private, and none), and so on. If they are interested in the insurance status of black males under age 65, they need to have a relatively large sample to make sure sufficient cases will be included. Sometimes, the population elements that fit into a particular category may be too few to be selected in simple random sampling. Then, stratified sampling may be considered as a method to sample the subcategories or strata separately.

The number of variables to be analyzed at one time also influences the sample size. Typically, in quasi-experimental research, relevant variables have to be controlled statistically because groups differ by factors other than chance. The more variables that need to be analyzed simultaneously, the larger the sample size should be to make sure the investigator will have sufficient cases representing the variables considered. Therefore, before deciding upon the sample size, researchers should also know the type of analysis they are going to conduct with the data. A rule of thumb is to include at least 30 to 50 cases for each subcategory.

Precision of Estimates

The precision of the estimates the investigator wishes to achieve also influences sample size. As has been shown before, the precision, or accuracy, of a sample estimate may be indicated by its standard error, the standard deviation divided by the square root of the sample size $(\sigma / \sqrt{N})$. The more precise the estimates, the larger the sample size required. Generally, the level of accuracy of estimates hinges on the importance of the research findings. If important decisions, those that have serious and costly consequences, are going to be based on research findings, then decision makers demand a very high level of confidence in the data and estimates. In such cases, a larger sample size would be needed. On the other hand, if there are few, if any, major decisions to be based on the research findings or only rough estimates are required by the sponsor, then the sample size would be correspondingly small.

Available Resources

Resources available to the researcher also influence sample size. Important resources include money, time, and staff support. Sometimes, the sample size is prespecified by the sponsor through available funding. Regardless of the theoretical sample size decided upon, the amount of the budget may dictate the upper limit of a sample. The budgeted research funding is not merely for data collection. It is also needed for research preparation, data analysis, and reporting. The time element is important if decisions based on the research have to be made at a certain time. Then research activities have to be planned around this deadline. Compromises have to be made that may include having a smaller sample size. Staff support is particularly important in interview surveys where the number of interviewers available is directly correlated with the number of subjects that can be studied given a particular time period, or the speed at which data can be collected given the number of interviews to be conducted.

Study Design

Different study designs tend to have different demands for sample size. In experiments where variables are controlled, researchers can use a relatively smaller sample size. In quasi-experimental designs, a larger sample size is generally required to statistically control for extraneous factors. For the same reason, stratified, cluster, and quota sampling methods generally require a smaller sample size than simple random or systematic sampling methods.

Response Rate

Often, the ideal and the actual sample sizes are different because of less-than-perfect response rates. Respondents may refuse to be studied. They may turn in illegible or unusable questionnaires. It may not be possible to locate them. Even among usable questionnaires, not all questions are answered. Some items may be left blank or answered improperly. Therefore, the final sample size, especially related to a particular questionnaire item, is always smaller than the initial plan. Researchers need to anticipate these factors and make necessary adjustments at an early stage. For example, if the ideal sample size is 500, and past experience indicates that the average response rate for this questionnaire is 65 percent minus 5 percent for ineligible questionnaires (e.g., those with too many missing values), then, to achieve the target sample size of 500, researchers may need to start with 810 [500/(0.65 − 0.05 × 0.65)].

The response rate also has an impact on the validity of the research. If a systematic bias exists that affects the response, then the results of the study may not be generalizable to the whole population. To evaluate the extent of nonresponse bias, researchers should gather information about nonrespondents (e.g., demographics and geographic locations) so that comparisons can be made between respondents and nonrespondents. These comparisons and possible bias are then included in reports of the study.

Calculation of Sample Size

As this chapter discussed, determining the appropriate sample size for any given study is shaped by several factors, including population characteristics, analysis plans, the level of precision of sample estimates, the availability of resources, the study design, and the anticipated response rate. With these considerations in mind, statistical formulas exist to estimate sample size. While closely related, these formulas differ depending on the type of research question asked and the nature of the data collected.

The first formula applies to binomial data, which is collected to answer a research question regarding the proportion of the population that has a particular trait, experiences a particular phenomenon, or expresses a particular preference, and so on. Binomial data is yes–no data. The formula used to calculate the sample size needed in order to produce an estimate for a population proportion with a certain level of precision is:

$$n = p(1 - p)(Z_{1-\alpha/2}/E)^2$$

where n = the sample size estimate, p = the population proportion, $Z_{1-\alpha/2}$ = the level of confidence (usually 95 percent), and E = the margin of error (Browner, Newman, Cummings, and Hulley, 2001; D'Agostino, Sullivan, and Beiser, 2002).

When data from previous studies or from a pilot study is available, p may be estimated. For instance, if a pilot study found 45 percent of patients visiting the emergency department for asthma attacks lacked health insurance, the value of p for determining the sample size needed for a larger-scale study of this phenomenon would be 0.45. In the absence of previous data, the most conservative sample size estimate would be obtained by setting p equal to 0.5.

Typically, the value of $Z_{1-\alpha/2}$ is 1.96, which reflects a 95 percent confidence interval for the true proportion of all emergency room asthma patients who lack health insurance. The margin of error term, E, reflects the maximum percentage of error (regarding the difference between the researcher's estimate and the true population proportion) that the investigator is willing to risk. In other words, if the researcher wants his or her estimate of the proportion of emergency room asthma patients without health insurance to be within 5 percent of the true proportion, he or she will set E at 0.05. Solving for n produces the minimum number of research subjects needed to estimate the true proportion of emergency room asthma patients without health insurance and to ensure a margin of error equal to E with the confidence interval specified by $Z_{1-\alpha/2}$.

If the research question shifts to determine the mean number of emergency room visits for asthma patients without health insurance, a different formula for sample size exists:

$$n = (Z_{1-\alpha/2}\sigma/E)^2$$

where n = the sample size estimate, $Z_{1-\alpha/2}$ = the level of confidence (usually 95 percent), σ = the standard deviation of the population characteristic, and E = the margin of error (Browner, Newman, and Cummings, 2001; D'Agostino et al., 2002).

In this example, σ (i.e., standard deviation) is the only variation from the formula for binomial data described above. The value of the standard deviation may be known from previous studies. If the value of σ is unknown, the researcher may wish to conduct a pilot study to generate an estimate, or she may wish to generate an educated guess using this formula:

Standard Deviation (estimated) = Range/4

where the range is the difference between the minimum and maximum values of the mean number of emergency room visits by asthma patients without health insurance. The margin of error, E, is expressed in the same units as the mean number of emergency room visits. In this case, the researcher may wish the margin of error to be three emergency room visits, so 3 becomes the value of E. Solving for n, the researcher is able to determine the minimum number of study participants required to determine the mean number of emergency room visits by patients with asthma who lack health insurance, with the confidence interval specified by $Z_{1-\alpha/2}$, and the margin of error expressed by E.

In addition to using formulas to estimate the sample size requirement, researchers may obtain the required sample size by using tables for sample size calculation (see Figure 11.2 for a sample size selection chart). For example, for an infinite population (use 100,000 for population size), with the relative precision (e) of 10 percent and the confidence level of 95 percent, a sample size of 100 would be needed. With the relative precision (e) of 5 percent and the confidence level of 95 percent, a sample size of 398 would be needed.

Another way to calculate sample size is the use of computer software such as STATA, SAS, Epi-Info, Sample, Power and Precision, and nQuery Advisor.

Population Size	Sample Size 5%	Sample Size 10%	Population Size	Sample Size 5%	Sample Size 10%
10	10		275	163	74
15	14		300	172	76
20	19		325	180	77
25	24		350	187	78
30	28		375	194	80
35	32		400	201	81
40	36		425	207	82
45	40		450	212	82
50	44		475	218	83
55	48		500	222	83
60	52		1000	286	91
65	56		2000	333	95
70	59		3000	353	97
75	63		4000	364	98
80	66		5000	370	98
85	70		6000	375	98
90	73		7000	378	99
95	76		8000	381	99
100	81	51	9000	383	99
125	96	56	10000	385	99
150	110	61	15000	390	99
175	122	64	20000	392	100
200	134	67	25000	394	100
225	144	70	50000	397	100
250	154	72	100000	398	100

Figure 11.2. Example of a sample size selection chart

Calculation of Power

Power is a concept closely linked to sample size. Conceptually, the power of a research study is that study's probability of rejecting a null hypothesis (i.e., the probability of making a correct decision). The higher the power, the better. As a rule of thumb, it is desirable to achieve a study power of 0.80 (Browner, Newman, Hearst, and Hulley, 2001).

Power is represented as $(1 - \beta)$. Beta (β) is the probability of a Type II error, which is the failure to reject a null hypothesis when it is false. Therefore, power $(1 - \beta)$ is the probability of rejecting a null hypothesis when it is false.

Power is dependent on the sample size, the significance level, and the estimated effect size of a study. Usually, the significance level of a study is set at 0.05 (which corresponds to a 95 percent confidence interval, as discussed in the previous section) or 0.01 (which corresponds to a 99 percent confidence interval). Effect size is defined as the strength of the relationship between the independent and dependent variables (Gliner, 2000, p. 177). The effect size (d) of a study comparing an intervention and a control group can be calculated using this formula:

$$d = (\overline{X}_1 - \overline{X}_C)/s_{pooled}$$

where $\overline{X}_1$ is the mean of the intervention group, $\overline{X}_C$ is the mean of the control group, and s_{pooled} is the pooled standard deviation of both groups. Effect size may also be expressed as the correlation coefficient, r. Computer statistical packages usually produce r as an output, but not d. Another means of estimating effect size is reviewing previous studies that have reported the effect size for similar interventions.

Once a researcher determines the sample size, the significance level, and the estimated effect size, the power of his or her study can be determined by using a power chart (see Figure 11.3 for a power chart). The power chart lists the sample size for each group on the x-axis and power on the y-axis. The curves on the chart correspond to different levels of effect size. This particular power chart is applicable for studies with a significance level of 0.05.

If the power level of a study is determined before the sample size is calculated, the power chart may also be used to determine the sample size. For instance, if a researcher wants his or her study to have a particular level of power, effect size, and significance, he or she can use the power chart to determine what size sample will be required.

Computer software can be used to calculate power for a given sample size. For example, under SAS 9.1, the procedures PROC POWER and PROC GLM-POWER are specifically designed to compute power for a variety of statistical designs including one- and two-sample t tests, correlations, and proportions, as well as regression and one-way ANOVAs, among others. Web-based sample size and power calculators are widely available on the Internet.

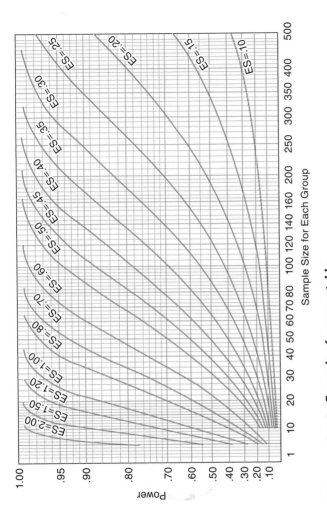

Figure 11.3. Example of a power table
Source: Gliner and Morgan (2000)

SUMMARY

In sampling, researchers select a subset of observations from the population and make inferences about the population based on sample characteristics. Sampling is necessary because of efficiency, accuracy, and access considerations. Commonly used probability sampling methods, where all sampling units in the study population have a known, nonzero probability of being selected in the sample, include simple random sampling, systematic sampling, cluster sampling, and stratified sampling. Nonprobability sampling methods, where the probability of selecting any sampling unit is not known because units are selected through nonrandom processes, include convenience sampling, quota sampling, purposive sampling, and snowball sampling. In determining the sample size required for the study, researchers consider such factors as the characteristics of the population, the nature of the analysis, the desired precision of the estimates, the resources available, the study design, and the anticipated response rate. For a given sample size, the power of the estimate may be calculated.

REVIEW QUESTIONS

1. Why is sampling used?
2. What are the differences between probability and nonprobability sampling? When is one more appropriate than the other?

3. Among probability sampling methods, what kinds of research conditions are more appropriate for each sampling method?

4. Among nonprobability sampling methods, what kinds of research conditions are more appropriate for each sampling method?

5. How does a researcher decide on the appropriate sample size for a given study?

REFERENCES

Babbie, E. (2006). *The Practice of Social Research* (11th ed.). Belmont, CA: Thomson/ Wadsworth.

Browner, W. S., Newman, T. B., Cummings, S. R., and Hulley, S. B. (2001). Estimating sample size and power: The nitty-gritty. In S. B. Hulley, S. R. Cummings, W. S. Browner, D. G. Grady, N. Hearst, and T. B. Newman (Eds.), *Designing Clinical Research* (2nd ed.). Philadelphia: Lippincott.

Browner, W. S., Newman, T. B., Hearst, N., and Hulley, S. B. (2001). Getting ready to estimate sample size: Hypotheses and underlying principles. In S. B. Hulley, S. R. Cummings, W. S. Browner, D. G. Grady, N. Hearst, and T. B. Newman (Eds.), *Designing Clinical Research* (2nd ed.). Philadelphia: Lippincott.

D'Agostino, R. B., Sullivan, L. M., and Beiser, A. S. (2002). *Introductory Applied Biostatistics*. Pacific Grove, CA: Brooks/Cole.

Fowler, F. J. (2002). *Survey Research Methods* (3rd ed.). Thousand Oaks, CA: Sage.

Gliner, J. A., and Morgan, G. A. (2000). *Research Methods in Applied Settings: An Integrated Approach to Design and Analysis*. Mahwah, NJ: Lawrence Erlbaum Associates.

Henry, G. T. (1990). *Practical Sampling*. Newbury Park, CA: Sage.

Kish, L. (1965). *Survey Sampling*. New York: Wiley.

Patton, M. Q. (2002). *Qualitative Evaluation and Research Methods* (3rd ed.). Thousand Oaks, CA: Sage.

Rubin, H. J. (1983). *Applied Social Research*. Columbus, OH: Charles E. Merrill.

Measurements in Health Services Research

KEY TERMS

concurrent validity
construct validity
content validity
double-barreled questions
face validity
internal consistency reliability
interrater reliability
interval measures

leading questions
loaded questions
measurement
measurement errors
measurement reliability
measurement validity
nominal measures
ordinal measures

parallel forms reliability
predictive validity
ratio measures
reliability
split-half reliability
test-retest reliability
validity

LEARNING OBJECTIVES

- To identify the ways concepts can be measured and the levels of measurement.
- To understand the ways to improve measurement validity and reliability.

- To construct a research instrument for data collection.

DEFINITION

Health services researchers and practitioners often talk about health status, quality of care, patient satisfaction, access to care, and so on. These are concepts that cannot be observed directly. We cannot see health status or quality of care in the same sense that we can see a house or tree. They need to be specified or operationalized before research can be conducted on them. **Measurement**, then, is the process of specifying and operationalizing a given concept.

In specifying a concept, we identify its particular dimensions and the indicators for these dimensions. For example, we may identify four aspects of quality of care: structure, process, outcome, and satisfaction. For each, we can further specify a series of indicators. The structural indicators may be facility licensure, certification of physicians, availability of certain medical equipment, and the like. Process indicators include diagnostic procedures, laboratory tests, drugs prescribed, operations, and so forth. Outcome indicators consist of readmission rate, recovery rate, death rate, infection rate, and the like. Satisfaction indicators may contain patients' attitudes toward physicians, the hospital, the treatment outcome, and so on.

The indicators need to be operationalized to complete the measurement process. Specifically, researchers need to specify the procedures for measuring indicators and deciding upon what questions to ask, the response categories, and then how to ask the questions and assign answers to particular response categories. For example, the structural indicator facility licensure may be measured by asking administrators to submit a copy of the license certificate. The response categories can be yes (referring to those who submit a license) and no (referring to those who are unable to submit a license). The process indicator diagnostic procedures may be measured by examining patient records. The specific diagnoses may be coded into International Classifications of Diseases categories or their relevant DRGs. The outcome indicator readmission rate can also be assessed through an examination of patient records, say after 60 days of patient discharge. The readmission diagnoses can be compared with the previous diagnoses. If there is a match, researchers may define this as an admission for the same condition. If the diagnoses are different, investigators may define this as an admission for a different condition. Patient attitudes toward the physician, a satisfaction indicator, may be measured by asking the patient directly about overall satisfaction level. The answer categories may be coded as very satisfied, somewhat satisfied, somewhat dissatisfied, and very dissatisfied.

All concepts should and can be measured. They should be measured because without so doing researchers cannot conduct empirical studies. Research can be measured because measurement is simply a process of defining and describing the dimensions or categories of concepts and their related indicators or variables (Babbie, 2006). To the extent that people can talk about and describe a concept, they should be able to measure it. To claim that all concepts are measurable is not to say that they can all be measured with comparable ease and accuracy, or in the same way. Some concepts are certainly more difficult to measure than others. Many researchers, going through the conceptualization and measurement phases of research, find a great deal of confusion within their mental images. Since research is cumulative, before designing their own measures, investigators typically review the measures used by those who have previously conducted similar research, and use them as references. The final measures adopted are frequently the result of numerous revisions.

Although ideally researchers would like to agree on how a particular concept should best be measured, in practice this is seldom accomplished. One reason for differences in measurement has to do with whether the research community has some explicitly agreed-upon criteria for certain measurements. Few investigators would argue about the proper measures for body weight, temperature, height, and blood pressure because these measures are explicitly established and accepted, whether it be a scale, a thermometer, a ruler, or a monitoring device. Researchers have little concern about using these measures because when properly employed, they generally produce accurate results that are almost universally accepted.

The difficulty of reaching commonly agreed-upon criteria may be due to the different situations researchers face and to the evolving nature of setting- and expectation-specific concepts. Research on quality of care at a long-term care facility probably emphasizes the caring aspect rather than treatment. Research on quality of care in an acute care setting may emphasize the treatment aspect more than the caring aspect. Also, different cultures may have different interpretations of quality.

Concepts themselves may evolve over time in accordance with changing social values, expectations, and technological advancements. To the extent that society is highly medicalized, the public's demand for medical services will rise and expectations increase. The rapid advancement of medical technology and highly publicized miracles in medicine further raise the level of expectation and correspondingly provide impetus to the expansion of quality indicators. However, difficulty in reaching commonly acceptable measurement criteria should not prevent the research community from trying to develop new and better ways to measure conceptual dimensions. At a minimum, core dimensions and indicators of concepts should be decided upon, reviewed, and revised every now and then. Consistent measurement is needed to ensure that accurate or valid studies are performed and that different studies based on the same concepts can be compared.

Another reason that researchers may use different measures for the same concepts has to do with the constraints different research methods face. Secondary study, for example, is limited by available variables. If certain dimensions of a concept are not represented by existing variables, researchers may have to work without them. It is also possible that certain indicators, although important, are difficult, expensive, or too time consuming to collect.

The choice of measures is also dictated by the research population. Can research subjects supply the information investigators are requesting? Are the measures compatible with their levels of literacy? The range of response categories

is also influenced by the expected distribution of attributes among the subjects under study.

Despite differences and incompleteness in measures, the measurement process is still valuable because, while investigators may disagree on the dimensions used, indicators chosen, and operational procedures, they are at least clear about the measures used. The measures are specific and unambiguous, even though incomplete or imprecise. At least investigators know how to interpret the results and criticize the study based on the measures used.

There are various procedures a researcher can use to operationalize indicators or variables of interest. These include relying on existing measures, observations, and self-reports. Often, the research method used plays a significant role in the choice of a particular procedure. Existing measures refer to commonly agreed-upon or frequently used measures. Using existing measures is intrinsic to secondary analysis. It is also common in primary research. If the research community has already agreed upon certain measures, then investigators should try their best to use or at least adapt them in their studies. To find out whether those measures exist, researchers may need to conduct a thorough literature review of relevant studies and consult with experts on the topic.

Researchers can also approach organizations specializing in health-related research for available instruments. For example, the Medical Outcomes Trust distributes a number of surveys related to health status, including the Short Form-36 (SF-36) Health Survey, the SF-12 (a shorter version of the SF-36), the Child Health Questionnaire (CHQ), the Sickness Impact Profile (SIP), the Primary Care Assessment Survey (PCAS), and the Quality of Well-Being Scale (QWB) (http://www.outcomes-trust.org). The National Health Interview Survey, administered by the National Center for Health Statistics, Centers for Disease Control and Prevention, also contains several questions related to health status, including people's capacities to undertake activities of daily living (ADL) and instrumental activities of daily living (IADL). Both ADLs and IADLs are discussed more thoroughly in Chapter 2.

Sometimes, even if there are no explicitly agreed-upon criteria for measuring certain concepts, researchers should still try to find existing measures from available, similar studies. There are many advantages to using existing measures. In addition to savings in time and money, using existing measures is consistent with the cumulative nature of scientific inquiry and gives investigators the benefit of other people's experience. Existing measures have already been tried out and their reliability and validity may have been documented. **Reliability** is the ability to repeat research and replicate findings, which is a necessary aspect of validating scientific knowledge. The **validity** of a measure is the extent to which it actually assesses what it purports to measure.

Observation is a direct method researchers may use to examine indicators or variables of interest. Targets that can be observed include behaviors, attitudes, clothing, conversations, relationships, feelings, events, surroundings, and the like. Qualitative research methods, and field research in particular, generally favor observation. Observations can also be used to complement quantitative research methods such as structured face-to-face interviews by noting the demeanor of the interviewee as a measure of personality and the type of household and neighborhood as a measure of social class. An experiment can also include observations to assess the impact of interventions.

Self-report refers to respondents' answers to questions in questionnaires or interviews. Self-report can be used to measure both objective and subjective variables, including demographics (age, sex, race), socioeconomic indicators (income, education, occupation), knowledge (awareness of certain concepts, facts, events, people), behaviors (frequency of doctor visits and hospitalization), attitudes (opinions about health care reform), feelings (satisfaction with care received), and beliefs (viewpoint about life events). With certain limitations, self-reports can include both past events and future intentions. Self-report is most commonly used in survey research. Qualitative research can also include self-report in the form of focus group studies or in-depth interviews.

Regardless of the operational procedures used, each measure should exhibit two important qualities: it should be exhaustive and mutually exclusive. The response categories that represent each indicator should be exhaustive so that all observations or sampling elements can be classified using the response categories. If, at the initial stage, researchers are uncertain about the variations among the subjects, they may want to design more categories than are eventually needed. Later, in analyzing the data, if needed, they can always combine precise attributes into more general response categories. Response categories should also be mutually exclusive so that each observation or sampling element can be classified into only one of the response categories.

LEVELS OF MEASUREMENT

Once the dimensions and indicators have been specified and the procedure to collect data determined, as part of the operationalization process, researchers need to decide what level of measurement to use for the response categories of the indicators or variables. The four levels of measurement are nominal, ordinal, interval, and ratio (Babbie, 2006; Singleton and Straits, 2005).

Nominal measures classify elements into categories of a variable that are exhaustive and mutually exclusive. The categories represent characteristics or attributes of a variable. For example, sex can be classified into two categories, male and female, which are both exhaustive (there can be no other categories of sex) and mutually exclusive (being classified as a male precludes one from being classified as a female). Nominal measures are the lowest level of measurements. There is no rank-order relationship among categories and the investigator cannot measure the distance between categories. When numbers are assigned to the categories, they mainly serve as codes for the purpose of data collection and analysis but have no numerical meanings. In other words, Category 2 is not twice as many as Category 1.

Ordinal measures refer to those indicators or variables whose attributes may be logically rank-ordered along some progression. For example, the variable *satisfaction with the medical treatment* may be categorized as very satisfied, somewhat satisfied, somewhat dissatisfied, and very dissatisfied. There is an obvious rank order among those categories, with very satisfied ranked first and very dissatisfied ranked last. Another use of ordinal measures is respondents' ranking of certain items in terms of their preference. For example, patients may be asked to indicate their health insurance preferences by rank-ordering their options according to, say, high premium and no deductible, low premium and low deductible, and no premium and high deductible. Ordinal measurement is more advanced than nominal measurement. In addition to the rank-order function, it contains all the characteristics of a nominal measure including classification, exhaustiveness, and exclusiveness.

Interval measures refer to those variables whose attributes are not only rank-ordered but are separated by equal distances. The often-used example is the Fahrenheit or the Celsius temperature scale. The difference, or distance, between 65 degrees and 75 degrees is the same as that between 35 degrees and 45 degrees, which is 10 degrees. We can feel not only that 35 degrees is cooler than 45 degrees (rank-order function) but how much cooler it is (interval function). Interval measures are more advanced than either nominal or ordinal measures and contain all the properties of the others. Interval measures do not have a true zero, and zero is merely arbitrary. For example, zero degrees does not indicate no temperature. (In fact, it is a very cold temperature.) Because of this arbitrary-zero condition, there are very few interval measures in health services research. Very often, interval measures are mixed together with ratio measures, called *interval-ratio measures*, and the arbitrary-zero requirement is ignored.

Ratio measures are similar to interval measures except that ratio measures are based on a nonarbitrary or true zero point. For example, the variable *number of years of education* is a ratio measure because zero years of education has a true meaning: no education whatsoever. The true-zero property of ratio measures makes it possible to divide and multiply numbers meaningfully and thereby form ratios. Other examples of ratio measures include age (measured in years), income (measured in dollars), and hospitalization (measured in days). Like interval measures, ratio measures are a higher level of measurement than nominal and ordinal measures and contain all their properties.

To the extent possible, researchers should try to measure their indicators or variables at a higher level rather than a lower level. The level of measurement chosen has significant implications for analysis. Most statistical techniques, including the most powerful ones, are designed for interval-ratio variables. Therefore, to make full use of statistical techniques and improve data analysis, researchers should construct interval-ratio measures whenever possible. Of course, some variables are inherently limited to a certain level. Another reason that interval-ratio measures are preferred is that even if later on the investigator decides to analyze the variable in different ways, the interval-ratio measure can always be recoded into ordinal or nominal measures. For example, age can be recoded into old, middle, and young (an ordinal measure); or working population (18–64) and nonworking population (less than 18 or greater than or equal to 65) (a nominal measure). You will not be able to convert measurements in the other direction, from a lower-level measure to a higher-level one.

MEASUREMENT ERRORS

After an operationalization of a concept has been applied to sampling elements, we notice that there are certain differences or variations among sampling elements with respect to the response categories. Part of the observed differences are true differences among elements that we wish to observe through the measurement process. Indeed, a valid measure should account for most of the variations in observed differences.

In addition to true differences, certain portions of the observed variations may be the result of measurement errors. **Measurement errors**, then, refer to sources of differences observed in the elements that are not caused by true differences among elements. Researchers classify measurement errors into two types: systematic and nonsystematic, or random, errors. Systematic errors refer to certain biases consistently affecting the measurement process. Nonsystematic, or random, errors refer to certain biases affecting the measurement process in haphazard, unpredictable ways.

Systematic errors may be caused by inaccurate operationalization of the concept of interest. Important dimensions or categories of the dimensions of the concept may be missing so that there is only a weak link between the categories used and the concept they try to measure. Sometimes, too few items are used to measure one particular concept so that it is difficult to assure their accuracy. For example, when only one item is used to measure an attitude, it is open to errors of interpretation and formulation of a response. When questions are improperly or ambiguously formulated, they may induce biased responses.

Systematic errors may also occur because of the research experience itself. When respondents act differently in front of researchers from their usual behavior, then observations may be biased. For example, when the data collection process is nonanonymous and/or nonconfidential, people may give socially desirable but not necessarily truthful responses. They may give inaccurate responses to sensitive questions or simply leave them blank. Certain people may choose not to participate in the research or drop out in the middle of the study. Low response or high attrition may present significant distortions to the study outcome because participants and nonparticipants or dropouts are typically different.

Random errors occur when certain characteristics of individuals, respondents, or investigators affect the measurement process. Respondents may have fluctuations in mood as a result of illness, fatigue, or personal experiences. Certain individuals may not understand the wording of a questionnaire item or may wrongly interpret the item. Certain questions may be too complicated for some respondents. Sometimes, individuals may not know the contents of the item being asked and either ignore the item or give a spontaneous response. This is particularly common with attitude and opinion questions. Not everyone has formed an opinion about everything. In addition, respondents may be too tired to think through the question, or their responses may be affected by people, noises, and other distractions present.

Random errors originating from investigators may include improper interview methods such as not following instructions, changing the wording of questions or the order in which they are asked, asking leading questions, or making subjective interpretations of respondents' answers. These biases are especially common when certain results are likely to benefit the investigators or are consistent with their beliefs. Interviewers may also omit instructions due to fatigue or lack of interest.

Both respondents and investigators may be turned off by each other due to their demographics, attitudes, or demeanor. A lack of trust on either side could affect how the questions are asked, responded to, or recorded. Both are also prone to classification errors. Respondents may erroneously choose a category or select a rating. Interviewers may check the wrong boxes. Keypunchers may strike the wrong key while inputting data. Programmers and analysts may make mistakes in modeling and calculation.

Systematic errors are serious threats to study validity and reliability. Researchers should make great efforts to reduce sources of systematic error. In contrast, unsystematic, or random, errors do not present a great threat to research, although they may also affect study reliability. Their impacts are unpredictable and tend to cancel each other out with sufficient sample size. There are so many sources of measurement errors that they are almost impossible to eliminate. Researchers should take into account those sources and try their best to reduce their impacts. At a minimum, their impacts should be studied so that measurement validity and reliability can be assessed.

VALIDITY AND RELIABILITY OF MEASUREMENT

Measurement validity refers to the extent to which important dimensions of a concept and their categories have been taken into account and appropriately operationalized. In other words, a valid measure has response categories truly reflecting all important meanings of the concept under consideration. For example, a measure of quality of care that includes the structure, process, outcome, and satisfaction dimensions is more valid than one that only includes one of these dimensions.

Measurement reliability refers to the extent to which consistent results are obtained when a particular measure is applied to similar elements. Thus, a reliable measure will yield the same or a very similar outcome when it is reapplied to the same subject or subjects sharing the same characteristics. For example, estimating a person's age or weight by checking his or her birth certificate or weighing him or her is more reliable than asking directly, which is more reliable than asking others.

A valid measure is usually also reliable, but a reliable measure may not be valid. For example, checking a birth certificate is both a valid and reliable measure of one's age but is not a valid measure of work experience since current age does not necessarily reflect years spent in the labor force. An unreliable measure cannot be valid; when the results fluctuate significantly, how can the measure capture the true meaning of a concept? The credibility of one's research will be influenced by the perceived validity and reliability of the measures used. Therefore, researchers, as a common practice, include in their report an assessment of the validity and reliability of their measures.

Validity Assessment

Even though there is no direct way of confirming the validity of a measure—otherwise there would be no need for the measure—there are many indirect methods researchers use to establish the validity of their measures. These include face validity, construct validity, content validity, concurrent validity, and predictive validity.

Face Validity

Face validity is exactly what it sounds like. If a measure has face validity, it appears to be appropriate for its intended purpose. On its "face," the measure seems valid. Face validity alone is not an adequate measure of validity, but it is a first step in such assessments.

Construct Validity

Construct validity refers to the fact that the measure captures the major dimensions of the concept under study. For example, a measure of quality of care should include questions about each of the major dimensions of quality, structure, process, and outcome (which includes satisfaction). Construct validity may be strengthened in a number of ways. If agreed-upon criteria exist in terms of measuring a particular concept, then those criteria should be reflected in the measures. Literature review and checking with experts allow investigators to find out whether there are established ways of measuring certain concepts. The construct validity of a measure can also be enhanced by establishing a high significant level of correlation with other measures of the same concept, or other theoretically related variables (this is called convergent evidence), or a low correlation with measures of unrelated concepts (this is called discriminant evidence). If investigators know for sure that some elements possess the construct of interest, they can enhance construct validity by including those elements in their measurement. Construct validity can be measured using factor analysis, a statistical technique that indicates whether the clustering of items chosen to be part of a particular measure have been grouped together appropriately. Factor analysis is discussed in greater detail in Chapter 14.

Content Validity

Content validity refers to the representativeness of the response categories used to represent each of the dimensions of a concept. For example, to sufficiently represent the outcome dimension of quality of care, the researcher may have to include questions about recovery rates, functional status, complication rates, morbidity, mortality, disability, mental well-being, and so on. After establishing construct validity, taking into account all major dimensions of a concept, the constructs or dimensions have to be translated in terms of specific categories that reflect how things actually work. Content validity is strengthened when all facets of a dimension have been taken into account. Again, expert knowledge, prior literature, and existing instruments are good sources to help identify different facets or components of a particular dimension.

Concurrent Validity

Concurrent validity may be tested by comparing results of one measurement with those of a similar measurement administered to the same population at approximately the same time. If both measurements yield similar results, then concurrent validity can be established.

Concurrent validity may be tested with items included in the same instrument. For example, to check the validity of a certain scale (e.g., items related to satisfaction), the investigator may hypothesize the relations of the scale to other variables (e.g., a question directly asking satisfaction level) in the instrument. Confirmation of the hypothesis (e.g., when the scale and the question are highly correlated) produces evidence in support of the validity of the scale.

Predictive Validity

Predictive validity may be examined by comparing the results obtained from the measurement with some actual, later-occurring evidence that the measurement aims at predicting. When there is a high degree of correspondence between the prediction and the actual event—the predicted event actually takes place—then predictive validity is established. The predictive validity of the Graduate Record Examination or the Graduate Management Admission Test, for example, lies in the extent of correlation between higher scores attained and better graduate school performance.

Reliability Assessment

While validity is related to systematic errors, reliability has to do with random errors. When a measure yields consistent or similar results from one application to the next, then we know it does not have too many random errors and we become more comfortable about its reliability. Reliability assessment mainly involves the examination of the consistency level of the measurement. There are many indirect ways researchers use to establish the reliability of their measures. Commonly used methods for reliability assessment include test–retest, parallel forms, internal consistency (including split-half, Kuder–Richardson 20, and Cronbach's alpha), and interrater reliability.

Test–Retest Reliability

Test–retest reliability involves administering the same measurement to the same individuals at two different times. If the correlation between the same measures is high (usually greater than 0.80), then the measurement is believed to be reliable. However, in using the test–retest approach, researchers should beware of the potential impact of the first test on the second test. If the first test can potentially affect responses on the second test, then the second test result will be different from that of the first. Sufficient time should elapse before the second test so that memory of the first has diminished. At the same time, researchers should not wait for too long lest real changes take place during the interval. The general procedure is to wait a minimum of two weeks before the second test (Netemeyer, Bearden, and Sharma, 2003). Of course, the applicability of this method and the actual time spacing depend on the particular measurement under study.

Parallel Forms Reliability

To avoid potential testing effects associated with test–retest reliability measures, one can create a parallel (or alternative) form of the test to be used for the second testing. To establish **parallel forms reliability** (i.e., the level of correlation between the original test and the parallel test), a group of participants completes both tests with little time in between. Similar to test–retest reliability, parallel forms reliability is established when the correlation coefficient for the two sets of scores is at least 0.80.

Internal Consistency Reliability

The **internal consistency reliability** of the items in a test can be determined in several ways. First, **split-half reliability**, as the name implies, involves splitting the test into two halves and correlating one half to the other. There are many ways to split the test in two, the most suitable method being randomly sampling half of the test items and comparing them with the remaining items. Most computer statistical software packages include split-half reliability assessments.

If each item on a test is scored dichotomously (i.e., yes–no, pass–fail, true–false), the proper method for determining internal consistency reliability is the Kuder–Richardson 20. In contrast, if each item on a test has multiple choices, Cronbach's alpha is the appropriate method. Both the Kuder–Richardson 20 and Cronbach's alpha methods are commonly available in computer statistical software packages.

Interrater Reliability

Interrater reliability involves using different people to conduct the same procedure, whether it be an interview, observation, coding, rating, or the like, and comparing the results of their work. To the extent that the results are highly similar, interrater reliability has been established. This form of reliability is particularly useful when subjective judgments have to be made, for example, in inspecting and rating a health care facility. Interrater reliability is commonly measured using percentage agreement methods, intraclass correlation coefficients, or the Kappa statistic (Gliner and Morgan, 2000).

Measures to Improve Validity and Reliability

To improve the validity and reliability of a measurement, researchers can proactively take a number of steps, including using established measures, ensuring confidentiality, improving the research instrument design, training the research staff, conducting a pretest or a pilot study, and validating the instrument.

When possible, efforts should be made to obtain existing measures that are well established. Only when no relevant measures are available or accessible may investigators then construct their own measures.

Confidentiality will help reduce biases associated with questions that are embarrassing, sensitive, or have a response set (e.g., social desirability). To ensure confidentiality, investigators should assure anonymity where possible and, in the case of interviews, establish a rapport with the subjects so that the promise of confidentiality can be trusted. The names of the interviewees should be replaced by codes when inputting data, and the original instrument should be locked away and only made accessible to core research staff. The interviews should be conducted in quiet, private settings.

Improving instrument or questionnaire design is important to reducing many response biases. Not only should investigators avoid asking leading, loaded, ambiguous, or too complex questions, but sometimes in dealing with sensitive topics, they may also have to use indirect questions. The sequence of questions and response categories within questions may also affect how the questions are answered. Great care should be given to questionnaire arrangement, by varying the arrangement and the ways questions are asked. To avoid response set, which is the tendency for respondents to be very agreeable or stick to a particular pattern of response, investigators can use two different items opposite in meaning to measure the same concept, and compare responses to these items to see whether they were answered differently. Questionnaire construction will be considered in detail in the next section.

Properly training the research staff is crucial to ensuring a high level of reliability in research. Items of training include how to conduct an interview, make observations, follow instructions, and record and input data. In addition to training, close supervision is necessary in the course of all phases of research activities. For example, in telephone interviews, the supervisor may either listen in or call a subsample of respondents to verify selected items in the questionnaire. In field research, the supervisor may accompany new investigators to the settings or interviews at an early stage of the process. The supervisor can routinely check the inputted data against the original instrument.

Before formally using one's own measures, a pretest or a pilot study will help identify those words, phrases, terms, sentences, response categories, and definitions that are ambiguously worded, unknown, or irrelevant to the respondents. Revisions can be made accordingly, and the final measures should be sufficiently clear, relevant, and understood.

Instruments, especially newly created, need to be validated. The validation process allows researchers to test the reliability and validity of the items included in the instrument, providing feedback for further modifications.

RESEARCH INSTRUMENT DESIGN

When no relevant measurement exists or is accessible, researchers will have to construct their own measurement. Sometimes there is access to some existing measurements but not others. Then the remaining measures will still need to be constructed. A research instrument contains the operational definitions of all measures related to the research and is primarily used to collect data. When a research instrument contains only questions and statements to be answered by respondents, it is called a questionnaire. Be aware that the term *questionnaire* implies a collection of questions but in reality may contain statements as well.

Before putting together the research instrument, investigators should have already identified the study objectives, the major concepts to be investigated, the major dimensions of these concepts, and their representative categories. If they are still unclear about any of these elements, investigators should conduct more research to find out about them before constructing the instrument. In the process of designing the research instrument, researchers make decisions about frame of reference, time, response format, composition of questions, instrument assembly, and pretesting.

Frame of Reference

Frame of reference is related to the respondents' particular perspectives. Before writing up the questions, investigators must find out about the general characteristics of their respondents. What is their general educational level? What words, phrases, terms, or languages are familiar to them? How well informed are they about particular issues? What kinds of general experience do they have? Do they have a particular perspective that must be taken into account? Knowledge about these characteristics will help in choosing the right words and asking relevant questions. If investigators do not have prior knowledge of the frame of reference of the research population, they have to conduct a pilot test of their instrument before finalizing it. More definitions and examples may be given to make sure respondents understand exactly what is meant by each question and how they are supposed to answer each one.

Time Frame

In designing an instrument, researchers can ask questions about the past, present, or future. Current questions generally produce more accurate answers than either past or future questions. The longer the time span from the present, the less accurate the answers become. Answering questions about the past is affected by memory, and significant differences exist among people in terms of what they recall. In addition, the ability to remember things is also influenced by the importance of the event. People are more likely to remember their hospitalization experiences than their doctor visits, presumably because hospitalization is usually related to a more serious health event, which is a rare occurrence. Even when we remember an important event, we may still place it on a wrong date. A common memory problem is what Bradburn, Sudman, and Wansink (2004) have termed "telescoping," the tendency to recall the timing of an event as having occurred more recently than it actually did. Answering questions about the future involves guesswork on the part of the respondents and tends to be even less reliable than recalling past events. When the time frame is improperly extended into the past or future, the responses are likely to be inaccurate.

A variety of methods exist to improve the accuracy of responses related to memory problems. Where possible, respondents should be encouraged to check with the records they possess before answering certain questions. Examples include hospital bills (when asking about hospital costs), birth certificates (when asking about the ages of children), payroll stubs (when asking about income), school records (when asking about time of education, courses taken, and degrees obtained), financial records (when asking about expenditures), diaries (when asking about health events or other activities), and so forth.

Another method to aid recall is to provide a list of response categories so that subjects have some references to think about. For example, patients may be presented a list of services and asked which ones they have had. Providing lists is not only useful for recalling past events but also helpful for remembering current events. For example, to find out the insurance coverage of patients, investigators can list all the insurance programs available in the region to aid patients in identifying the programs to which they subscribe.

Paying attention to question formulation will also reduce memory problems. In addition to detailed lists of items, questions can be worded more specifically and include specific contexts. Where possible, visual aids may be used in either interviews or mailed questionnaires. Recall periods should be reduced to a reasonable level, usually within two weeks. For example, while it may be reasonable to ask patients about their hospitalizations during the past year, it may make more sense in terms of doctor visits to focus on the past few weeks or months. In general, the importance and frequency of the events dictate how long a period a person can reasonably recall.

Response Format

In terms of response format, the researcher must make the choice between open-ended questions and close-ended questions. Open-ended questions require the respondents to provide their answers using their own words. Open-ended questions can have quantitative as well as qualitative answers. Quantitative open-ended questions require respondents to provide numerical answers that are often categorized as interval ratios. Since interval-ratio measures provide the most advanced measurement and are most suitable for statistical analysis, researchers should try their best to include as many quantitative open-ended questions as feasible in their instruments. Examples include questions about age, income, education, number of children, and the like, which can be analyzed directly. Table 12.1 provides some commonly used examples. Qualitative open-ended questions require respondents to answer the questions using their own words.

Close-ended questions provide answer categories for the respondents to choose based on their own characteristics. The following is an example of a question asked in both open-ended and close-ended ways.

- What type(s) of health insurance plans do you have?
  [*Qualitative open-ended*]

- What type(s) of health insurance plans do you have?
  (*Check all those that apply.*)
  ( ) Medicare
  ( ) Medicaid
  ( ) Blue Cross/Blue Shield
  ( ) HMO/prepaid plan

Table 12.1. Commonly used quantitative open-ended questions

- How old are you now? _____ years of age
- How many years of education have you received from educational institutions? _____ years
- What is your annual salary or wage plus bonus? $ _____
- How many children do you have? _____ number of children
- How often did you visit the doctor during the past three months? _____ times
- How often were you hospitalized during the past two years? _____ times
- What is the number of licensed beds in your hospital? _____ beds
- What was the occupancy rate in your hospital last year? _____ %
- How many patients with congenital heart failure (ICD-9 Code 42800) did your hospital have last year? _____ number of patients
- What is the average length of stay for patients with congenital heart failure (ICD-9 Code 42800) in your hospital? _____ days

( ) Other private insurance (specify ——)
( ) Other public insurance (specify ——)
( ) No insurance
( ) No charge
[*Close-ended*]

While quantitative open-ended questions should be used wherever possible, the choice between qualitative open-ended and close-ended questions is based on many factors including the knowledge of the subject matter, depth of information required, sample size, desired response and completion rates, desired level of standardization, length of questionnaire, data analysis techniques, and the amount of time to complete the research.

Knowledge of the subject matter is critical for close-ended questions. If the researcher does not know the subject area well enough, he or she cannot identify the important dimensions, their associated categories, and the range of possible answers. A qualitative open-ended format will have to be used, as in qualitative research, to explore the dimensions, categories, and range of answers. Therefore, an open-ended qualitative pilot study may be conducted prior to a large-scale close-ended survey. Even in close-ended questions, researchers cannot always be sure that the response categories are exhaustive. Often, an "Other (specify ——)" category is included after the listing of known items.

The depth of information required also plays a significant role in the choice between qualitative open-ended and close-ended questions. Open-ended questions provide greater depth than close-ended questions, giving respondents the opportunity to describe their unique experiences, rationales, anecdotes, opinions, feelings, attitudes, beliefs, logic, and thought processes. Frequently, unanticipated things may be revealed and the strength of the feeling detected. These results, often in respondents' own words, provide a rich context for the research description and supporting evidence for summary statistics. Therefore, open-ended questions are necessary in a qualitative study to explore research issues and categories, but they are also useful in a quantitative study to support and expand on summary findings. It is common to include both open-ended and close-ended questions in survey research.

Expected sample size affects the choice between qualitative open-ended and close-ended questions. Open-ended questions are more appropriate for small sample sizes and close-ended questions for large sample sizes. Since open-ended questions generally have to be converted, or recoded, into close-ended categories before quantitative analysis can be performed, it would be too time consuming to recode many open-ended questions in large-scale surveys. Furthermore, the results of recoding may be biased. The fact that some respondents have not mentioned certain categories does not necessarily mean they are not relevant to them. They may not have thought about them at the time and, if provided with these choices, they might well have selected them. Other potential sources of bias include the difficult task of analyzing responses and classifying them into different categories, and dealing with ambiguous responses and missing data.

There are also differences in response and completion rates between qualitative open-ended and close-ended questions. The response rate has to do with the proportion of research subjects who actually send back the questionnaire or participate in the interviews. Completion rate refers to the proportion of questions within the research instrument, whether it be a questionnaire or interview guide, that get answered by the responding subjects. Open-ended questions demand greater effort and time on the part of the respondents and are likely to cause relatively low response and completion rates. Moreover, respondents are likely to be different from nonrespondents in that they tend to be more interested in the research topic than nonrespondents. Completion rates have an educational bias. Those with higher levels of education are likely to complete more questions and write more per question than those with lower levels of education. Because of the extra demand on time, effort, and educational level, open-ended questions can turn off potential respondents who are either busy, find the topic less interesting or relevant, or have less education.

Respondents are not the only people affected by open-ended questions. Interviewers who administer open-ended questions need to be trained so that appropriate probing can be used to draw out responses. The interview time for open-ended interviews tends to be much longer than for close-ended interviews. In order to achieve higher response and completion rates, it is recommended that a very limited number of open-ended questions be used and placed near the end of the instrument so that even if they were not answered the earlier close-ended questions would have been completed.

Qualitative open-ended and close-ended questions also differ in the level of standardization in responses. Close-ended questions, by providing the same frame of reference and options to all respondents, generate more standardized responses than do open-ended questions, in which individuals differ in terms of their interpretation of questions, perspectives, experiences, and ability to put their thoughts into words.

There is a close relationship between the choice of qualitative open- versus close-ended questions and the length of the questionnaire. Open-ended questions, due to their difficulty and time demand, require the questionnaire to be relatively short. Close-ended questions, because of their ease of use, enable the questionnaire to be relatively long. While the length of a questionnaire is inversely related to the response and completion rates, a longer questionnaire with many open-ended questions has significantly lower response and completion rates than a longer questionnaire with mostly close-ended questions.

The methods of data analysis also determine the choice between qualitative open- and close-ended questions. Most of the statistical techniques are used for quantitative data elements derived from quantitative open-ended or close-ended questions, which can be transferred directly into computer format. Qualitative open-ended questions first have to be recoded into close-ended categories.

Finally, the amount of research time may dictate the number of qualitative open-ended questions to be included. Open-ended questions take longer to answer, code, and analyze. More interviewers are required to complete the surveys on time. Methods of coding and analysis cannot be predetermined and have to be thought out after data collection. More time is spent on training interviewers and coders to ensure the validity and reliability of the results. If research time is very limited, a close-ended format will be more appropriate than an open-ended one.

Once researchers have decided to use close-ended questions, they need to make additional decisions about specific close-ended formats that are most suitable for the research. These formats include contingency questions, two-way questions, multiple-choice questions, ranking scale questions, fixed-sum scale questions, agreement scale questions, Likert-type format questions, semantic differential scale questions, and adjective checklist questions.

Contingency Questions

Contingency questions are those questions whose relevance depends on responses to a prior question. The use of contingency questions makes it possible for some respondents to skip questions that do not apply to them. Special care should be given to the design of contingency questions and clear instructions provided for the skip pattern. Below are two examples of the use of contingency questions.

■ Example 1:
Have you ever been hospitalized?
( ) Yes (*Please answer questions 8–11.*)
( ) No (*Please skip questions 8–11. Go directly to question 12 on page 3.*)

■ Example 2:
Do you currently smoke cigarettes?
( ) Yes
( ) No ↓

If yes: About how many cigarettes do you smoke a day?
( ) Less than 5 a day
( ) 5–10 a day
( ) 11–20 a day
( ) Greater than 20 a day

Two-Way Questions

Two-way questions include a question or statement followed by two dichotomous, realistic alternatives. Terms used to designate the alternatives include yes–no, agree–disagree, for–against, approve–disapprove, true–false, favor–oppose, like–dislike, and so on. Sometimes, a third alternative, "don't know" or "no opinion," is included to make the choices more realistic. The following are two examples of two-way questions.

■ Example 1:
Have you had a mammogram in the past 12 months?
( ) Yes

( ) No
( ) Don't know

■ Example 2:
What is your attitude toward universal health care?
( ) Agree
( ) Disagree
( ) No opinion

Multiple-Choice Questions

Multiple-choice is among the most frequently used formats for close-ended questions. There are two types of multiple-choice questions: multiple-choice single-response and multiple-choice multiple-response. In multiple-choice single-response questions, respondents are presented with a question or statement followed by a list of possible answers from which they are asked to select the one most appropriate to their situation. In multiple-choice multiple-response questions, respondents are presented with a question or statement followed by a list of possible answers from which they are asked to select as many as are relevant or applicable to their situation. Multiple-response questions are also called checklist questions because a list of all relevant items are provided for respondents to check off. In constructing multiple-choice questions, the investigator should make sure that each alternative answer contains only one idea (mutually exclusive), that the alternatives are balanced, and that they convey all important ideas of the question (all inclusive). Often, an "other" category is included to let respondents fill in information not available in the items listed. The following are two examples of multiple-choice questions.

■ Example 1:
Please check *one* race or ethnic origin you belong to.
( ) White
( ) Black
( ) Asian/Pacific Islander
( ) Native American/Eskimo/Aleut
( ) Other   *[Single-response]*

■ Example 2:
In which of the following settings do you currently provide services to your patients? (*Please check all those that apply.*)
( ) Hospital inpatient
( ) Hospital outpatient
( ) Group practice office
( ) Solo practice office
( ) Public health department
( ) Community/migrant health center
( ) Free clinic
( ) Other   *[Multiple-response]*

Ranking Scale Questions

A ranking scale, also called a forced ranking scale, asks respondents to rank a number of items in relation to one another. A forced ranking scale generally provides more information than multiple-choice questions because it not only allows multiple selections (as in multiple-choice multiple-response questions) but also obtains the sequence of the ranking in terms of importance or relevance to the respondent. It parallels many life situations where choices among programs, services, treatments, decisions, ideas, and so forth have to be made. However, a ranking scale is more difficult to respond to than other scales because respondents have to assess all items relative to one another. Therefore, in order to facilitate response, researchers should limit the number of items to be ranked to generally no more than five items, unless they are easy to compare. The following are two examples of ranking scale questions.

- Example 1:

  The following are conditions listed alphabetically that are often cited as influential to the provision of care to patients with HIV/AIDS. Please rank them in the order that you would most prefer to see them improved. Assign the number 1 next to the one you prefer most, number 2 to your second choice, and so forth.

  ( ) Additional training
  ( ) Better community and social services support
  ( ) Higher reimbursement
  ( ) Limited liability
  ( ) Specialty backup

- Example 2:

  A person can obtain information about AIDS through the following sources. Given your situation, please rank these sources in terms of their relevance to you. Put the number 1 next to the source most relevant to you, number 2 next to the second most relevant source, and so forth.

  ( ) Newspapers
  ( ) Radio
  ( ) Television
  ( ) Books
  ( ) Workplace/school
  ( ) Friends
  ( ) Relatives
  ( ) Family members
  ( ) Other

Fixed-Sum Scale Questions

Fixed-sum scale asks the respondents to describe what proportion of a resource (e.g., time, money, efforts, activities) has been devoted to each of the listed items. In designing fixed-sum scale questions, the researcher should clearly state the total sum when all proportions have been added. To facilitate response and calculation, the researcher should limit the number of items to be considered, generally no more than 10, and the activities described should be very familiar to the respondents. Below are two examples of fixed-sum scale questions.

- Example 1:

Among your current patients with health insurance, what percentage of them have the following insurance?

(*Please be sure to make the total equal to 100%.*)

Medicare only ＿＿ %
Medicaid only ＿＿ %
Medicare plus Medicaid ＿＿ %
Private third-party insurance ＿＿ %
HMO/prepaid ＿＿ %
Other insurance ＿＿ %
Total 100 %

- Example 2:

As a nursing home administrator, how much time do you spend per week on the following activities?

Resident care ＿＿ hours/week
Personnel management ＿＿ hours/week
Financial management ＿＿ hours/week
Marketing/public relations ＿＿ hours/week
Physical resource management ＿＿ hours/week
Laws/regulatory codes/governing boards ＿＿ hours/week
Quality assurance ＿＿ hours/week
Family relations ＿＿ hours/week
Other ＿＿ hours/week
Other ＿＿ hours/week
Total ＿＿ hours/week*

(*<35 part-time, 35–45 full-time, >45 overtime*)

Agreement Scale Questions

An agreement scale presents a statement and asks respondents to indicate their level of agreement or disagreement. When a series of such statements is used, it is called the Likert scale, named after its creator Rensis Likert. The agreement scale differs from the two-way dichotomous question in that it has more gradations of agreement and hence is more detailed. There are typically five ordinal response categories: "strongly agree," "agree," "undecided," "disagree," and "strongly disagree." The following are two examples of agreement scale.

- Example 1:

How much do you agree or disagree with health care reform that stresses universal coverage?

( ) Strongly agree
( ) Agree

( ) Undecided
( ) Disagree
( ) Strongly disagree

- **Example 2:**
  The following statements describe your experience as a physician in the community. Please indicate your degree of agreement with each of these statements by circling the number most applicable to your condition.

	Strongly Agree	Agree	Undecided	Disagree	Strongly Disagree
1. I am a valuable contributor to the community's health.	5	4	3	2	1
2. I appreciate what the community offers me.	5	4	3	2	1
3. The local physicians accept me as "one of them."	5	4	3	2	1
4. I was well prepared for the realities of living in this community when I first came.	5	4	3	2	1
5. I am pleased with the backup support and referral system in the community.	5	4	3	2	1

[Likert scale]

Likert-Type Scale Questions

The Likert-type format can be used not only for agreement questions, but also for many other types of questions, by modifying the ordinal response categories. For example, the response categories for the verbal frequency scale are "always," "often," "sometimes," "seldom," and "never." When using the frequency scale, the researcher should provide some indication of how to interpret the terms in the scale. For example, once a day can mean often, once a month seldom, and so on, so that respondents have a common frame of reference. The response categories for an evaluation scale are "excellent," "good," "fair," and "poor." The response categories for a satisfaction scale are "very satisfied," "somewhat satisfied," "somewhat dissatisfied," and "very dissatisfied." As can be seen, the middle neutral category may be omitted to force respondents to make a choice. The decision to include or omit the neutral category should be based on a consideration about reality. If respondents truly might not have an opinion or attitude, the middle neutral category should be included. Another variation of the Likert-type scale is the number of response categories used. Although five is most frequently used, one may choose to use fewer (e.g., three) or more (e.g., seven) categories to obtain the most appropriate level of gradations. The following are two examples of Likert-type scales.

■ Example 1:
How would you rate your general health status?
( ) Excellent
( ) Good
( ) Average
( ) Fair
( ) Poor
( ) Don't know

■ Example 2:
On average, about how often do you visit a doctor, HMO, or clinic?
( ) Less than once a year
( ) Yearly
( ) More than once a year, but less than once a month
( ) Monthly
( ) More than once a month, but less than once a week
( ) Weekly
( ) More than once a week

Generally, when a Likert-type scale is used, a series of statements or items are included that measure different dimensions of a particular concept. Each item should express only one idea. Jargon and colloquialism should be avoided. A total score for a scale is calculated by adding the numbers associated with responses to each item. Negatively worded items are reverse scored so that two opposite items will not cancel out in the total score. The formula used for reverse scoring is: $(H + L) - I$, where H is the largest number, L the smallest number, and I a particular response to an item. For example, when a respondent circles 2 for the following question, the reverse score becomes $4 [(5 + 1) - 2 = 4]$.

	Strongly Agree	Agree	Undecided	Disagree	Strongly Disagree
The pay is inadequate for my job.	5	4	3	2	1

Table 12.2. Commonly used adjective pairs for constructing semantic differential scale

Negative	Positive
angry	calm
bad	good
biased	objective
boring	interesting
closed	open
cold	warm
confusing	clear
cowardly	brave
dirty	clean
dull	lively
irrelevant	relevant
old	new
passive	active
prejudiced	fair
reactive	proactive
sad	happy
sick	healthy
slow	fast
static	dynamic
superficial	profound
tense	relaxed
ugly	pretty
uninformative	informative
weak	strong
worthless	valuable
wrong	right

Semantic Differential Scale Questions

The semantic differential scale uses a series of adjectives and their antonyms listed on opposite sides of the page and asks the respondents to indicate their positions about a statement using the adjectives provided. Semantic differential scale questions are often related to measuring people's attitudes, opinions, impressions, beliefs, or feelings about certain events, organizations, behaviors, and the like. The adjective pairs used must truly be antonyms. Table 12.2 lists examples of some of these. Below are two examples of semantic differential scale questions.

■ Example 1:

Below are a number of adjectives used to describe a person's feeling toward his or her job. Please pick a number from the scale (1 to 7) to indicate your feeling about your job.

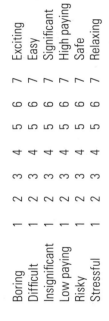

Boring	1	2	3	4	5	6	7	Exciting
Difficult	1	2	3	4	5	6	7	Easy
Insignificant	1	2	3	4	5	6	7	Significant
Low paying	1	2	3	4	5	6	7	High paying
Risky	1	2	3	4	5	6	7	Safe
Stressful	1	2	3	4	5	6	7	Relaxing

▪ Example 2:

How important do you think each of the following characteristics is to being a successful hospital administrator? Please circle the *one* number that best represents your feeling.

	Least Important				*Most Important*		
Analytical skills	1	2	3	4	5	6	7
Business skills	1	2	3	4	5	6	7
Communication skills	1	2	3	4	5	6	7
Decision-making skills	1	2	3	4	5	6	7
Entrepreneurial skills	1	2	3	4	5	6	7
Financial skills	1	2	3	4	5	6	7
Human resource skills	1	2	3	4	5	6	7
Goal oriented	1	2	3	4	5	6	7
Health care background	1	2	3	4	5	6	7
Leadership skills	1	2	3	4	5	6	7
Networking skills	1	2	3	4	5	6	7
Planning skills	1	2	3	4	5	6	7

Adjective Checklist Questions

The adjective checklist questions present a statement about a topic followed by a list of adjectives and ask respondents to check off as many as are relevant to their situation. Unlike the semantic differential scale, adjectives in the checklist do not have to be antonyms, although some representation of both positive and negative expressions will facilitate the response process. These questions can provide more descriptive information about a topic of interest and can be used to reinforce or illustrate quantitative findings. Simplicity, directness, and economy are the major strengths of these types of questions. Below are two examples using the adjective checklist.

▪ Example 1:

Please check any words or phrases below that describe your current job.

( ) Boring   ( ) Dead-end   ( ) Difficult   ( ) Easy
( ) Exciting   ( ) High paying   ( ) Insignificant   ( ) Low paying
( ) Pleasant   ( ) Rewarding   ( ) Risky   ( ) Safe
( ) Satisfying   ( ) Significant   ( ) Stressful   ( ) Technical

- Example 2:

  Below are words and phrases describing interactions a person might experience at the hospital. Please check those most appropriately reflecting your own experience as a patient along each of the aspects measured.

	Physicians	Nurses	Other (Specify ____)
caring	( )	( )	( )
effective	( )	( )	( )
inconsiderate	( )	( )	( )
indifferent	( )	( )	( )
ineffective	( )	( )	( )
responsive	( )	( )	( )
tardy	( )	( )	( )
timely	( )	( )	( )

Questionnaire Composition

A research instrument or questionnaire may contain a variety of questions, such as background, knowledge, experience, behavior, feeling, opinion, attitude, values, intentions, or plans. Background questions are generally related to the demographic characteristics of the individual being studied. Examples include age, sex, race, education, occupation, and residence. Knowledge questions are asked to find out what factual information the respondent has. Examples include the respondent's income or awareness of a particular event, term, issue, law, and the like. Experience questions are related to what a respondent has gone through or is still going through. Examples include sickness, tiredness, stress, and so forth. Behavior questions are concerned with what a respondent does or has done. Examples include visiting a doctor or hospital, undergoing an operation, and the like. Feeling or attitude questions aim at understanding the emotional state of the respondent with respect to particular issues. Examples include satisfaction, anxiety, happiness, and so on. Opinion, attitude, or value questions try to find out what a respondent thinks about some particular issue. Examples include attitudes toward health care reform, values regarding universal coverage, opinions about managed care plans, and so on. Intentions and plans are generally future-oriented questions. Since they contain a high degree of speculation, their reliability is generally less than for questions about the past and present. Examples include the number of nurse-practitioners to be hired by community health centers in the next three years, conditions necessary to quit smoking, and so forth.

In formulating questions for the instrument, researchers should pay particular attention to content validity. An instrument valid in content is one that has drawn representative questions from a universal pool (Cronbach, 1971). A Delphi method can be used which includes experts in the field to review the questions until a consensus is reached about their representativeness.

In addition to maintaining content validity, in writing specific questionnaire items, researchers should avoid biases wherever feasible and pay special attention to certain types of questions. Below are a number of popular reminders for questionnaire formulation.

Avoid Loaded Questions

Investigators use words and phrases that reflect their perception of a particular issue or event in **loaded questions**. The questions are biased because they suggest certain beliefs that could influence respondents' answers. An example of a loaded question is: "What is your opinion toward a socialist one-payer health care system?" The question is loaded because it implies that the one-payer system is necessarily the product of socialism. Respondents may be negatively or positively influenced by their attitudes toward socialism regardless of the merits of a one-payer system.

Avoid Leading Questions

A question with particular wording that suggests or demands a particular answer is a **leading question**. They are biased because they hint at a desired answer rather than finding out what the respondent feels. An example of a leading question is: "The U.S. president believes that universal access to care is an essential element of health care reform. Do you agree that universal access should be mandated?" The question is leading because it uses the president to establish the legitimacy of the claim for universal access. Then, presenting only "Do you agree . . ." may suggest that the respondent ought to concur with the statement.

Avoid Double-Barreled Questions

Two separate questions in one statement are **double-barreled questions**. They are biased because respondents may have different answers for each of the two questions. An example of a double-barreled question is: "Do you think the treatment you received from the doctor was costly and ineffective?" Respondents may agree that the treatment was costly but disagree that it was ineffective. The question is also leading because only negative concepts are conveyed.

Use Appropriate Words

The words used to form questions should be appropriate to the respondents. If the respondents have little education, then researchers should use very simple vocabulary. If the respondents do not know a particular event or term, a definition should first be provided so that they understand what is being asked. Providing definitions is also important for words that have different meanings to different people. For example, respondents often have varying interpretations of the words "often," "frequently," "seldom," "occasionally," "a lot," "a few," "rarely," and the like. They should be defined so that everyone will have the same frame of reference.

The use of appropriate words further means that the words used should be very specific rather than abstract. Their meanings should be clear to the respondents.

Finally, appropriate wording is crucial for sensitive questions. For example, to ask about socially undesirable conduct, such as smoking, alcohol consumption, and drug abuse, researchers may want to start with a statement that implies that these behaviors are somewhat common before asking respondents to reveal their experiences.

To test whether words are appropriate, researchers may employ the cognitive laboratory method, which assists in the understanding of respondents' thought processes as they respond to questions. This approach is used regularly by federal agencies involved in the collection of survey data. These agencies include the Bureau of the Census, the Bureau of Labor Statistics, the National Center for Health Statistics, and the National Center for Education Statistics. The cognitive laboratory method allows researchers to determine why respondents answer questions in certain ways. Is it because they lack mastery of a subject area or skill related to the question? Or is it because they may not know a word or phrase that is relevant to the test item, thereby inhibiting their ability to comprehend the question? Without cognitive lab data in such cases, questionnaire developers would be unaware that certain words or phrases were placing some respondents at a disadvantage, or that some test items were unnecessarily complicated.

Write Short Questions

If possible, the researcher should try to keep each question to under 20 words. Short questions are usually easier to read and answer than longer questions, which tend to become ambiguous and confusing. Indeed, both well-educated and poorly educated people prefer short questions to longer ones. Respondents are usually unwilling to study a question or statement for too long before answering it. Short questions are also less likely to be double-barreled.

Write Simple Questions

To write simple questions, researchers should try to limit the number of complex concepts in one question and use words with three or less syllables, unless they are certain the vocabulary is familiar to the respondents. They should try to ask questions directly and positively. Indirect questions may confuse some respondents. Negative words in questions may be overlooked. If the researcher must ask negative questions, the negative word can be underlined to draw the respondents' attention to it. Investigators should always avoid asking double-negative questions, that is, questions having two negative words. An example of a double-negative question is: "Do you disagree with the statement that the United States does not have a coordinated health care system?" Instead, one could ask: "Do you agree with the statement that the United States has a coordinated health care system?"

Item-Analyze the Scale

As discussed in the reliability assessment section, use of item analysis to ensure internal consistency is essential when several statements are used to produce one scale. The purpose is to ensure that items included in the instrument form an internally consistent scale, and to eliminate those that do not. By internal consistency, we mean the items measure the same construct. If several items reflect the same construct, then they should also be interrelated empirically. Internal consistency may be tested by administering the scale with a sample of respondents (100–200) and examining the intercorrelations among items representing the scale. Items that represent a common underlying construct (sometimes referred to as a latent construct) are significantly intercorrelated. A given item that is not related to other items should be dropped from the scale. On the other hand, if a very strong relationship is found between two items, then only one may be needed in the scale because it also conveys the meaning of the other.

According to Specter (1992), an item–remainder coefficient can be calculated for each item. It is the correlation of each item with the sum of the remaining items. For example, for a scale with 10 items, the item–remainder coefficient for Item 1 can be calculated by correlating responses to Item 1 with the sum of responses to Items 2 through 10. The item–remainder coefficient for Item 2 can be calculated by correlating responses to Item 2 with the sum of responses to Item 1 and Items 3 through 10. Only items with sufficiently high item–remainder coefficients (e.g., >0.40 and <0.95) are retained. If this criterion leaves too many items, then those with the largest coefficients are chosen. If the number of items is insufficient, then new items need to be constructed and reexamined. Researchers should be aware of an inherent trade-off between the number of items and the magnitude of item–remainder coefficients. The more items included, the lower the coefficients can be and still yield a good, internally consistent scale. Another important concern in selecting items is to make sure that they can produce sufficient variations in responses.

In addition to item–remainder coefficients, Cronbach's coefficient alpha can be calculated, which measures the internal consistency of a scale. Cronbach's coefficient alpha ranges from 0 to 1.0 and is a direct function of both the number of items and their magnitude of intercorrelations. It is available in most computer statistical programs. For a scale to reach a sufficient level of internal consistency, the coefficient alpha should reach at least 0.7. Further revisions of items may be needed if the coefficient alpha is too low. As discussed in the measurement reliability section, Cronbach's alpha may be used if each item on a scale has multiple-choice answers. If each item has dichotomous answers (yes–no, true–false, and so on), the Kuder–Richardson 20 should be used in place of Cronbach's alpha.

After the best have been selected, investigators then decide whether to assign different weights to the items in the scale. Generally, all items are weighted equally unless there are strong reasons to believe certain items should be given greater weights. One reason is the lack of balance in the items included. If there are fewer items chosen to represent one aspect of the concept than another, then these items may be given higher weights to make the results more balanced. For example, for a scale with three items, if Items 1 and 2 represent the same dimension and Item 3 represents a different dimension, then Item 3 may be assigned a weight of two and the other items a weight of one each. Weighting can also be based on the relative importance of the different dimensions of a particular concept.

Another issue in summarizing scale items is dealing with missing values. When the sample size is large and only a few cases have missing values, the researcher may simply exclude these cases from analysis. When the sample size is small, the investigator may want to replace the missing values with the sample average values. This is usually a conservative approach and works against significant findings.

Assembling

Assembling a questionnaire is like packaging a product. The quality of the paper and appearance of the pages all create impressions on potential respondents and may affect the response rate. In general, white paper is used to facilitate reading. A typeface that can produce a photocopied instrument resembling a printed copy is recommended. The pages of the questionnaire should not appear too crammed. Questions and statements should be spread out and uncluttered. Sufficient space should be available for answering every question, particularly openended ones. Cramming many questions on fewer pages is not the way to shorten the length of a questionnaire. In addition to paper and appearance, assembly also means the sequencing of questions and writing instructions that facilitate questionnaire administration.

The growing popularity of web and e-mail surveys in health services research presents additional design and assembly considerations. For instance, when designing e-mail and web surveys, the researcher must be careful to present the questions in a format that is compatible with multiple types of servers, browsers, and operating systems. The capacity for creativity with graphics increases when using e-mail or web surveys, and the researcher should use this to his or her advantage, through the use of welcoming, motivational colors and fonts. However, the researcher should beware of using too many graphics, or varying the graphics from one screen to the next, which may overwhelm or confuse the respondent (Dillman, 2000). Moreover, researchers should resist the urge to create long, burdensome online surveys simply because they are inexpensive.

Also, online surveys give researchers the ability to offer respondents multiple text sizes and language translations, which may increase the reach of the instrument to different populations. However, this capacity must be balanced with careful assessment of the appropriateness of survey questions for these different populations. For instance, translation of a survey from English into Spanish requires a nuanced understanding of the meaning of particular phrases and words that may not translate well. Instructions to the respondent may be more involved in online surveys than in paper surveys, because the instructions must include technical pointers for how to correctly complete the survey electronically. The researcher must also consider whether respondents will print out their answers or send them electronically, and how to ensure privacy and confidentiality in either situation (Dillman, 2000).

Sequencing

Questionnaire sequencing differs between self-administered instrument and interviews. In the self-administered questionnaire (including paper, e-mail, and web surveys), it is usually proper to start with interesting but relatively easy questions so that respondents are motivated to answer them. Routine questions, such as background questions, are usually placed at the end. In interviews, however, background questions, such as those related to demographics, are usually asked in the beginning after a general introduction about the nature of the study. The purpose is to gain a rapport so that answers to later questions can be facilitated.

Both self-administered questionnaires and interviews require a certain logic in the order of questions. Subheadings may be used to divide the questionnaire into logical sections. Early questions should be easy and interesting and subsequent questions should flow naturally and logically from earlier ones. Difficult, sensitive, or potentially embarrassing questions should be placed near the end when respondents have already committed time and effort and are more likely to complete them. However, if the questionnaire is lengthy, the difficult questions should be placed at a point early enough that respondents are not too tired when they get to them. In general, knowledge, experience, and behavior questions are easier to answer than questions related to feeling, opinion, attitude, or value. As a rule of thumb, qualitative open-ended questions should be placed at or near the end of a questionnaire so that even if respondents do not answer them they will have completed the earlier, close-ended portions. As Aday and Cornelius (2006, p. 303) suggest, "We should view the questionnaire completion process in the same way we view a conversation: starting with an introduction and then moving from general questions to specific questions and sometimes to sensitive questions."

The sequencing of questions should also consider the possibility of reactivity, in which earlier questions affect responses to later ones. For example, in interviews, earlier questions about the relationship between smoking and lung cancer as well as other diseases may affect later questions relating to respondents' smoking behavior. In general, to reduce reactivity, researchers should place behavior- and experience-related interview questions before attitude and value questions. In self-administered questionnaires, since respondents may go back and change previous responses, one should avoid including questions that may cause a particular response set.

Instructions

Questionnaires, whether self-administered or conducted by interviewers, must include clear instructions that facilitate their completion. A cover letter often accompanies a self-administered questionnaire, as is the case with surveys administered online. It specifies the purpose, significance, and sponsor of the research; the benefits of completing the instrument; and the length and return method of the questionnaire. In interviews, the contents of the cover letter are read to the respondent by the interviewer.

Knowing the purpose of the study gives potential respondents a sense of the type of research they are participating in. People are generally more willing to complete the questionnaire if the study purpose is of interest to them. Likewise, a person's likelihood of responding hinges on how important the research is. The significance section should be carefully worded to make a connection between the targeted respondents and the study objective. The research sponsor is the funder, a person or organization, who has supported the research. When the sponsor is familiar and influential to the research population, the response rate can be improved.

The benefits of completing the questionnaire may be financial or nonfinancial. Financial benefit means respondents receive monetary compensation upon completing and returning the questionnaire. In most situations, nonfinancial benefits are promised. Examples include the improvement of social programs, medical practices, productivity, efficiency, or effectiveness, or an advancement in theories. Respondents may also receive a summary of results upon the completion of the study.

The approximate time for completing the questionnaire is suggested so that respondents can plan this activity accordingly. In general, a shorter length is preferred, and respondents are prompted to complete it as soon as possible. Delay in completing a questionnaire often means no response. Finally, the method of returning the completed instrument needs to be specified. Generally, a postage-paid, addressed envelope is provided to the respondent, who is encouraged to use it to return the completed questionnaire as soon as possible. For e-mail surveys, respondents may either reply to the e-mail or (less commonly) print out their surveys and mail them to the researcher. For web surveys, respondents simply submit the survey electronically.

Within the questionnaire, instructions and explanatory statements are provided where appropriate. The beginning of each section may include a short statement ("In this section, we would like to . . .") indicating the objective and major content of the section to create a proper frame of reference for the respondents. At the end of the section, a transitional statement may be used to smoothly direct the respondents to the next section.

For each question, basic instructions should be given in terms of how to complete it. Instructions are particularly important when there are variations in response formats. For close-ended questions, respondents can be asked to indicate their answers by placing a check mark or an X in the box beside the appropriate response category or by writing answers when called for. For open-ended questions, guidance needs to be provided as to the length of the response. If researchers are interested in elaboration to close-ended questions, they should clearly state so and leave sufficient space for written-in answers. Another element sometimes included in survey instructions is a skip pattern, which is a statement clarifying that the respondent should move on to the next question or next section if the current question or section is not applicable.

If a single answer is desired, this should be made perfectly clear in the question: "From the list below, please check the *primary* reason that explains why you do not have any health insurance." Or the question may be followed by a parenthetical note: "Please check the *one* best answer." If multiple answers are expected from the respondent, this should also be made clear in the questions or instructions: "Please check as many answers as apply."

When questions are difficult to respond to, examples can be given as guidance in addition to general instructions. For example, ranking questions should illustrate how ranking is to be performed besides indicating whether single or multiple answers are desired: "Please write *1* beside the most important factor, *2* beside the next most important factor, and so forth until you finish ranking all the listed factors."

For interviews, instructions not only provide guidance to the respondents but also serve the purpose of standardizing the administration of the instrument, thus reducing interviewer biases. For this reason, separate sheets of instructions are provided to the interviewers that detail the background and purpose of the study, administrative matters, rules on what to say and how to say it, when to call, how to decide about personal appearance, and how to handle different situations. Further, more transitional statements and probing are included in questionnaires to be administered by interviewers so that ad-libbing becomes unnecessary. Transitional statements are included to make the interviewing proceed in a smooth and logical fashion. Examples include: "Hello, my name is . . ." and "That completes our interview: thank you for . . ." Probes are necessary when responses are incomplete or vague or when respondents ask for further clarification. Examples are: "What do you mean by . . ." and "Can you explain that a little more?" In writing instructions for interviews, one should differentiate the formats between those to be read out loud and those not to be read. For example, parenthesis or capital letters may be used for words not to be read aloud ("IF THE RESPONDENT IS HOSTILE IN ANSWERING THIS QUESTION, THEN . . .").

Pretesting

After the questionnaire has been assembled satisfactorily, the next step is to conduct a pretest. Pretesting is usually conducted among a relatively small number of respondents (say, 10–20) who closely resemble the research population. Purposive sampling is used to select as heterogeneous a sample of respondents as the research population.

The purpose of pretesting is to find out whether additional revisions of the questionnaire are necessary. Specifically, researchers are interested in knowing the actual time it takes to complete the questionnaire; whether the level of language matches respondents' knowledge; which words, terms, phrases, or sentences are still confusing, ambiguous, or misunderstood; whether response categories are truly mutually exclusive and all inclusive; which questions generate a relatively high nonresponse rate; whether current instructions are understood or additional instructions are needed; and whether responses to open-ended questions are given in the way intended. Those who participate in pretesting may be contacted to talk about their general feelings, interpretations, and comments about the questionnaire items.

SUMMARY

Measurement is the process of specifying and operationalizing a given concept. Various procedures can be used for operationalization, including existing measures, observation, and self-report. The four levels of measurement into which concepts may be operationalized are nominal, ordinal, interval, and ratio. To ensure that a measurement is valid and reliable, researchers examine a particular measure in terms of its face, construct, content, concurrent, and predictive validity and its test–retest, parallel forms, internal consistency, and interrater reliability. In designing a research instrument, researchers take into account the frame of reference, time span covered, questionnaire response format, question composition, instrument assembly, and completed instrument pretesting.

REVIEW QUESTIONS

1. What are the levels of measurement? What are their characteristics?
2. What are the differences between systematic errors and random errors in measurement?
3. What measures can be taken to ensure measurement validity and reliability?
4. In designing a research instrument for data collection, what considerations must be taken into account prior to writing the questions?
5. Design a questionnaire on a topic of interest to you using as many of the response formats illustrated in this chapter as possible.

REFERENCES

Aday, L. A., and Cornelius, L. J. (2006). *Designing and Conducting Health Surveys: A Comprehensive Guide* (3rd ed.). San Francisco: Jossey-Bass.

Babbie, E. (2006). *The Practice of Social Research* (11th ed.). Belmont, CA: Thomson/ Wadsworth.

Bradburn, N., Sudman, S., and Wansink, B. (2004). *Asking Questions: The Definitive Guide to Questionnaire Design for Market Research, Political Polls, and Social and Health Questionnaires* (Rev. ed.). San Francisco: Jossey-Bass.

Cronbach, L. J. (1971). Test validation. In R. L. Thorndike (Ed.), *Educational Measurement* (2nd ed.). Washington, DC: American Council on Education.

Dillman, D. A. (2000). *Mail and Internet Surveys: The Tailored Design Method* (2nd ed.). New York: Wiley.

Gliner, J. A., and Morgan, G. A. (2000). *Research Methods in Applied Settings: An Integrated Approach to Design and Analysis*. Mahwah, NJ: Lawrence Erlbaum Associates.

Netemeyer, R. G., Bearden, W. O., and Sharma, S. (2003). *Scaling Procedures: Issues and Applications*. Thousand Oaks, CA: Sage.

Singleton, R. A., and Straits, B. C. (2005). *Approaches to Social Research* (4th ed.). New York: Oxford University Press.

Specter, P. E. (1992). *Summated Rating Scale Construction: An Introduction*. Newbury Park, CA: Sage.

CHAPTER 13 ❖

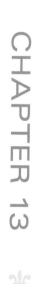

Data Collection and Processing in Health Services Research

KEY TERMS

acquiescence
auspices
code sheet
codebook
coding
computer-aided personal
interviewing (CAPI)
computer-assisted telephone
interview (CATI)

data cleaning
data dictionary
fixed-column format
Health Insurance
Portability and
Accountability Act
(HIPAA)

medical chart review
mental set
prestige
social desirability

LEARNING OBJECTIVES

- To describe the various data collection methods used in health services research.

- To identify situations where some methods are more appropriate than others.

- To specify the measures that can be taken to improve response rates.

- To learn how to prepare a codebook for a research instrument.

Data collection in HSR takes place only after many other research stages have been satisfactorily completed, including conceptualizing the research topic, preparing for research, determining the research method and design, sampling, and constructing the measurement. This chapter describes various methods of data collection, placing emphasis on the most commonly used methods in HSR: mail questionnaire surveys and face-to-face and telephone interviews. The chapter compares their relative strengths and weaknesses and discusses choices among various methods. It further examines ways to improve both the response rate and the quality of responses. Since a data collection instrument may be precoded (i.e., coded before data are collected), this chapter also introduces coding concepts and the components of a codebook. Finally, it presents the concepts and procedures of data processing.

DEFINITION

Figure 13.1 displays various data collection methods that can be used in HSR. Research data may be collected either empirically or from existing sources. As presented in Chapter 5, studies based on existing data use what is called secondary analysis. Existing data come from both published and unpublished sources.

Published data may be ordered directly from the publisher or obtained from university libraries, mostly in the documents section. Federal, state, and local governments regularly publish various kinds of data. Those of particular interest to health services researchers include official vital statistics abstracted from birth, death, marriage, and divorce certificates (*Vital Statistics of the United States* from the National Center for Health Statistics: http://www.cdc.gov/nchs/datawh/statab/unpubd/natality/natab2000.htm). Also of interest are data on population demographics prepared from census data (*Statistical Abstract of the United States* from the U.S. Bureau of the Census: http://www.census.gov/compendia/statab/2006/2006edition.html). In addition, health services investigators rely heavily on health statistics, health survey results, and mental health statistics of the type that can be found through the following:

- *Publications and Information Products* from the National Center for Health Statistics: http://www.cdc.gov/nchs/products.htm

- *Health, United States, 2006*, from the National Center for Health Statistics: http://www.cdc.gov/nchs/hus.htm

- *Morbidity and Mortality Weekly Report* from the Centers for Disease Control and Prevention: http://www.cdc.gov/mmwr

- *Mental Health, United States, 2002*, from the National Mental Health Information Center: http://www.mentalhealth.samhsa.gov/publications/allpubs/SMA04-3938/default.asp

The American Medical Association and the American Hospital Association periodically publish data on physicians and health services institutions, respectively.

Unpublished data can be directly obtained from institutions or investigators. The national-level health surveys described in Chapter 3 can be purchased from the federal agencies sponsoring the surveys. Hospitals, insurance companies, and other health services institutions routinely collect data on their patients and clients. Many private foundations, research institutes, and individual researchers have conducted studies on a range of health-related topics. Researchers may negotiate with institutions or individuals to gain access to their data. Official documents kept by agencies can also be important sources of information, particularly in qualitative research.

Access to unpublished data, particularly administrative and patient records that are created for nonresearch purposes, is subject to regulatory constraint. For example, the **Health Insurance Portability and Accountability Act (HIPAA)**, enacted by the U.S. Congress in 1996, requires the establishment of national standards for electronic health care transactions and national identifiers for providers, health insurance plans, and employers. Provisions of the HIPAA also address the security and privacy of health data, establishing minimum federal standards for protecting the privacy of individually identifiable health information (as published in the *Federal Register*, August 14, 2002). These include an individual's rights to access and amend their personal health information and to obtain a record of when and why this information has been shared with others. Institution Review Board approval of studies is also required.

Figure 13.1. Health research data collection methods

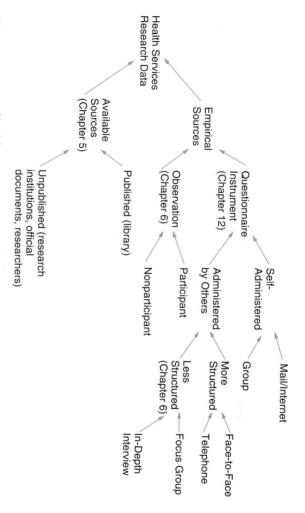

Restrictions stipulated by the HIPAA have affected the ability of investigators to perform retrospective, chart-based research as well as their ability to prospectively evaluate patients by contacting them for follow-up. In addition, informed consent forms for research studies are now required to include extensive detail on the benefits versus harm to study participants, rights of anonymity and confidentiality, and how the participants' protected health information will be kept private. While such information is important, the addition of a lengthy, legalistic section on privacy may make these already complex documents even less user friendly for patients who are asked to read and sign them. Thus, the HIPAA privacy rule, as currently implemented, may be having a negative impact on the cost and quality of medical research (Armstrong et al., 2005; Fisher Wilson, 2006).

Empirical data originate with the research and may be collected either with a data collection instrument (e.g., questionnaire) or through observational methods. As is presented in Chapter 6, the purpose of observational methods is to learn about things firsthand. Observation can occur in many settings: homes, communities, organizations, programs, and so on. Observational data help describe the research setting, the activities that took place in that setting, the people who participated in these activities, and the meaning of what was observed from the perspective of those observed (Patton, 2002). Observation may be conducted either as a participant or nonparticipant. A participant-observer is one who is immersed in the research setting, learning to think, see, feel, and sometimes act as an insider (Powdermaker, 1966, p. 9). A nonparticipant-observer describes the program to outsiders as an insider. A nonparticipant-observer is an onlooker who sees what is happening but does not become involved. There are, however, many variations along the continuum between participation and nonparticipation.

Collecting data with a prepared instrument is the most common method of data collection in HSR. The issues regarding the construction of research instruments were covered in Chapter 12. The data collection instrument may be self-administered by subjects who fill it out themselves, or administered by researchers. The mail questionnaire survey is the most common self-administered data collection method. The questionnaire, containing a list of information or opinion questions, is mailed to potential respondents representative of the research population. The respondents are asked to complete the questionnaire and return it by mail.

As discussed in Chapter 8, the use of the Internet to deliver self-administered questionnaires is growing in popularity. Further, Internet-based surveys save time and money. Questionnaires may also be self-administered in group settings, where the questionnaire is distributed to group members who are asked to complete and return the instrument either right away or sometime later. Examples of groups include classroom students, workplace employees, and association and club members.

When researchers or trained staff administer questionnaires to respondents, they may do so in a more or less structured manner. The more structured methods include face-to-face interviews and telephone interviews. In the face-to-face interview, the interviewer administers a highly structured questionnaire with a planned series of questions to a respondent. The interviewer records the respondent's answers by checking off relevant categories in close-ended questions and taking notes in open-ended questions. In the telephone interview, researchers first locate potential respondents by telephone before administering the prepared research instrument. Almost all residences in the United States now have telephones. The probability of social-class bias due to telephone availability has greatly diminished (Groves, 1980). With the increasing availability of telephones, the telephone survey is fast becoming a popular data collection method. However, an increasing number of people, particularly those from upper-income households, choose not to list their numbers. Researchers may use random digit dialing, which selects telephone numbers based on tables of random numbers. With random digit dialing, even unlisted numbers have an equal probability of being selected.

The less-structured data collection methods include focus group studies and in-depth interviews. As described in Chapter 6, both are common qualitative research methods. While the in-depth interview refers to a one-on-one interview, the focus group study involves several respondents at a time. In both methods, rather than strictly following the predetermined questions from a questionnaire instrument, interviewers encourage respondents to freely discuss their thoughts, asking questions spontaneously based on the flow of conversation. Often researchers come into the interview with a topic in mind and an interview guide, which may be modified in the course of the interview.

COMPARISONS

Each data collection method has its own strengths and weaknesses. This section compares data collected using the various sources presented earlier. Tables 13.1 and 13.2 summarize the comparisons. It should be pointed out that the relative strengths and weaknesses are based on general observations and may not apply to each individual study.

Available versus Empirical Sources

Using available sources generally saves money, effort, and time. It is also a more efficient way of achieving a large sample size. When the research budget is limited, using available data may be the only viable choice. Data collected empirically, however, tend to be more relevant to the research topic because researchers can design studies according to the intended purpose. Access can be a problem for both available and empirical sources and is an important consideration in determining data sources. Table 13.1 summarizes these differences in column 1.

Table 13.1. Comparison of data collection methods

	(1)		(2) Available Sources		(3) Empirical Sources	
	Available Sources	Empirical Sources	Published	Unpublished	Instrument	Observation
Data collection costs	+	−	+	−	+	−
Data collection time	+	−	+	−	+	−
Data collection effort	+	−	+	−	−	+
Sample size for a given budget	+	−	−	+	+	−
Data usability	−	+	−	+	?	?

Note: "+" indicates a relative strength; "−" indicates a relative weakness; "?" indicates uncertainty.

Published versus Unpublished Sources

Among available sources, using published sources saves time and money and allows relatively easy access. A fundamental weakness of published sources is that often only aggregate summaries are presented, making secondary analysis difficult and sometimes impossible. Unpublished sources are generally more helpful to the researcher, offering raw data and large sample sizes, but gaining access may be difficult, particularly when the data set contains sensitive questions or is considered confidential. Table 13.1 summarizes these differences under column 2.

Instrument versus Observation Sources

Research based on a prepared instrument generally saves time and cost in data collection, thus increasing the sample size for a given budget. The data collected tend to be more uniform, thus facilitating analysis. However, gaining access to respondents is a potential challenge. Observational methods, on the other hand, have relatively few problems with access but involve a greater time commitment. They are more appropriate for finding out how people behave in public, but less appropriate for learning how people behave in private, or what people think. However, observation approaches focus on reality rather than on perceived reality. Table 13.1 summarizes these differences under column 3.

Instrument-Based Data Collection Methods

Table 13.2 compares data collection methods using research instruments, including self-administered mail, Internet, or group surveys; face-to-face or telephone interviews; focus group studies; and in-depth interviews. The following paragraphs summarize the principal strengths and weaknesses concerning their impact on research projects, respondents, interviewers, and instruments. Again, these comparative strengths and weaknesses are based on general observations and may not apply to each individual study.

Table 13.2. Comparison of data collection methods using research instruments

	Self-administered			Administered by others		
	Mail	Internet	Group	Face-to-Face Interview	Telephone Interview	Focus Group
Research project						
Data collection costs	+	+	+	−	−	−
Data collection time	−	+	+	−	+	−
Data collection effort	+	+	−	−	−	+
Sample size for a given budget	+	+	−	−	−	−
Data usability	−	−	−	+	+	−
Respondents						
Dispersed sample	+	+	−	−	+	−
Low literacy level	−	−	−	+	+	+
Degree of privacy	+	+	+	−	−	−
Rate of nonresponse	−	−	+	?	?	+
Interviewer						
Need interaction with respondents	−	−	−	+	?	+
Presentation of visual aids	+	+	+	+	−	+
Degree of interview bias	+	+	+	−	+	−
Degree of fieldwork training	+	+	−	−	−	+
Instrument						
Length of survey	−	−	−	+	−	+
Response to sensitive questions	+	−	?	−	−	+
Check other sources for information	+	+	+	−	−	+
Independent work	+	+	+	−	−	+
Uniformity of questions	+	+	+	+	+	−
Sequencing of questions	−	−	−	+	+	−
Completion rate	−	−	−	+	?	+

Note: "+" indicates a relative strength; "−" indicates a relative weakness; "?" indicates uncertainty.

Impact on Research Projects

Data Collection Costs

Self-administered data collection methods such as mail, Internet, and group questionnaires have the lowest overall costs. Most of the costs are incurred in such categories as postage, printing, web interface design, and supplies. The significant savings is in labor. Interview methods have relatively higher costs in all phases of their operation: staff recruiting, training, supervision, travel, the interview itself, and sometimes lodging and meals. Focus group studies and in-depth interviews are potentially most costly due to their labor-intensive nature. Face-to-face interviews, although requiring interviewers as well, are less costly because the interview is more structured and takes considerably less time. Telephone interviews are even less costly due to savings in travel and related expenses, including personnel and gasoline (Groves and Kahn, 1979; Lavrakas, 1993). The telephone interview also saves money spent on staff supervision. Rather than sending numerous supervisors to the field to monitor face-to-face interviews, telephone interviews allow one supervisor to oversee several interviewers calling from the same office. In addition, callbacks are made more easily and economically than with the face-to-face interview.

Data Collection Time

The group self-administered questionnaire offers the greatest savings in time spent on data collection. Web-based surveys and e-mail questionnaires are also very time efficient, as the electronic data from the respondent is collected automatically (Dillman, 2000). The mail questionnaire tends to be most time consuming mainly due to processing and transit times. The telephone interview saves travel time compared to the face-to-face interview. Additional time is saved with the use of a **computer-assisted telephone interview (CATI)** system, in which survey questionnaires are displayed on computer terminals for interviewers, who type respondents' answers directly into the computer. The focus group method, although involving travel, collects data from a number of people simultaneously, thus saving time on a per-respondent basis when compared with in-depth interviews.

Data Collection Effort

While all data collection methods require researchers to devote a lot of energy, focus groups and in-depth interviews demand the greatest effort on the part of interviewers. Face-to-face and telephone interviews require less, though still significant, effort from interviewers. Self-administered methods, on the other hand, require the least effort. The group method calls for greater effort than mail or Internet surveys because of the required physical presence of the researcher should questions arise.

Sample Size

For a given budget, self-administered methods can achieve the greatest sample size, mainly due to savings in labor. Focus groups and in-depth interviews yield the smallest sample size because of added labor costs and lengthy interviews. Telephone interviews yield a larger sample than do face-to-face interviews because of the savings in travel costs.

Data Usability

If data usability is measured by the validity of respondents' statements, then qualitative methods achieve higher usability than quantitative methods. This is because qualitative methods allow for the truly in-depth exploration of important issues. Quantitative methods, such as mail and Internet surveys, achieve relatively low quality because response validity depends on the ability and willingness of respondents to provide information. Respondents who have trouble understanding and interpreting questions cannot receive any help from researchers, and researchers cannot observe which respondents are reluctant or evasive in answering certain questions. Among qualitative methods, in-depth interviews have higher validity than focus groups. While the in-depth interview can better ensure privacy and confidentiality, the focus group is more suitable for assessing the impact of group interactions.

If data usability is measured by the reliability of responses, then focus groups and in-depth interviews may present the greatest problem because they are not readily susceptible to codification and comparability. Open-ended questions need to be coded, and careful independent observers should establish the validity and reliability of the coding. Other methods have greater uniformity in the manner in which questions are posed.

Impact on Respondents

Dispersed Sample

When potential respondents are geographically dispersed, mail and Internet surveys and telephone interviews are the preferred methods because they afford wider geographic contact by reaching people who are difficult to locate and interview. Indeed, it costs no more to conduct a national mail survey than a local one. Group and other interview methods can be difficult because respondents may have to travel a long distance to the researcher, or vice versa. The cost of a national interview survey would be far greater than one conducted at the local level.

Literacy Level

When potential respondents cannot read and write, self-administered methods are automatically excluded from consideration. Among the remaining methods, the telephone interview poses greater problems than does the personal interview because of long-distance communication and lack of in-person contact.

Privacy

When proper precautions are taken, mail and Internet surveys afford the greatest privacy to respondents. Questionnaires administered in group settings also provide significant privacy because responses can be given anonymously. The focus group interview is the least private because each participant is heard by other participants, in addition to the interviewer. Other interview methods have comparatively greater privacy: only the interviewer knows who the respondents are and what they say.

Response Rate

High nonresponse rates are perhaps the greatest problem of the mail survey method (and increasingly for web-based surveys). Furthermore, it is difficult to separate bad addresses from nonresponses. In contrast, personal interviews generally have higher response rates. Since respondents of the group method are generally a captive audience (e.g., students, employees, members, patients, conference participants), response rates tend to be high. Telephone interviews yield higher responses than mail surveys but lower than personal interviews. The telephone interview requires greater effort in training interviewers, introducing the study to respondents, and monitoring the interview procedures (Groves and Kahn, 1979, p. 217). Higher nonresponse rates in telephone versus personal interviews reflect the difficulty in establishing a rapport between respondents and interviewers over the telephone. Further, it suggests that respondents find such interviews to be less rewarding and more of a chore than personal interviews. The proliferation of bogus telephone surveys (i.e., telemarketing in the guise of research), the use of answering machines as screening devices, and the ease with which people can hang up also contribute to a low rate of response.

A low response rate is not a problem in itself. Questionnaires can be sent to a greater number of people to achieve the desired sample size. What is problematic is that respondents and nonrespondents are generally significantly different with respect to the research interest. Typically, responses are bimodal, with those for and against the issue responding and those who are indifferent not responding. Such an unrepresentative sample will likely produce biased results.

Impact on Interviewers

Interaction with Respondents

Mail and Internet surveys do not allow any interaction between researchers and respondents. Group surveys allow some interaction when researchers help clarify a particular statement. Telephone interviewers may also clarify misinterpretations, but the phone interview affords limited interaction due to lack of in-person contact. Personal interviews, particularly focus group studies and in-depth interviews that are not constrained by predominantly close-ended questions, afford significantly greater interaction.

Direct interviewer–respondent interaction has many advantages. In addition to clearing up seemingly inaccurate answers by restating or explaining the questions, interviewers can control which individuals answer the questions, secure more spontaneous reactions, ensure that every relevant item is answered, and collect valuable supplementary information about respondents' personal characteristics and environment. Interaction also improves responses to open-ended questions because interviewers can elicit fuller, more complete responses than questionnaires requiring respondents to write out answers. This is particularly true with respondents whose writing skills are weak or who are less motivated to make the effort to respond fully.

Visual Aid

Telephone interviews cannot use visual aids to help explain questions. With all other methods of data collection, visual material can be presented to various extents. Mail and Internet surveys can use pictures in the questionnaire, whereas personal interviewers can show various kinds of visual aids, including videos, photos, drawings, cards, objects, and so on. Cards showing response options are useful when the options are difficult to remember or when respondents may feel embarrassed to say the options aloud.

Bias

Unfortunately, interviews may also introduce biases as a result of interactions with respondents. Biases may originate from either the interviewer or respondent. Interviewers may fail to follow the interview schedule in the prescribed manner or may suggest answers to respondents. Bias also may be introduced through a respondent's reaction to the interviewer's gender, race, manner of dress, or personality. Common sources of respondent-originated bias include social desirability, acquiescence, auspices, prestige, and mental set. **Social desirability** refers to responses based on what is perceived as being socially acceptable or respectable, positive or negative. **Acquiescence** involves responses based on the respondent's perception of what would be desirable to the interviewer. **Auspices** are responses dictated by an opinion or image of the sponsor, rather than the actual question. Responses intended to improve the image of the respondent in the eyes of the interviewer are known as **prestige. Mental set** refers to responses to later items influenced by perceptions based on previous items.

Biases are more likely to be introduced in focus group studies and in-depth interviews. Interviewers with certain biases may unconsciously ask questions so as to secure confirmation of their own views. In face-to-face and telephone interviews, the effect is lessened because the instrument is more structured and there is less opportunity for interviewers to ad-lib.

Training

To reduce interviewer biases, interview methods, whether conducted face-to-face or by telephone, require well-trained personnel. Interviewers need to be trained to build a rapport with respondents and to conceal personal values or avoid letting their values affect the interview process. Building a rapport over the telephone is particularly challenging because the respondents are called to the telephone unexpectedly and asked to do something they are not prepared for or do not fully understand. They may be in the middle of other activities (e.g., preparing meals, looking after children, or watching television). They may not be in the mood to talk to strangers. Interviewers may have to prove their legitimacy and the worth of the time granted to them by reluctant respondents. It is even harder to train facilitators for focus group studies and in-depth interviews. Interviewers not only need to know the proper way of conducting interviews so as not to introduce biases, but they also need to be very familiar with the research topic so that they can ask the right questions.

Potential interviewers should have a good command of both the spoken and written language. They must understand and believe in the purpose of the study, and they need to be familiar with the specific questionnaire items. Desirable qualities of good interviewers include being tactful, careful, sensitive, polite, accurate, adaptable, consistent, interested, honest, assertive (but sensitive enough to know when to be less assertive), persevering, and able to withstand tiring and sometimes boring work. Evening and weekend work is often necessary. Part-time work may be preferable due to the repetitive nature of interviews.

Interviewer training includes instructions on how to contact a respondent to obtain an interview, how questions must be asked (e.g., order, meaning, and probing), and behaviors to avoid that tend to inhibit respondents (e.g., interrupting, disagreeing, and frowning). Before beginning fieldwork, trainees should observe trained interviewers and practice interviews. Role-playing simulations may be set up in which prospective interviewers interview each other with the instructor commenting on proper procedures and mistakes. An interview manual should be prepared that covers techniques specific to the study, including neutral probes and instructions on how to handle problems. For example, in dealing with reluctant respondents, interviewers should be patient and explicit, explaining what will be required and offering some sample questions. The following summarizes the common dos and don'ts for interviewers (Bailey, 1994; Miller and Salkind, 2002).

Do's

- dress formally to legitimize your role as an interviewer, and unobtrusively to avoid attention being diverted to your appearance
- introduce yourself and your sponsor to the respondent
- explain the purpose of the study, its significance, and the expected length of the interview
- tell how the respondent was chosen, assure confidentiality, and ask for permission to conduct the interview
- follow the interview guide closely by asking questions as worded, maintaining the same sequence, and using similar inflection and intonation
- use neutral probes when respondents ask for clarification or express confusion by restating the question, repeating the answer, and explaining the meaning of certain words and phrases in the same manner to all respondents
- record respondents' answers exactly as given
- thank the respondent for his or her time and leave the name and telephone number of the contact person in case there are questions

Don'ts

- do not provide false information concerning the purpose of the study, its expected length, or its benefits to respondents
- do not alter the questionnaire by omitting certain questions or changing question wording
- do not use biased probing by asking leading questions or offering suggestive answers

- do not interpret or modify respondents' answers
- do not assume respondents' answers before asking the questions
- if you made any promise to respondents such as sending them the study results, do not forget to follow through

During fieldwork, interviewers should be monitored from time to time to maintain quality control. Regular meetings should be held to collect questionnaires, answer questions, review completed questionnaires, share problems and solutions, and improve morale.

Impact on Instruments

Length

Compared with interviews, when using self-administered methods, shorter questionnaires are generally preferred. Among interview methods, telephone surveys, which offer the least control over respondents' behavior, require a relatively short instrument. In face-to-face interviews, the length of the interaction usually does not affect refusal rate once respondents agree to the process. Focus group studies and in-depth interviews are usually much longer than structured face-to-face interviews.

Sensitive Questions

When sensitive questions are posed, the in-depth interview is most likely to obtain truthful responses. In group-based methods, obtaining frank responses can be quite a challenge given the lack of confidentiality. Methods that make establishing a rapport with respondents difficult, including mail and telephone interviews, also are less appropriate for sensitive questions unless complete confidentiality is assured.

Checking Other Sources

When the goal of research is to collect specialized information, the mail survey is the most appropriate choice because it provides the opportunity for more considered answers and for respondents to check and secure information or consult with others. Methods that require respondents to provide answers spontaneously are less suitable for questions that demand more specialized knowledge. The focus group method is relatively less problematic because presumably someone within the focus group knows the answers.

Independent Work

When the goal is to find out whether the respondent possesses a particular piece of knowledge or information, methods requiring spontaneous answers are more suitable than mail or Internet surveys, where the intended respondent may not be the actual respondent. The focus group method is not appropriate for knowledge questions because the person responding to a question may or may not be the only person who knows the answer.

Uniformity

Highly structured data collection methods yield more uniform answers than less-structured methods, such as focus group studies and in-depth interviews. Among structured methods, interviews, whether face-to-face or by telephone, yield less uniform results than mail, Internet, or group surveys because of the potential for interviewer effect.

Sequencing

When sequencing of questions is important, interview methods are more appropriate than mail, Internet, or group surveys because interviewers can control the order in which questions are asked. Mail or group surveys cannot prevent respondents from reading ahead or changing earlier answers based on later information. However, Internet surveys can control for this by not allowing a respondent to move to the next screen until he or she completes the first screen. In addition, both face-to-face interviews and Internet surveys may use a question-skip format, in which certain questions are passed over when they do not apply to a particular respondent. Such a format could be confusing for respondents completing a questionnaire.

Completion Rate

Completion rates are highest among personal interview methods where interviewers have greater control and can be trained to elicit responses to every question. In mail or group survey methods, respondents have greater control and can skip questions if they want. Tedious or sensitive items can be passed over easily. Thus, there are usually more missing values in self-administered methods than there are in interviews. The problem of missing items may be alleviated somewhat by instructions stressing the need to answer every item, assuring confidentiality, and making items easy to understand.

Choices Among Methods

In deciding which data collection methods to use, researchers compare the strengths and weaknesses of these methods with their unique research situation and select those that optimally match their situation. Sometimes it is obvious which method should be used. If many respondents are illiterate, then interview methods rather than self-administered questionnaires have to be used. When research funding is limited, a cheaper method, such as a mail or an Internet survey, may be the only viable choice. The nature of the questions also dictates which method should be chosen. If many of the questions are sensitive, greater honesty and validity of response may be obtained through self-administered methods, which, compared with interviews, offer greater anonymity and confidentiality. Many situations, however, are not so clear-cut. Researchers have to weigh the pros and cons of various methods and select the most appropriate ones. To facilitate choosing the right method, researchers should be familiar with the conditions most appropriate to each data collection method.

The conditions required for a self-administered mail questionnaire include: (1) literate respondents, (2) relatively simple and straightforward questions and instructions, (3) nonspecific ordering of questionnaire items, and (4) validity of responses unaffected by the use of outside sources for information. In addition, the self-administered mail questionnaire is most appropriate when the research budget is limited, when a large sample size is desired, when a sampling list representative of the study population is readily available, when the sample is more dispersed, when privacy is important, and when respondents have to check other sources to give appropriate responses.

The conditions necessary for administering an e-mail or web survey are similar to the conditions necessary for a self-administered mail questionnaire. An obvious additional condition for an Internet survey is that the respondents have access to a computer and to the Internet. Internet surveys are preferable when: (1) respondents are spread across a broad geographic area, (2) respondents are computer-literate and have easy access to the Internet, and (3) rapid data collection is desired.

The conditions for a self-administered group survey are as follows: (1) respondents can be gathered in the same setting, (2) the gathered respondents are representative of the research population, and (3) the ordering of questionnaire items is not important. The self-administered group survey can be used for respondents who are less educated than those in a mail survey situation. With the assistance of the researcher, survey questions and instructions can be relatively more difficult. The method is appropriate when research budget and time are both limited, and consultation with other sources for information is not allowed.

The conditions for a face-to-face interview include: (1) researchers have access to respondents or organizations in which respondents are located, (2) interviewers are adequately trained to perform the interview in an unbiased manner, and (3) a sufficient budget exists for performing an adequate number of interviews. The face-to-face interview is preferred when: (1) respondents are illiterate or have little education and interviewers have to do the recording, (2) interaction with the respondents is required, (3) the sample size is relatively small, (4) respondents are concentrated in a confined geographic area, (5) the order of the questions is important, (6) the questions are relatively complex and difficult, (7) the questions are not so sensitive that respondents feel threatened or embarrassed about answering them, (8) visual aids have to be used, (9) the research instrument is relatively lengthy, and (10) checking other sources for information is not allowed.

A telephone interview requires that a telephone directory or other lists serve as a representative sample frame and interviewers are properly trained to establish a rapport with respondents within a short time. The telephone interview is preferred when: (1) respondents are spread out geographically, (2) rapid data collection is needed, (3) the questionnaire is relatively short and easy, (4) question sequence is important, (5) questions are somewhat sensitive and anonymity of response is desired, (6) no visual aid is required, (7) respondents are not permitted to receive help in answering questions, (8) respondents are illiterate or have little education, and (9) the research setting is unimportant.

Both the focus group and the in-depth interview may be used either at the initial stage of research, to identify issues and measures to be used in the survey instrument, or after the survey research, to collect additional information that explores the factors and details associated with survey findings. Both methods are time consuming and require a small sample size. They are the most valid ways to collect qualitative data and sensitive information. Both demand greater interviewer skill with the language and techniques that encourage respondents to speak frankly and at length. Interviewers and facilitators should also have considerable knowledge about the research topic. However, quantitative analysis of the collected information is difficult. The data elements obtained can vary significantly among subjects depending on their interests and the approach adopted by the interviewer or facilitator. It is difficult to code and use these data in a quantitative way.

However, focus groups and in-depth interviews also differ in significant ways. While the focus group is a good medium for getting an exhaustive inventory of reactions, feelings, ideas, issues, or aspects of a problem or topic out on the table, it is less successful in measuring the frequency or intensity of attitudes or perceptions. This is due to a number of factors including the operation of group dynamics and interpersonal influence processes whereby some ideas are expressed and others repressed due to the personalities of individuals. There are also conformity pressures that may cause people to change or adjust their ideas based on others in the group. With a good rapport and measures to ensure confidentiality, the face-to-face interview can garner very high-quality data in terms of what people think and feel.

In many situations, researchers may combine different data collection methods in the same research. For example, the focus group study may be used first to explore important issues related to the topic that may be incorporated in the research instrument. Mail surveys may be used in combination with telephone and personal interviews to improve the response rate. Telephone interviews may be used as a screening method to determine study eligibility before face-to-face interviews. On the other hand, respondents may be notified via mail, with follow-up taking the form of a telephone interview. An in-depth interview may be used to obtain more thorough understanding of the topic.

IMPROVING RESPONSE RATES

A high response rate is critical for research results to be valid. Many researchers believe an adequate response rate should be at least 50 percent (Babbie, 1990). Major national surveys such as the National Health Interview Survey and Medical Expenditure Panel Survey have consistently achieved response rates of more than 90 percent. A high response rate can mean that those who answered the questionnaire differ significantly from nonrespondents, thereby biasing the sample. In most situations, nonrespondents tend to be less educated, less wealthy, or less interested in the research topic. Research thus has an inherent bias toward overrepresenting the better-educated population and underrepresenting the poor and minorities. As a minimum effort, researchers should take care to assess how nonrespondents compare with respondents. Examples include using registered letters, telephone calls, personal interviews, and so on (Wallace, 1954).

More important, researchers should incorporate various means of improving response rates in the data collection process. The following, as summarized in Table 13.3, presents these measures as well as their relative need for different data collection methods.

Follow-up Efforts

Intensive follow-up efforts are the best means to increase returns. When completed questionnaires are returned, they should be assigned serial identification numbers so that researchers can keep track of returns and facilitate follow-up. Follow-up is particularly important for mail surveys and telephone interviews. Often, more than one follow-up may be needed. In their comprehensive reviews of published studies, Herberlein and Baumgartner (1978) found that the average response rate for the initial mailing was 48 percent (based on 183 studies). The response rate increased by an additional 20 percent with a second mailing (based on 58 studies), 12 percent with a third mailing (based on 40 studies), and 10 percent with a fourth (based on 25 studies).

Table 13.3. Methods of data collection and means to improve response rate

	Self-Administered			Administered by Others			
	Mail	Internet	Group	Face-to-Face Interview	Telephone Interview	Focus Group	In-Depth Interview
Follow-up	5	5	3	2	4	1	1
Sponsor	5	5	5	4	5	4	4
Length	5	5	4	2	4	1	1
Introductory letter	5	5	2	3	4	1	1
Types of questions	5	5	3	1	4	1	1
Inducement	3	3	3	4	4	5	5
Type of population	5	5	3	3	4	2	1
Anonymity/confidentiality	5	2	3	3	4	1	5
Time of contact	4	4	4	3	5	1	1
Method of return	5	1	1	1	1	1	1

Note: A Likert-type scale ranging from 1 to 5 is used, with 5 indicating the most effective approach to improving response rate and 1 indicating the least effective.

Telephones can often be used effectively for follow-up. Researchers can find out if a respondent needs another copy of the questionnaire to replace the original one, which may have been destroyed or misplaced. The telephone may be used to collect information directly from respondents, especially when the questionnaire is relatively short and the respondent has lost the form. Waves of mailed questionnaires and a final telephone interview can generate a very high response rate. The research experience of Community and Migrant Health Center administrators indicates that a second mailing after a three-week interval improves the response rate from 50 to 70 percent (Shi, Samuels, and Glover, 1994). Then contact by telephone, after the second mailing, improves response rate by an additional 15 percent.

Sponsor

The appeal of the sponsor is an important factor in improving the response rate. Preferably, the sponsor should be a person or agency that the respondents know and respect. Examples of legitimate sponsors are scientific organizations, government agencies, universities, professional associations, and well-known nonprofit agencies. A cover letter from the prestigious and respected sponsor making an appeal to respondents can significantly influence returns. The sponsor factor is important for all data collection methods, particularly those where little or no direct personal contact is involved and where establishing a rapport with respondents is difficult.

Length

The length of a questionnaire is critical with respect to response rate, particularly when it comes to mail surveys and other methods where researchers have no or limited personal contact with respondents. For these methods, the shorter the questionnaire, the higher the response rate (Berdie, 1973). For face-to-face interviews, the length of the instrument is less critical. Respondents who have agreed to be interviewed generally do not mind if the questionnaire is somewhat lengthy.

Introductory Letter

An introductory or cover letter explains the nature and purpose of the research and stresses its importance. A good cover letter is short and concise. It should not exceed one page in length. The letter ends with a solicitation to participate. Use of an actual signature on the cover letter is more appealing than using copies of a signed cover letter. The personalization of large numbers of letters can be accomplished with word processing software using the Replace command so that the respondent's name and address can be inserted into the body of the text.

An introductory letter is particularly important for survey methods where researchers have the least control over respondents' behavior, and respondents have the greatest need for motivation. An introductory letter may be sent by mail prior to the telephone interviews to explain the study and inform recipients that a representative will call soon. This way they are not caught by surprise. Just like a consent form, the content and structure of a cover letter are often strongly determined by the researcher's IRB, as appropriate.

Types of Questions

With respect to response rate, the questions used for mail surveys are more critical than the ones used for other methods. In general, respondents are more likely to complete questions that are interesting, relevant, or judged as salient to them. Questionnaires asking for objective information receive a better response rate than those asking for subjective information. Those containing simpler questions receive better returns than those with difficult questions or ones that require consultation with additional sources. The response rate drops substantially if questions probe areas regarded by respondents as private, sensitive, and/or a threat to them or their immediate groups. Examples of sensitive questions include those that ask about sexual behavior, deviant behavior (e.g., drug use and smoking), income, and education level. Questionnaires using a complex format also receive lower responses. A survey with many contingency items is too confusing for the average respondent. Complex questionnaires may be used in an interview when interviewers have been given extensive training in the format and skip patterns. Finally, clean, neat, less-cluttered, and straightforward questionnaires improve response rates.

Inducement

Researchers may offer certain inducements to enhance response rates. Inducements can be financial or nonfinancial. Financial incentives are provided particularly when the questionnaire or interview is lengthy and research results are important (Armstrong, 1975). The problem with offering financial inducement, besides its costliness, is that some respondents will be offended that the researcher considers their time to be worth so little.

Nonfinancial inducements include sending reports of study results to respondents, enclosing a souvenir such as a ballpoint pen, emphasizing study significance, or making an altruistic appeal. Nonfinancial means are preferred if monetary inducement is insignificant. Using a deadline is another nonfinancial inducement. Its advantage is that respondents can plan to complete the questionnaire based on the deadline. Its disadvantage is that once the deadline is passed, respondents may assume it is too late to return the survey and throw it away instead.

Type of Population

Response rates vary significantly with the type of population surveyed or interviewed. Response generally varies with education, income, and occupation. Better-educated people are more likely to return surveys, and among the educated, professionals and those who are wealthier are more likely to return them (Herberlein and Baumgartner, 1978). Minority populations have lower response rates than white populations. Ensuring accurate and appropriate translation or interpretation services helps improve response in non-English-speaking populations (Bowling, 1997).

Anonymity/Confidentiality

Among data collection methods, only self-administered methods and telephone interviews are capable of maintaining anonymity. The anonymous nature of surveys enhances the response rate, particularly when questions are sensitive. The downside of anonymity is that follow-up is not possible. An alternative is to send everyone a second questionnaire with the instruction to disregard it if they have already completed and returned the first one. However, this method is expensive, particularly when the sample size is large. Questionnaires using identification codes to track responses are not truly anonymous because they can be traced to individual respondents. Another method for identifying non-respondents while maintaining anonymity involves mailing a postcard with the questionnaire to the respondents. The postcard contains the respondent's name and address. Respondents are asked to return the postcard when they complete the questionnaire. The questionnaire is mailed back separately with no name or identification code (Babbie, 1990, 2006; Bailey, 1994). Because of the difficulty and deficiency of anonymity, most researchers promise complete confidentiality rather than anonymity to improve the response rate.

Time of Contact

The time chosen to contact respondents for interviews or to send questionnaires in mail surveys can play a significant role in returns. When respondents are working, they are best located at the end of the day or during weekends. The questionnaire, if sent home, should arrive near the end of the week. When sending questionnaires to administrators in organizations, summer or near a holiday season is the worst time because many people are gone for vacation.

Method of Return

The method of returning completed questionnaires may be psychologically important to respondents. Including a stamped (preferably with a new commemorative stamp), self-addressed envelope adds a personal touch and produces better results than business-reply or metered envelopes. If the questionnaire is short and simple, double postcards may be used as a convenient way to secure returns. A double postcard contains the questionnaire as well as the return address so that respondents, upon receiving the postcard, can easily fill out the questionnaire, fold it up, and mail it back to the researcher.

QUESTIONNAIRE CODING

Coding consists of assigning numbers to questionnaire answer categories and specifying column locations for these numbers in the computer data file. Such standardization and quantification of data is necessary in order to permit computer storage, retrieval, manipulation, and statistical analysis. Coding is a critical part of data preparation.

In general, data should be coded into relatively more categories to maintain details. Code categories can always be combined during data analysis if it is deemed that less-detailed categories are more desirable. Conversely, if too few categories are used, it is impossible to capture the original detail. Code categories should be both exhaustive and mutually exclusive. Every data element should fit into one, and only one, category. Code categories may be determined before data collection (i.e., precode) or after data collection (i.e., postcode or recode). A codebook is usually prepared after data collection.

Precoding

Precoding assigns numbers to data categories and indicates their column locations prior to data collection. Precoding is also called deductive coding because previous knowledge or theory was used to construct response categories (Bowling, 1997). Assigning columns may be unnecessary if data are directly entered into a statistical program or spreadsheet that assigns a field instead of columns to each variable. Precoding can be prepared when the questionnaire is being written so that coding categories and column locations appear in the questionnaire instrument itself. Because data collected by surveys are typically transformed into some type of computer format, it is usually appropriate to include data-processing instructions on the questionnaire itself. These instructions indicate where specific pieces of information will be stored in the machine-readable data files.

Figure 13.2 presents a precoded questionnaire studying respondents' attitudes toward a single-payer health care system. Precoding appearing in the margin of a questionnaire is also called edge-coding. Note the numerical codes in the right-hand margin of the questionnaire, which indicate the column location for the questions. For example, Question 6 requires respondents to check only one answer. The number in the right-hand margin, 20, indicates the column of the computer data file in which the code for Question 6 is to be entered.

When a code for a particular variable is greater than nine, then two columns must be used to code one variable. Question 1, for example, requires respondents to record their age. Unless we expect a respondent to be 100 years old or more, two columns will be sufficient to capture all variations in respondents'

age. Question 4 asks about respondents' annual income and uses six columns. More columns may be used if you suspect higher income levels.

When multiple answers to a single question are needed, as in Question 5, they cannot be coded into a single column. Rather, separate columns should be allotted for every potential answer. Such coding is equivalent to transforming one variable containing five different response categories into five variables. Each of the variables now becomes binary, coded either as present (when respondent checks off the response) or absent (when respondent leaves the response blank). For example, suppose a respondent checks off Medicare and Blue Cross/Blue Shield; then the researcher will enter one in column 15, zero in column 16, three in column 17, and zero in columns 18 and 19.

Precoding is also often used in **medical chart review**, which abstracts critical patient and treatment information based on the medical records of the patients. Physicians, nurses, and technicians are required to record in the medical record all information on a patient's current tests, procedures, vitals, and more.

RECORD 1

1. Your current age _____   5–6/

2. Your sex: male (1) female (2)   7/

3. Your race: White (1) Black (2) Asian (3) Other (4) _____   8/

4. What was your annual income last year? $ _____   9–14/

5. Which of the following health insurance plans do you currently have?

   (Check all that apply)

   Medicare   ___ (1)   15/

   Medicaid   ___ (2)   16/

   Blue Cross/Blue Shield ___ (3)   17/

   Other (specify ___)   ___ (4)   18/

   No insurance   ___ (5)   19/

6. Indicate your agreement with a single-payer health care system.   20/

   (Check one only)

   Strongly agree   ___ (1)

   Agree   ___ (2)

   Unsure   ___ (3)

   Disagree   ___ (4)

   Strongly disagree   ___ (5)

Figure 13.2. Mini survey: Single-payer system preference

Diagnostics, medicines, and treatments are also recorded. Medical chart review helps identify the answers to "What happened?" In addition to research questions, legal, personal, medical, and insurance questions can also be answered by medical chart review. Likewise, hospital procedures and medical recommendations benefit from the results of a chart review. During billing processes, medical chart review can prevent unwarranted charges for tests not performed or services not received. The medical chart review can note specific tests were ordered, but not completed. For an example of a medical chart abstract form, refer to the National Ambulatory Medical Survey (http://www.cdc.gov/nchs/data/ahcd/namcs-30_2006.pdf). In addition to medical records, abstracting can also be conducted with health information systems that capture patient care experiences. Figure 13.3 shows a medical encounter abstracting form designed for a patient information system.

Using precoding has two time-saving advantages. In face-to-face interviews, respondents can tell the interviewer the numerical codes for response categories rather than remembering the complete categories and repeating the appropriate one to the interviewer. In self-administered surveys, respondents can jot down the numerical codes in the appropriate spaces rather than writing out the answers. The second time-saving advantage to using precoding is avoiding having to code respondents' answers again. The actual questionnaire can also serve as a codebook that defines the meaning of each numerical code and specifies its column location. Data entry can be accomplished by reading directly from respondents' questionnaires and entering their responses into the computer according to the column locations specified in the right-hand margins. In addition to the saved time from compiling a new codebook and transferring data from the questionnaire to a transfer sheet, using precoded questionnaires also reduces the number of errors made in data transfer.

However, precoding can only be used when questions are close-ended. When researchers cannot predict what answer categories or how many additional "other" categories exist for a given question, open-ended questions have to be used. Postcoding then becomes necessary.

Postcoding

Postcoding assigns numbers to data categories and indicates their column locations after data collection, that is, after respondents have answered the questions in the questionnaire. Postcoding is also called inductive coding because the code is designed after analyzing a representative sample of answers to survey questions (Bowling, 1997). Postcoding is necessary mainly for open-ended questions for which researchers cannot anticipate response categories. For example, the following open-ended question may be added to the single-payer survey as Question 7: "Why are you in favor of, unsure about, or opposed to the 'single-payer' system?" Since we are not certain about all the possible answers to this question, we have to leave it as open-ended. After reviewing the actual responses from respondents, we can decide the number of categories to use and assign numerical codes accordingly.

1. **Unique encounter identifier**
   - Available in IS? (1 = yes, 2 = no)
   - If yes, how is this identifier created? (free text)

2. **User identifier**
   - Available in IS? (1= yes, 2 = no)
   - If yes, how is this identifier created? (free text)
   - Is this identifier unique across PC-Sites? (1 = yes, 2 = no)
   - If there are multiple PCOs, is the identifier unique across PCOs? (1 = yes, 2 = no)

3. **PC-Site identifier**
   - Available in IS? (1 = yes, 2 = no)
   - If yes, how is this identifier created? (free text)
   - If there is more than one PCO, can this identifier be linked to a specific PCO? (1 = yes, 2 = no)

4. **Practitioner identifier**
   - Available in IS? (1 = yes, 2 = no)
   - If yes, how is this identifier created? (free text)
   - Is this identifier unique across PC-Sites? (1= yes, 2 = no)

5. **Diagnosis codes**
   - For each encounter, how many are available in your IS? (count)
   - Does your IS link diagnosis codes to procedure codes in the same record? (1 = yes, 2 = no)

6. **Procedure codes**
   - For each encounter, how many are available in your IS? (count)

7. **Date of service**
   - Year (4 digits), month (2 digits), day (2 digits)
   - Available in your IS? (1 = yes, 2 = no)

8. **Optional item: Medications**
   - Does your IS include medication information? (1 = yes, 2 = no)
     i. If yes, does the IS list medications ordered during an encounter? (1 = yes, 2 = no)
     ii. If yes, are medications linked to a specific diagnosis code? (1 = yes, 2 = no)
   - If your IS does not currently include medication information, would you be willing to collect medication data related to the care of patients with diabetes and related comorbidities? (1 = yes, 2 = no)

Figure 13.3. Medical encounter abstracting form

Questions with "other" as a response category may also need to be postcoded if many people have chosen it as their choice. For example, the "other" category in Question 3, Figure 13.2, may generate many responses from Hispanics. Similarly, the "other" category in Question 5 may generate many answers such as HMO, PPO, or other managed care arrangements. New response categories may be needed to better represent the research population. A rule of thumb is to add new categories when the "other" response accounts for 10 percent or more of the total responses.

Since open-ended questions are the principal reason for postcoding, and postcoding is more labor intensive and time consuming, researchers often use open-ended questions in small-scale exploratory research or qualitative research where the sample size is small. These questions help identify not only the right questions to ask, but also the most common categories for a given question. These findings pave the way for the design of a close-ended and precoded questionnaire instrument to be used for large-scale survey research.

Recoding

Recoding serves to change earlier coding assignments of the attributes of a variable. Similar to postcoding, recoding is done after data have been collected. However, rather than assigning numerical codes to attributes before data analysis, as is the case with postcoding, recoding is generally done after some preliminary data analysis so that researchers have some feel for the nature of the data. Data recoding is also known as process editing, which involves using a computer to edit the data so that the analysis can proceed in the most meaningful manner.

For example, the variable *age* in our single-payer survey may be recoded from a continuous variable into a categorical one (e.g., over 65: old age, 45–64: middle age, under 45: young age) to compare people within different age groups and their attitudes toward a single-payer system. In addition to collapsing categories, other forms of recoding include adding together the responses to several items to form an index, and creating new variables based on combinations or mathematical transformations of existing variables (e.g., creating a dummy variable by assigning one to all those with any form of insurance and zero to those without). The number of variables to be recoded is limited only by the needs of data analysis and the knowledge of researchers.

As another example, the variable *race* is initially obtained using the following categories: Aleut, Eskimo, or Native American; Asian/Pacific Islander; Black; White; Other; Multiple race; and Unknown. "Race" can then be recoded in a number of ways depending on analysis needs. For example, "race1" can be coded as White (1), Black (2), or Other (3). "Race2" can be coded as White (1) or Non-White (2). "Race3" can be coded as Black (1) or Non-Black (2).

Codebook

A **codebook** is a document that describes the locations of different variables and lists the numerical codes assigned to represent different attributes of the variables (Babbie, 2006). Its primary purpose is to assist in the coding process. Like a dictionary, a codebook guides researchers to find the right code for each answer category and to record the code either on a coding sheet or directly into the computer. It may also contain instructions on how to code missing values or errors, such as when two answers are circled for a single-response question.

Table 13.4. Code sheet for mini survey: Opinion toward single-payer system

	RECORD 1 Column Location
Q1. _____	5–6/
Q2. _____	7/
Q3. _____	8/
Q4. _____	9–14/
Q5.1. _____	15/
Q5.2. _____	16/
Q5.3. _____	17/
Q5.4. _____	18/
Q5.5. _____	19/
Q6. _____	20/

Another purpose of a codebook is its utility as a guide in locating variables and interpreting results in data analysis.

When data are assembled from multiple places, a data dictionary may be created. A **data dictionary** contains a list of all files in the database, the number of records in each file, and the names and descriptions of each field. Most database management systems keep the data dictionary hidden from users to prevent them from accidentally destroying its contents. Data dictionaries do not contain any actual data, only bookkeeping information for managing the database. Without a data dictionary, a database management system cannot retrieve data from the database.

Table 13.4 is a **code sheet** for the single-payer survey questionnaire. The code sheet may be called a data transfer sheet because responses from the instrument are recorded or transferred onto the code sheet before they are entered into the computer. A code sheet is usually necessary for a questionnaire with open-ended questions, for which it is impossible to precode. Reading responses from the questionnaire and checking the correct code from the codebook could lead to numerous errors in data entry. Transfer sheets are used to reduce the number of errors. For a precoded questionnaire, as in Table 13.4, a code sheet is usually not necessary because data recorded on the questionnaire can be entered directly into the computer following the column location instructions.

Note that the word *record* indicates the row of the responses. Since our survey example has only six questions, only one record will be needed for each respondent. Lengthier questionnaires require more records per respondent because the number of columns per record is limited.

Table 13.5 presents the codebook for the single-payer survey questionnaire. The codebook is required primarily for open-ended questions. If a questionnaire can be completely precoded, as with our example, the questionnaire itself can be used

Table 13.5. Codebook of mini survey: Opinion toward single-payer system

Question/Statement	Column Location	Variable Name	Codes
	RECORD 1		
Respondent ID	1–3	RESPID	001–200
Coder ID	4	CODERID	1—John
			2—Mary
			3—David
1. Your current age.	5–6	AGE	99—Missing
			Precoded
2. Your sex.	7	SEX	1—male
			2—female
			9—missing
3. Your race.	8	RACE	1—White
			2—Black
			3—Asian
			4—Other
			8—Don't know
			9—Missing
4. What was your annual income last year?	9–14	INCOME	Precoded
			888888 — Don't know
			999999 — Missing
5. Which of the following health insurance plans do you currently have?			
5.1. Medicare	15	MEDICARE	1—Yes
			0—No
5.2. Medicaid	16	MEDICAID	2—Yes
			0—No
5.3. Blue Cross / Blue Shield	17	BLUES	3—Yes
			0—No
5.4. Other	18	OTHER	4—Yes
			0—No
5.5. No insurance	19	NONE	5—Yes
			0—No
6. Indicate your agreement with a single-payer health care system.	20	SINGLPAY	1—Strongly agree
			2—Agree
			3—Unsure
			4—Disagree
			5—Strongly disagree
			9—Missing

as a codebook. Or, if a questionnaire contains predominantly close-ended questions with only one or two open-ended questions near the end, a partial codebook can be prepared separately for the open-ended postcoded questions, and data from close-ended questions can still be entered directly from the questionnaire.

Note that a codebook usually contains the following information: questions or statements, column location, variable name, and codes. Questions or statements are exactly the same as they appear in the questionnaire, serving as a linkage between the questionnaire and the codebook. Column location specifies the exact location in a data file that responses to a particular question or statement are to be placed. Storing information for each variable in the same column of the computer data file for all respondents is known as a **fixed-column format**. The variable name is the abbreviated name of the question or statement and usually contains fewer than eight characters. To facilitate data analysis at a later stage, researchers can assign names that easily remind them of the particular questions or statements. Codes refer to the numerical assignments of the attributes of a given question or statement.

While missing data are usually unavoidable in research, too many missing data points reflects deficiencies in the choice of the data collection method and threatens the validity of the research findings. Missing data is a particularly common problem with mail surveys, where researchers have the least control. Missing data is the result when respondents refuse to be interviewed or fail to answer all the questions in an interview, or when participants drop out of an experiment or program, particularly from the control group, in which little or no benefit is derived. The attrition rate is likely to be higher in longitudinal than in cross-sectional studies.

When nonresponses are received, researchers should devise a consistent scheme for coding them so that they can be easily singled out in data analysis. Investigators should avoid leaving missing values blank because some computer programs may treat blanks as zeros or change the original format of the data file. A conventional solution is to represent missing values with nines, so long as nine is not a legitimate response. For example, if one of the respondents is 99 years old, it would be necessary to use three columns for the variable *age* in order to represent missing values (i.e., 999). Similarly, eights are used to indicate "don't know" responses and sevens are used to indicate "not applicable" responses.

DATA ENTRY

Because health services research typically uses large sets of data, computers, ranging from mainframes to personal computers, are becoming indispensable for data analysis. Increasingly, software is used in data collection to simplify and streamline the process of data collection, entry, processing, and analysis. **Computer-aided personal interviewing (CAPI)** allows for the conducting of the interview by means of a computer rather than a paper questionnaire. With CAPI, the interview is conducted face-to-face, usually employing a laptop computer. The interviewer is prompted with the questions by the computer and response codes are keyed in directly according to the respondent's answers. A routing protocol uses these codes to determine which question is presented next. Since the data are entered directly into the computer, analyses can be produced quickly.

Online survey software allows researchers to easily design, program, and manage web surveys of any size, from small patient satisfaction surveys to large multi-country and multi-lingual tracking studies. Multiple question formats can be designed using animation, split screens, skip patterns, and advanced logic. The CATI software increases interviewer productivity and call-center efficiency through its fast, intuitive interviewer and supervisor interfaces, multiple dialing modes, and robust, user-friendly panel management tool. This personal interviewing software can be used to monitor productivity (e.g., by tracking interview length, dialing reports, and project progress), manage interviewers (e.g., supervise performance and provide timely feedback), report a disposition (e.g., schedule appointments, update contacts, and add notes or comments to the call history), and even provide simultaneous analyses (e.g., set up report formats and analysis filters and provide real-time updates of findings).

The development of portable computers, or laptops, has revolutionized the data collection process. Direct data entry is no longer limited to telephone interviews. The interviewer can easily carry a laptop to the respondent's residence or workplace, read questions off the screen, and record the answers directly into the computer. In addition, computers may be used for self-administered questionnaires where respondents can be asked to sit at computer terminals and enter their own answers to the questions that appear on the screen. Data may be stored on computer disks, and at least one backup copy should be made of the data set.

There are many statistical software packages into which data can be directly entered. These include SAS, SPSS, SYSTAT, Minitab, Statview, Microstat, Stat-Pro, and JUMP, to name just a few. An easier alternative is to enter the data into a spreadsheet package, such as Excel. Data can also be entered into Access and then uploaded into SPSS or other statistical software for analysis. Direct data entry not only saves the time incurred in transferring data from the questionnaire to the electronic data file (a computer file that contains only raw data), but also reduces the chance for data-transfer errors. In addition, data entry in the field, either by interviewers or respondents, is less tedious compared to data entry after collection.

Indeed, data entry is often considered the least glamorous aspect of research. However, "probably at no other stage is there a greater chance of a really horrible error being made" (Davis and Smith, 1992, p. 60). Sources of error include incorrect reading of written codes, incorrect coding of responses, incorrect column location assignment, missed entry, repeated entry, and so forth. Unlike nonresponses or missing values, data entry errors are largely avoidable. Since a mail questionnaire survey still relies on data entry after collection, great effort should be made to reduce error. This effort includes screening personnel so that careless people are weeded out. Those assigned to transfer or enter the data must be trained so that they carry out their tasks to minimize simple clerical errors. Incentives should be built into data entry to promote accurate work.

Data entered must be checked for accuracy. The process of checking for and correcting errors related to data coding, transfer, and entry is often called **data cleaning**. Common methods include having another person re-enter the data and using a verifier to check for errors. When noncompatible entries are noted, the source document (i.e., the respondent's questionnaire) is consulted and the errors are then corrected.

Another method is to visually examine the data file to see if all records have the same pattern and whether blank entries can be found. If a fixed-column format is used, any aberration in the pattern of a record indicates the presence of coding errors from mistakes in column assignments. Data from the case containing the record should be re-entered to correct the errors. Blank entries also indicate entry errors since even missing values have codes.

Another method is to use the computer to do the cleaning. Since every variable has a specified range of legitimate numerical codes assigned to its attributes, the computer can be used to check for possible code violations. Many data entry or text editor packages (e.g., EPI-INFO) can be programmed to accept only legitimate codes for each variable. They check for errors automatically as the data are being entered and will beep when wrong codes are being entered. Even if one does not have such a program, a frequency distribution analysis can easily be performed to examine if the categories are legitimate for each variable. If errors are discovered, a cross tabulation between the variable *respondent ID* and the variable with the coding error can be performed. This will help identify the cases where coding errors occur. Next, the researcher should go to the source document and correct the errors accordingly.

Finally, more complicated surveys may use a process called consistency checking to examine whether responses to certain questions are logically related to responses to other questions (Sonquist and Dunkelberg, 1977, p. 215). For example, coding errors are suspected if one finds a respondent who is 25 years old and has Medicare insurance. Consistency checking is usually accomplished through computer programs using a set of if-then statements (e.g., "if MEDI-CARE, then AGE $\geq$ 65").

SUMMARY

Data used for health services research may be collected either from existing sources or empirically. Existing data come from both published and non-published sources. Empirical data may be collected by the researcher either with a data collection instrument (e.g., questionnaire) or through observational methods. More-structured data collection methods include face-to-face interviews and telephone interviews. Less-structured methods include focus group studies and in-depth interviews. Each data collection method has its own strengths and weaknesses. In choosing the most appropriate method, researchers compare the impact on the research project (e.g., cost, time, effort, sample size, and quality), the respondents (e.g., nature of the sample, literacy, privacy, and response rate), the interviewer (e.g., interaction, visual aids, biases, and training), and the instrument (e.g., length, sensitive questions, knowledge questions, uniformity, sequencing, and completion rate). They then select the methods that optimally match their situation. A number of measures have proven effective in improving response rate. These include intensive follow-up, sponsorships, shorter length, introductory letters, questionnaire design, inducements, maintaining anonymity, time of contact, and method of return. Once data have been collected, they need to be coded before analysis. A codebook may be prepared that assists in data coding and analysis.

REVIEW QUESTIONS

1. What are the methods of data collection used in health services research? Describe their characteristics.
2. What do researchers take into account in selecting a data collection method?
3. Compare the strengths and weaknesses of mail questionnaire surveys and personal and telephone interviews. What situations are most suitable for each of these methods?
4. What measures can be used to improve both the quantity and quality of responses?
5. Find an existing questionnaire either constructed by yourself or others. Design a codebook for that questionnaire.
6. What are the components in data processing?

REFERENCES

Armstrong, D., Kline-Rogers, E., Jani, S. M., Goldman, E. B., Fang, J., Mukherjee, D., et al. (2005). Potential impact of the HIPAA privacy rule on data collection in a registry of patients with acute coronary syndrome. *Archives of Internal Medicine*, 165, 1125–1129.

Armstrong, J. S. (1975). Monetary incentives in mail surveys. *Public Opinion Quarterly*, 39, 111–116.

Babbie, E. (1990). *Survey Research Methods* (2nd ed.). Belmont, CA: Wadsworth.

Babbie, E. (2006). *The Practice of Social Research* (11th ed.). Belmont, CA: Thomson/Wadsworth.

Bailey, K. D. (1994). *Methods of Social Research* (4th ed.). New York: Free Press.

Berdie, D. R. (1973). Questionnaire length and response rate. *Journal of Applied Psychology*, 58, 278–280.

Bowling, A. (1997). *Research Methods in Health: Investigating Health and Health Services*. Buckingham, UK: Open University Press.

Davis, J. A., and Smith, T. W. (1992). *The NORC General Social Survey: A User's Guide*. Newbury Park, CA: Sage.

Dillman, D. A. (2000). *Mail and Internet Surveys: The Tailored Design Method* (2nd ed.). New York: Wiley.

Fisher Wilson, J. (2006). Health Insurance Portability and Accountability Act privacy rule causes ongoing concerns among clinicians and researchers. *Annals of Internal Medicine, 145*(4). 313–316.

Groves, R. M. (1980). Telephone helps solve survey problems. *Newsletter of the Institute for Social Research. 6*(1), 3. Ann Arbor: University of Michigan.

Groves, R. M., and Kahn, R. L. (1979). *Surveys by Telephone: A National Comparison with Personal Interviews*. New York: Academic Press.

Herberlein, T. A., and Baumgartner, R. (1978). Factors affecting response rate to mailed questionnaires. *American Sociological Review, 43*, 451.

Lavrakas, P. J. (1993). *Telephone Survey Methods: Sampling, Selection, and Supervision* (2nd ed.). Thousand Oaks, CA: Sage.

Miller, D. C., and Salkind, N. J. (2002). *Handbook of Research Design and Social Measurement* (6th ed.). Thousand Oaks, CA: Sage.

Patton, M. Q. (2002). *Qualitative Evaluation and Research Methods* (3rd ed.). Thousand Oaks, CA: Sage.

Powdermaker, H. (1966). *Stranger and Friend*. New York: W. W. Norton.

Shi, L., Samuels, M. E., and Glover, S. (1994). *Educational Preparation and Attributes of Community and Migrant Health Center Administrators*. Columbia: University of South Carolina Press.

Sonquist, J. A., and Dunkelberg, W. C. (1977). *Survey and Opinion Research: Procedures for Processing and Analysis*. Englewood Cliffs, NJ: Prentice-Hall.

Wallace, D. (1954). A case for—and against—mail questionnaires. *Public Opinion Quarterly, 18*, 40–52.

CHAPTER 14

Statistical Analysis in Health Services Research

KEY TERMS

bivariate analysis
causal modeling
chi-square
chi-square-based measures
distribution
econometrics
factor analysis
kurtosis
leptokurtic
logistic regression
mean
measures of central tendency
measures of variability/
dispersion

median
mode
multilevel analysis
multiple regression
multivariate analysis
normal/bell curve
odds ratio
path analysis
Pearson product–moment
  correlation coefficient
platykurtic
proportional reduction in
  error (PRE)

range
rate
ratio
relative risk ratio
simple regression
skewed
Spearman rank correlation
  coefficient
standard deviation
standard scores
univariate analysis
variance

LEARNING OBJECTIVES

- To explore and prepare data for analysis.
- To become aware of the common statistical methods used in research analysis.

- To identify appropriate statistical methods for the analysis of data at the nominal, ordinal, and interval-ratio levels.

Although data analysis follows data collection, planning for analysis comes before data collection. Analysis decisions are related to the research question or hypothesis, the level of measurement, the sampling method and size, and the computer programs used. If there is more than one research question or hypothesis, several statistical procedures may be performed. If the relationship between two variables is explored, some statistical measure of association is needed. If the differences between two groups are examined, the significance of the differences will be tested. If the impact of certain predictors on dependent variables is assessed, a multivariate procedure is usually required.

The choice of statistics is also determined by the level of measurement of the variables. Different statistics exist for nominal, ordinal, and interval-ratio measures. Sampling considerations are important because many statistics are founded on the randomized, probability sampling method. Indeed, inferential statistics, which deals with the kinds of inferences that can be made when generalizing from sample data to the entire population, are based on samples being randomly selected. Sample size influences analysis because the more variables that are analyzed simultaneously, the larger the required sample size.

One way to facilitate analysis decisions well before data collection is to construct dummy statistical tables, which represent the actual tables to be used for analysis when data are collected and frequencies or values are inserted in them (Miller and Salkind, 2002). For example, one may create a dummy descriptive table including all key variables used in the analyses, a dummy comparative table contrasting the key measures between the intervention and control groups, and a dummy multivariate table assessing the impact of key determinants on outcomes while controlling for critical covariates. These dummy statistical tables become the statistical plan. By setting them in advance, researchers can make a careful appraisal of the relevant statistics to be used, design the most appropriate research instrument, and select sampling and data collection methods pertinent to the analysis to be undertaken. Constructing dummy statistical tables enables data analysis to be projected in advance for appraisal and evaluation. Improvement of the study design can be made with minimum waste of time and money, and the risk of failure is also reduced.

Data analysis can seldom be performed without computer software. Among the statistical software packages most commonly used by health services researchers are SAS (Statistical Analysis System), SPSS (Statistical Package for the Social Sciences), STATA (Statistics/Data Analysis), BMD (biomedical computer programs), and LISREL (Analysis of Linear Structural Relationships by the Method of Maximum Likelihood). These programs generally have both mainframe and personal computer versions, and technical support is usually available from both the manufacturer and the researchers' institutional computer center.

This chapter describes the process of conducting data analysis and illustrates the most commonly used statistical measures. Specifically, this process involves data exploration, univariate analysis, bivariate analysis, and multivariate analysis (Singleton and Straits, 2005). Statistical measures can be based on one or more variables. **Univariate analysis** examines the characteristics of one variable at a time and often produces descriptive statistics. **Bivariate analysis** examines the relationship between two variables at a time. **Multivariate analysis** examines the relationship among three or more variables at a time. Throughout this chapter, the emphasis is placed on choosing the appropriate methods based on the nature of the variables and the level of measurement. The chapter is not a substitute for statistics textbooks. Readers who want in-depth descriptions and illustrations of the statistics described in this chapter are encouraged to consult current biostatistics and econometrics textbooks.

DATA EXPLORATION

After the collected data have been entered into the computer and the process editing completed, researchers often spend a considerable amount of time exploring the data before launching a formal analysis. One of the purposes of this exploration is to make sure all data elements are included in one data file. If a research project uses several data sources, the separate data files have to be combined and merged. The files can be merged based on shared variables but different cases, or on similar cases but different variables. Data can also be sorted in a different order based on the value of one or more variables. On the other hand, if the data file is too large for the research purpose, a subset of cases may be selected to restrict the analysis to that subset. The unit of analysis can also be altered by grouping cases together.

Another purpose of examining data carefully before analysis is to prepare it for hypothesis testing and model building. Researchers may display the data in tabular (e.g., frequency tables) or graphic (e.g., scatterplots, histograms, stem-and-leaf plots, or box plots) forms. Inspecting the distribution of values is important for evaluating the appropriateness of the statistical techniques to be used for hypothesis testing or model building. Since normal distribution is important to statistical inference, a normal probability plot may be used to pair each observed value with its expected value based on a normal distribution. If the sample is drawn from a normal distribution, the points will fall more or less on a straight line.

In such a case, a simple linear regression model may be needed. If the distribution does not appear to be normally distributed, data transformation might be necessary, or some nonparametric techniques can be used. If the plot resembles a mathematical function, that function may be employed to fit the data. For example, when the data do not cluster around a straight line, the researcher can take the log of the independent variables. If this does not coax the data toward linearity, a more complicated model of data transformation may have to be used. Some commonly used transformations include cube (3), square (2), square root $(\frac{1}{2})$, natural logarithm (0), reciprocal of the square root $(-\frac{1}{2})$, and reciprocal (-1).

UNIVARIATE ANALYSIS

Univariate analysis, which examines one variable at a time, may be conducted as part of data exploration, as a major component of descriptive analysis, or as a prelude to bivariate and multivariate analysis. As part of data exploration, univariate analysis is performed to help assess whether assumptions of statistical tests have been met (e.g., whether the data are normally distributed). Very large standard deviations often imply outliers, that is, extreme values that may disproportionately affect the statistics (Grady and Wallston, 1988, p. 152). Examination of variable distribution may reflect departures from normality and require the transformation of variables. Lack of variation in responses makes it more difficult to determine how differences in one variable are related to differences in another. Univariate analysis also helps in deciding whether to collapse categories of a variable.

When information on a group of individuals or other units has been systematically gathered, it needs to be organized and summarized in an intelligible way. As a major component of descriptive analysis, univariate analysis helps to profile a sample in terms of the variables measured. While research often goes beyond descriptive analysis, univariate analysis serves as a prelude to more complex analysis by providing a complete picture of the bases upon which conclusions are founded.

Commonly used univariate statistics include frequency and percentage distributions, measures of central tendency (e.g., mean, median, and mode), vari-

Table 14.1. Level of measurement and statistics for analyzing one variable at a time

Level of Measurement	Distribution	Statistics			
		Average	Dispersion	Shape	Standardized Score
Nominal	Frequency Percentage	Mode			Ratio Rate
Ordinal	Frequency Percentage	Mode Median	Range Maximum Minimum		Ratio Rate
Interval-Ratio		Mode Median Mean	Range Maximum Minimum Variance Standard Deviation	Skewness Kurtosis	z Score

ability or dispersion (e.g., range, standard deviation, and variance), shape (e.g., frequency or percentage polygon, skewness, kurtosis, leptokurtic, and platykurtic), and standard scores (z score, rate, and ratio). The choice of these statistics typically depends on the level of measurement of the variables (see Table 14.1).

Figure 14.1. Standard normal distribution

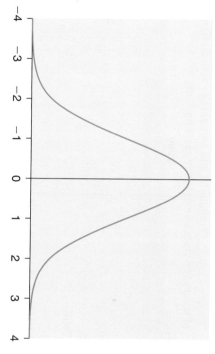

Distributions

A **distribution** organizes the values of a variable into categories. A graph representing the density function of the normal probability distribution is also known as a **normal curve** or a **bell curve** (see Figure 14.1). A frequency distribution, also known as a marginal distribution, shows the number of cases that fall into each category. Data measured at the nominal or ordinal level can be organized in terms of the categories of responses given. Interval-ratio-level data usually have to be grouped into a distribution in terms of categories that are convenient and substantively meaningful.

Another way of summarizing a variable is to report its percentage distribution, obtained by dividing the number or frequency of cases in the category by the total N, or by the corrected total if missing data are to be excluded, and then multiplying by 100 to convert to a percent. Thus, frequency distribution can easily be converted into percentage distribution. The advantage of percentage distribution is to facilitate comparisons across distributions based on different sample sizes since all numbers are converted to a base 100. The distribution of a variable can also be shown graphically to highlight certain aspects. Examples are bar charts, histograms, polygons, and pie charts.

Table 14.2 displays a frequency and percentage distribution of the insurance status of emergency room patients in a large urban county teaching hospital. When tables are used, it is necessary to present the data clearly so that readers

Table 14.2. Frequency and percentage distribution of insurance status emergency room patients

Insurance	Frequency	Percentage
Medicaid	16,130	29.4
Medicare	4,660	8.5
Private	16,882	30.8
No Insurance	17,161	31.3
Total	54,833	100.0

can easily understand it. Each table should stand by itself. It ought to be possible for the reader to understand a table without referring to the text that surrounds it. Each table should have a unique and detailed title describing what the variables are and what the cell entries are. Columns and rows should be clearly labeled. A table should also show the relevant sample size. If a percentage table is used, marginals are typically reported as well. Marginals refer to the frequency counts and percentages for the row and column variables taken separately. Footnotes may be used to indicate sources, explain symbols and missing values, or summarize procedures used.

Measures of Central Tendency

Measures of central tendency summarize information about the average value of a variable, a typical value around which all the values cluster. The three commonly used measures are mode, median, and mean. The **mode** is the value (or category) of a distribution that occurs most frequently. Although the mode can be reported for any level of measurement, it is most often used for nominal-level data. For grouped data, the mode may be affected by the way in which values are grouped into categories. Therefore, it is necessary to verify that the categories are of the same width, or else adjustments have to be made.

The **median** is the middle position, or midpoint, of a distribution. It is computed by first ordering the values of a distribution and then dividing the distribution in half; that is, half the cases fall below the median and the other half are above it. In general, researchers may find the observation that has the median value for an ordered distribution simply by computing $(N + 1)/2$.

The median is used for both ordinal and interval-ratio levels of measurement. It is a meaningless statistic for nominal data. Since the median is a stable measure of central tendency and is not affected by extreme values, it is typically used when there are extreme values in one of its ends (e.g., income data).

The most commonly used measure of central tendency is the **mean**, the arithmetic average computed by adding up all the values and dividing by the total number of cases. Where x_i equals the raw or observed values of a variable and N equals the total number of cases or observations, then the mean is calculated with the following formula:

Formula 14.1
$$\frac{\sum x_i}{N} \quad \text{or} \quad \frac{(x_1 + x_2 + x_3 + \cdots + x_N)}{N}$$

Mean is only used for the interval-ratio level of measurement. It is the preferred measure of central tendency because it has important arithmetic and other properties useful in inferential statistics. It is also a good summary measure because its computation utilizes every value of a distribution. However, extreme values do affect the mean. Therefore, for extreme distributions, it is best to report both the mean and the median to avoid misleading interpretations.

Measures of Variability

While measures of central tendency identify a single, most representative value of the distribution, **measures of variability/dispersion** refer to the spread or variation of the distribution. A simple measure of variability or dispersion is the **range**, the difference between the highest (maximum) and lowest (minimum) values in a distribution. Range can be used for both ordinal and interval-ratio levels of measurement. Since range only takes into account those minimum and maximum values in a distribution, it does not reflect the rest of the distribution.

Other distance-based measures of dispersion have been developed that are more informative about the middle of a distribution. One such measure is the interquartile range, which is the range of values in the middle half (50 percent) of a distribution. Such a measure is more sensitive to the way values are concentrated around the midpoint of the distribution, but it still only provides the difference between two values and tells little about the aggregate dispersion of a distribution.

A more informative characterization of dispersion is the extent to which each of the values of a distribution differs from the mean. The **variance** is such a measure and is defined as the average squared deviation from the mean.

Formula 14.2
$$\text{variance} = S^2 = \frac{\sum (x_i - \text{mean})^2}{N - 1}$$

However, variance does not have a direct interpretation for descriptive purposes. A more intuitive measure of variability is the **standard deviation**, defined as the square root of the variance. The standard deviation is expressed in the original unit of measurement of the distribution. Both the variance and standard deviation can be used only for the interval-ratio level of measurement.

Measures of Shape

When a distribution of observations lacks symmetry, that is, when more observations are found at one end of the distribution than the other, such a distribution is **skewed**, or is said to exhibit skewness. If the tail is skewed toward larger values, the distribution is positively skewed, or skewed to the right. Conversely, if the tail is skewed toward smaller values, the distribution is negatively skewed, or skewed to the left. **Kurtosis** refers to the extent to which cases or observations cluster around a central point. When cases cluster around the central point more than in a normal distribution, the distribution is called **leptokurtic**. When cases cluster around the central point less than in a normal distribution, the distribution is called **platykurtic**.

Statistics measuring skewness and kurtosis are generally automatically generated by computer statistical software in univariate analysis. If the observed distribution is normal, skewness and kurtosis measures will fluctuate around zero. A researcher may get some sense of possible skewness and kurtosis by examining a histogram. Both skewness and kurtosis measures can only be validly used at the interval-ratio level of measurement.

Standard Scores

Standard scores describe the relative position of an observation within a distribution. One standard score, the z score, uses both the mean and standard deviation to indicate where an observation falls: the number of standard deviations above or below the mean.

A positive z score indicates that a particular score is above the mean, whereas a negative z score indicates that a particular score is below the mean. The distribution of the z score has two important properties: the mean of the z score is always zero, and the standard deviation is always one. The z score is calculated by obtaining the difference between the value of a particular case x_i and the mean of the distribution, and then dividing this difference by the standard deviation. A normal distribution with a mean of zero and a standard deviation of one is also known as the standard normal distribution (see Figure 14.1).

Formula 14.3
$$z_i = \frac{(x_i - \text{mean})}{SD}$$

Suppose a student wants to see how his or her performance on two exams (90 in the first and 80 in the second) compared with that of the class. The distribution of scores on the first exam had a mean of 75 and standard deviation of 5. The distribution of scores on the second exam had a mean of 60 and standard deviation of 4. (Note that the second exam was harder, and there was less variation around the mean than for the first exam). The z scores for the two exams are 3 [(90 − 75)/5] and 5 [(80 − 60)/4], respectively, indicating that the student performed better in the second exam than the first one relative to the average score and variation in each of the class distributions. In other words, 90 is equivalent to three standard deviation units higher than the mean, but 80 is equivalent to five standard deviation units higher than the mean. The z score is used only with the interval-ratio level of measurement.

In addition to the z score, ratios and rates may be used to standardize and meaningfully compare across different numbers. Ratio and rate computations are called norming, or standardizing, operations. Both involve dividing one number (or a set of numbers) by another. A **ratio** is simply one number divided by another: the frequency of observations in one category is divided by the frequency in another category. A **rate** is similar to a percentage since it is computed by dividing the number of cases or events in a given category by the total number of observations. The resulting proportion is then expressed as any multiple of 10 that clears the decimal, usually 100 or 1,000. The formula is:

Formula 14.4 $\quad \text{rate} = \dfrac{\text{number of events during a time period}}{\text{total } N \text{ (or number of possible events)}} \times 100 \text{ (or 1,000)}$

For example, natality or birth rate is usually expressed as the number of births in a population per 1,000: if there are 10,000 births during a year, and the population at the middle of the year is 500,000, the crude birth rate is 50 births per 1,000 (10,000/500,000 × 1,000).

A rate of change is useful in comparing the distribution of a variable through time; say, before (Time 1) and after (Time 2) an intervention program. A positive result indicates the rate of gain whereas a negative result indicates the rate of loss. The result can be multiplied by 100 to remove the decimal and reflect percentage change. The formula is:

Formula 14.5 $\quad \text{rate of change} = \dfrac{\text{value at Time 2} - \text{value at Time 1}}{\text{value at Time 1}}$

BIVARIATE ANALYSIS

Bivariate analysis examines two variables at a time and may be conducted to determine the relationship between the two variables (i.e., a measure of independence), and, if a relationship exists, how much influence one variable has on the other (i.e., a measure of association). Commonly used bivariate procedures include the following: cross-tabulation, chi-square (χ^2), phi coefficient (ϕ), coefficient of contingency (C), Cramér's V, Goodman–Kruskal's lambda (λ), relative risk ratio, Kendall's tau (τ), Goodman–Kruskal's gamma (γ), ANOVA, Pearson correlation coefficient (r), and paired t test. The choice of these statistics depends on the level of measurement of the variables (see Table 14.3 for these and other statistics that may be used for bivariate analysis).

Bivariate analysis is commonly used in subgroup comparisons and as a preparation for multivariate analysis. In subgroup comparisons, the researcher can choose any stratification variable and describe each subgroup of that variable in terms of any other variable. The examination of the relationship between pairs of variables helps select appropriate variables in multivariate analysis.

The bivariate measure of association is a correlation usually ranging from −1 to +1 and assesses the strength and direction of the relation between two variables. A negative sign means that higher values of one variable are associated with lower values of another, and vice versa. When the statistic is close to zero,

Table 14.3. Level of measurement and statistics for analyzing two variables at a time

Level of Measurement	Statistics		
	Nominal	Ordinal	Interval-Ratio
Nominal	Cross-tabulation Chi-square (χ^2) Phi coefficient (ϕ) Coefficient of contingency (C) Cramér's V Goodman–Kruskal's lambda (λ) Relative risk ratio Fisher's exact test		

Ordinal	Cross-tabulation
	Chi-square (χ^2)
	Goodman–Kruskal's lambda (λ)
	Kruskal–Wallis test
	Median test
	Sign test
	Wilcoxon signed-rank test
	Somers's d
	Kolmogorov–Smirnov
	  two-sample test
	Runs test
		Cross-tabulation
		Chi-square (χ^2)
		Goodman–Kruskal's gamma (γ)
		Kendall's tau (τ)
		Spearman rank correlation
		  coefficient (r_s)	

Interval-ratio	Paired t test
	ANOVA
	F test
	Multiple comparison
	  procedures (Bonferroni
	  test, Duncan's
	  multiple range test,
	  Tukey's b, Scheffé test)
		Somers's d
		Simple regression
			Pearson correlation
			  coefficient (r)
			Simple regression
			F test

the variables are considered to be uncorrelated. Statistical tables are used to assess the probability that a correlation is significantly different from zero. The closer the number is to one (perfect correlation), the greater the magnitude of correlation or association.

Cross-Tabulation

The first step in determining the existence of a relationship between two variables is to cross-tabulate them, or to examine their joint distribution. In general,

Table 14.4. Contingency table: Hospital setting and patient gender

Hospital Setting	Gender		Total
	Male	Female	
Emergency Room	25,427	29,406	54,833
	(46.37%)	(53.63%)	
Inpatient	10,383	14,475	24,858
	(41.77%)	(58.23%)	
Outpatient	26,518	51,808	78,326
	(33.86%)	(66.14%)	
Clinics	19,060	53,850	72,910
	(26.14%)	(73.86%)	
Dental	2,523	4,365	6,888
	(36.63%)	(63.37%)	
Total	83,911	153,904	237,815
	(35.28%)	(64.72%)	

we study the influence of an independent variable on a dependent variable, or how the distribution of the dependent variable varies within the categories of the independent variable. The contingency table where cross-tabulation is presented is set up so that the categories of the independent variable are in the columns (i.e., across the top of the table) and the categories of the dependent variable are in the rows of the table. Three different percentages can be computed for each cell, each conveying a different meaning. Specifically, the column percentage divides the cell entry by the total for its column. The row percentage divides the cell entry by the total for its row. Table 14.4 is a contingency table about hospital setting and patient gender. The row percentage is displayed.

Chi-Square Test for Independence

For cross-tabulation, **chi-square** (χ^2) is a very common test for independence. It is based on a comparison between an observed frequency table with an expected frequency table, that is, the table one would expect to find if the two variables were statistically independent, or unrelated to each another. An expected frequency table is computed from the marginal frequency totals only and represents a frequency table showing no relationship between the variables. Table 14.5 presents the expected cell frequencies (derived from Table 14.4), assuming no relationship between gender and hospital setting. Table 14.5 also shows the derived bivariate percentage distribution with cell percentages the same as the marginals. The chi-square statistic may be calculated using the following formula:

Table 14.5. Frequency table: Hospital setting and patient gender

Hospital Setting	Frequencies Gender			Percentages Gender		
	Male	Female	Total	Male	Female	Total
Emergency Room	19,347	35,486	54,833	23%	23%	23%
Inpatient	8,771	16,087	24,858	11%	11%	11%
Outpatient	27,637	50,689	78,326	33%	33%	33%
Clinics	25,726	47,184	72,910	30%	30%	30%
Dental	2,430	4,458	6,888	3%	3%	3%
Total	83,911	153,904	237,815	100%	100%	100%
	(83,911)	(153,904)	(237,815)			

Formula 14.6

$$\chi^2 = \sum \frac{(O_{ij} - E_{ij})^2}{E_{ij}}$$

$$= \frac{(25427 - 19347)^2}{19347} + \frac{(10383 - 8771)^2}{8771} + \cdots + \frac{(4365 - 6888)^2}{6888}$$

$$= 45011$$

The calculated chi-square value is compared against the critical points of the theoretical chi-square distribution, and this corresponds to the preestablished level of significance and degrees of freedom. The degrees of freedom are $(r - 1) \times (c - 1)$, where r is the number of rows and c the number of columns. In this example, the degrees of freedom are $(5 - 1)(2 - 1)$, or 4, and the p value (i.e., significance level) is less than 0.001, indicating that gender and hospital setting are not independent. This should be obvious from the observed frequencies. For example, while males and females are relatively similar in emergency room visits (46.37% vs. 53.63%), there is a much larger difference in clinic visits (26.14% vs. 73.86%).

However, chi-square is a test of independence and provides little information about the strength of the association. Chi-square statistics depend on sample size and will increase as the sample size becomes larger. Conversely, when the expected cell frequencies are very small, the chi-square test statistic is not distributed exactly as the chi-square distribution. Thus, the rule of thumb is not to use the chi-square test for independence when the expected frequency (f_e) of the smallest cell is five or less.

Chi-Square–Based Measures of Association

Once the researcher has found a significant relationship, the next step is to examine its nature and magnitude. Measures of association refer to statistics that quantify the relationship between variables in cross-tabulation and indicate the magnitude or strength of that relationship. For nominal-level variables, several

chi-square-based measures can be used to assess the extent of the relationship. Since the significance of chi-square is closely and positively associated with sample size and degrees of freedom, these measures modify the chi-square statistics to reduce the influence of sample size and degrees of freedom and restrict the values between zero and one.

The phi coefficient (ϕ) divides chi-square by the sample size and takes the square root of the result:

Formula 14.7
$$\phi = \sqrt{\chi^2/N}$$

In our example, the phi coefficient is 0.44 (or r$45011/237815$). When the chi-square value is greater than the sample size, the phi coefficient lies beyond zero and one.

Pearson's coefficient of contingency (C) and Cramér's V are always between zero and one:

Formula 14.8 $C = \sqrt{\chi^2/(\chi^2 + N)}$

Formula 14.9 $V = \sqrt{\chi^2/[N(k-1)]}$

In our example, C and V are respectively 0.40 [or $\sqrt{45011/(45011 + 237815)}$] and 0.25 [or $\sqrt{45011/(237815 \times 3)}$]. Although chi-square-based measures of association can be used to compare magnitude or strength of association across different contingency tables, they are difficult to interpret due to the nominal nature of the variables.

PRE-Based Measures of Association

Proportional reduction in error (PRE) is a broad framework that helps organize a large number of measures for data at the nominal, ordinal, and even interval-ratio levels. PRE-based measures are typically ratios of a measure of error in predicting the values of one variable based on that variable alone and the same measure of error based on knowledge of an additional variable (Goodman and Kruskal, 1954). The logic behind this framework is that if prior knowledge about another variable improves the knowledge of this variable, then these two variables are related. PRE may be summarized below:

Formula 14.10

$$\mathrm{PRE} = \frac{\text{error using dependent variable only} - \text{error using independent variable}}{\text{error using dependent variable only}}$$

For example, Table 14.6 presents the one-day frequency distribution of patient race and insurance status. If we use only the distribution about insurance, we would predict private insurance (the mode) and be correct 52.5 percent of the time (105/200) and wrong 47.5 percent of the time [(55 + 40)/200].

However, if we also use the distribution of insurance within each racial category, we would predict Medicare/Medicaid when the sampled individual is black and be correct in 35 of 70 guesses (i.e., 35 errors). We would predict private insurance when the sampled individual is white and be right in 90 of 110 guesses

Table 14.6. Patient race and insurance status

| | Race | | | |
Insurance	White	Black	Hispanic	Total
Medicare/Medicaid	10	35	10	55
Private	90	10	5	105
No Insurance	10	25	5	40
Total	110	70	20	200

(i.e., 20 errors). We would predict Medicare/Medicaid when the sampled individual is Hispanic and be right in 10 of 20 guesses (i.e., 10 errors). When we do not know the person's race, we make 95 errors in 200 guesses. When we do know the person's race, we make only 65 errors in 200 guesses. That our predictions improve when we know ethnicity over the predictions we make when we do not indicates that race and insurance status are related. Applying the PRE formula, our predictions may be computed as follows:

$$PRE = \frac{95 - (35 + 20 + 10)}{95} = .32$$

Goodman–Kruskal's lambda (λ) is a measure of association for nominal-level data based on the PRE method. The computing formula for lambda is:

Formula 14.11

$$\lambda = \frac{\text{Sum of modal frequency for each category of } x - \text{modal frequency of } y}{N - \text{modal frequency of } y}$$

where x is the independent variable, y is the dependent variable, and N is the sample size. Applying this formula to the data in Table 14.6, we can calculate lambda as:

$$\lambda = \frac{(95 + 35 + 10) - 105}{200 - 105} = \frac{135 - 105}{95} = \frac{30}{95} = .32$$

This is the same as the proportional reduction in our guessing errors. Lambda ranges between zero and one. A value close to one indicates the independent variable closely specifies the categories of the dependent variable. When the two variables are independent, lambda is close to zero.

For measures of association for ordinal-level data based on the PRE method, we may use either Goodman–Kruskal's gamma (γ) or Kendall's tau (τ). For ordinal-level data, we can make our predictions not only based on the mode of a distribution, but also the rank-ordering of the categories. The computation of gamma is as follows:

Formula 14.12

$$gamma = \frac{s - d}{s + d}$$

Table 14.7. Patient education and income level

Income	Education			Total
	Elementary	Secondary	College	
Low	60	15	5	80
Medium	20	30	10	60
High	5	10	45	60
Total	85	55	60	200

where s is the number of same-ordered pairs, and d is the number of different-ordered pairs. To compute gamma, the table must be consistently ordered: both the column and row must be ordered either from low to high or from high to low. To find s, or the number of same-ordered pairs, we start with the upper left-hand cell and multiply the cell frequency by the sum of the frequencies of all the cells that are both to the right and below the reference cell. This procedure is repeated for each cell until all the cells to the right and below that cell have been included. We then sum up all those pairs to obtain s. To find d, or the number of different-ordered pairs, we start with the lower left-hand cell and multiply the cell frequency by the sum of the frequencies that are both to the right and above the reference cell. This procedure is repeated for each cell until all the cells to the right and above that cell have been included. We then sum up all those pairs to obtain d.

For example, Table 14.7 presents the distribution of patient education and income level. The values s and d may be obtained by summing up all same-ordered or different-ordered pairs, respectively:

$$60(30 + 10 + 45) = 5700 \qquad 5(15 + 5 + 30 + 10) = 300$$
$$15(10 + 45) = 825 \qquad 10(5 + 10) = 150$$
$$20(10 + 45) = 1100 \qquad 20(15 + 5) = 400$$
$$30(45) = 1350 \qquad 30(5) = 150$$
$$s = 8975 \qquad d = 1000$$

Gamma may then be calculated as:

$$\text{gamma} = \frac{8975 - 1000}{8975 + 1000} = .80$$

This means there is an 80 percent reduction in error if we predict ranking on income based on ranking on education, as opposed to predicting randomly.

Since gamma ignores all the tied pairs, it tends to overestimate the strength of association. Kendall's tau (τ) takes into account tied pairs and is:

Formula 14.13

$$\tau = \frac{s - d}{\sqrt{(s + d + t_x)(s + d + t_y)}}$$

where s is the number of same-ordered pairs, d is the number of different-ordered pairs, t_x is the number of pairs tied to the independent variable, and t_y is the number of pairs tied to the dependent variable. To compute t_x and when the categories of the independent variable are in the columns, we look for cells that are in the same column and below the referent cell. To compute t_y and when the categories of the dependent variable are in the rows, we look for cells that are in the same row and to the right of the referent cell. Using the same example in Table 14.7, t_x may be calculated as: $60(20 + 5) + 15(30 + 10) + 5(10 + 45) + 20(5) + 30(10) + 10(45) = 1500 + 600 + 275 + 100 + 300 + 450 = 3225$. t_y may be calculated as: $60(15 + 5) + 20(30 + 10) + 5(10 + 45) + 15(5) + 30(10) + 10(45) = 1200 + 800 + 275 + 75 + 300 + 450 = 3100$. Kendall's tau (τ) may then be calculated as:

$$\tau = \frac{8975 - 1000}{\sqrt{(8975 + 1000 + 3225)(8975 + 1000 + 3100)}} = .61$$

By adjusting for tied pairs, the measure of association is reduced from .80 to .61. Another ordinal measure of association is the **Spearman rank correlation coefficient** (r_s). To compute r_s, the two variables are rank-ordered, with each person having two ranks, one for each variable. The values of the two variables are ranked from the smallest to the largest for all cases. The difference between the pairs of ranks for each person is denoted by d. For example, if a person ranks first on one variable and fifth on another, the d score would be $4(5 - 1)$.

The values of r_s range from 1 (when $\sum d_i^2 = 0$ or all pairs of ranks are identical) to -1 (when no pairs of ranks are identical). The formula for r_s is:

Formula 14.14
$$r_s = 1 - \frac{6 \sum d_i^2}{N(N^2 - 1)}$$

When data are collected with interval-ratio-level measurement, researchers have the choice to convert interval-level data to ordinal and categorical variables, and then use measures of association appropriate to these levels. For example, income, if obtained as a dollar amount, can be converted into an ordinal-level (e.g., <$10,000, $10,000–$20,000, and so on) or nominal-level (e.g., above poverty line vs. below poverty line) measure, depending on the purpose of the research.

Alternatively, researchers may use measures appropriate only for interval-ratio. A commonly used measure of association is the **Pearson product–moment correlation coefficient** (r). As with most other measures, r ranges from 1 (perfect positive relationship) to -1 (perfect negative relationship). Zero indicates no relationship or independence between the two variables. The computation formula for r is:

Formula 14.15
$$r = \frac{N \sum xy - (\sum x)(y)}{[N \sum x^2 - (\sum x)^2][N \sum y^2 - (\sum y)^2]}$$

The correlation coefficient may be tested for statistical significance based on sample size. In general, a correlation coefficient may be interpreted as follows (Herman, Morris, and Fitz-Gibbon, 1987; Miller and Salkind, 2002):

.00 to .20: little or no positive correlation

.20 to .40: some slight positive correlation

.40 to .60: substantial positive correlation

.60 to .80: strong positive correlation

.80 to 1.00: very strong positive correlation

−.80 to −1.00: very strong negative correlation

−.60 to −.80: strong negative correlation

−.40 to −.60: substantial negative correlation

−.20 to −.40: some slight negative correlation

.00 to −.20: little or no negative correlation

However, statistical significance does not indicate substantive importance. Suppose that we find that two groups are significantly different at the .05 level. Our finding only means that there is a 5 percent chance that we would make a mistake in concluding that the two groups are not exactly equal; that is, the difference is zero. Thus, two groups can be significantly different in a statistical sense, even though the difference between them is very close to zero.

From a practical sense, statistically significant tests are highly sensitive to sample size. With a large-enough sample size, even a trivial difference will likely be statistically significant. Thus, statistical significance only expresses the degree of confidence in the conclusion. Being confident that there is a difference does not imply that the difference is either large or important. Substantive and theoretical considerations must be involved when decisions are based on statistical tests, particularly in applied health services research.

Other Bivariate Measures

Other commonly used measures of association include relative risk ratio or odds ratio, testing hypotheses about differences in sample means or proportions, and the simple regression procedure.

Relative Risk Ratio

The **relative risk ratio** can be used for two nominal-level measures. Specifically, it measures the strength of association between the presence of a factor (x) and the occurrence of an event (y). See Figure 14.2 for its calculations. Relative risk ratio is used in a prospective study, either a randomized clinical trial or a cohort study.

	Outcome		Risk rate of developing outcome	Relative risk (risk ratio) =	Relative risk reduction
	+	−			
Exposure +	a	b	Risk rate of developing outcome in exposed $a/(a+b)$	$\dfrac{(a/(a+b))}{(c/(c+d))}$	$\dfrac{(a/(a+b))-(c/(c+d))}{(c/(c+d))}$
Exposure −	c	d	Risk rate of developing outcome in nonexposed $c/(c+d)$		

Figure 14.2. Relative risk ratio calculation

For example, data have been collected on lung cancer (y) for those who smoke and those who don't (x). A two-by-two table may be created, as Table 14.8 shows. The relative risk ratio is the ratio of the incidence of disease (lung cancer) among the exposed (those who smoke) to the incidence of disease among the unexposed (those who don't smoke):

Formula 14.16

$$\text{relative risk} = \frac{\text{Incidence rate of disease in exposed group}}{\text{Incidence rate of disease in nonexposed group}} = \frac{ad}{bc}$$

The relative risk can be estimated by the cross-product of the entries in a two-by-two table. However, two assumptions are necessary to make such an estimate: (1) the frequency of the disease in the population must be small, and (2) the study cases should be representative of the cases in the population, whereas the controls should be representative of the noncases (Lilienfeld and Lilienfeld, 1994). The relative risk ratio for our example is 2.11. If the 95 percent confidence interval does not include one, then this ratio is significant.

For retrospective or case-control studies, the term *odds ratio* is often used in lieu of *relative risk*. **Odds ratio** may be defined as the ratio of two odds, that is,

Table 14.8. Smoking and lung cancer

	Smoking		
Lung Cancer	Yes	No	Total
Yes	100 (*a*)	900 (*b*)	1000
No	50 (*c*)	950 (*d*)	1000
Total	150	1850	2000

Figure 14.3. Odds ratio calculation

	Outcome			
		+	−	
Exposure	+	a	b	Odds of being exposed in cases
	−	c	d	Odds of being exposed in controls
		a/c	b/d	

Odds ratio = a/c ÷ b/d

the ratio of the probability of occurrence of an event to that of the nonoccurrence (Last, 2001). See Figure 14.3 for its calculations. In a rare condition, the odds ratio approximates the relative risk (or risk ratio).

Measures of Differences

The t test can be used when there is a single independent variable with only two categories (e.g., nominal level : male/female) and a single continuous dependent variable (e.g., interval-ratio : income). The t value may be calculated as follows:

Formula 14.17

$$t = \frac{x_1 - x_2}{\sqrt{(S_1^2/N_1) + (S_2^2/N_2)}}$$

where x_1 is the mean of one category, x_2 is the mean of another category, S_1^2, S_2^2 are the variances, and N_1, N_2 are the sample sizes for the two categories, respectively. The t value can be checked for its observed significance level from a statistics table (e.g., critical values for a student's t). If the observed p level is sufficiently small (e.g., less than 0.05, or 0.01), we can then reject the hypothesis that the means of the two categories are equal.

When there are more than two categories within a single nominal variable (e.g., race), the analysis of variance (ANOVA) method is used to test the differences among these categories in terms of the continuous dependent variable. The null hypothesis in ANOVA states that the means for the different categories or groups are equal in the population ($\mu_A = \mu_B = \mu_C$). The test statistic is the F ratio, which compares the variations in the scores from the different sources: variation between categories or groups (or treatment variation) and variation within categories or groups (or error variation). The variation between groups reflects the treatment and random error; the variation within groups reflects random error only. Thus, the F ratio can be conceptualized as follows:

Formula 14.18 $\quad F = \dfrac{\text{Treatment} + \text{Error}}{\text{Error}} = \dfrac{\text{Mean square between groups}}{\text{Mean square within groups}}$

The larger the F ratio, the more likely there is a true difference in means among various categories or groups. However, a significant F value only indicates that the means are not all equal. It does not identify which pairs of categories or groups appear to have different means. Post hoc or multiple comparison procedures can be used to test which means are significantly different from one another. Examples of multiple comparison procedures include the Bonferroni test, Duncan's multiple range test, Tukey's b, and the Scheffé test (SPSS Inc., 1997).

A test for significant difference between two proportions can be performed with the same logic as a test for significant difference between means. The computation formula is as follows:

Formula 14.19

$$z = \frac{p_1 - p_2}{\sqrt{(p_1 q_1 / n_1) + (p_2 q_2 / n_2)}}$$

where p_1 is the proportion of one group (e.g., male) with a particular characteristic (e.g., those who smoke), p_2 is the proportion of another group (e.g., female) with the same characteristic, $q = 1 - p$, and n is the sample size. If the z statistic is significantly large, then we reject the hypothesis that the proportion of one group with a particular characteristic is the same as that of another group.

Simple Regression Procedure

Another way to examine the relationship between two interval-ratio-level variables is to perform a **simple regression** procedure:

Formula 14.20 $y = \alpha + \beta_x + \text{random error}$

where y equals the variable to be predicted (or the dependent variable), x equals the variable to be used as a predictor of y (or the independent variable), α (alpha) equals the y-intercept of the line, and β (beta) equals the slope of the line.

The intercept (α) gives the predicted value of y when x is zero. In general, it is technically incorrect to extend the regression line beyond the range of values of x for which it was estimated, because the procedure produces the best-fitting (ordinary least squares) line through the observed data points. Other data points beyond the ones used as the basis of the calculations might change the nature and extent of the relationship drastically. For example, the relationship may be nonlinear if additional observations are included.

The regression coefficient (β) is interpreted as the change in y for a unit change in x. The procedure is referred to as the regression of y on x. If the coefficient is positive, a unit change in x produces an increase in y (i.e., the line slopes upward). If the coefficient is negative, a unit change in x produces a decrease in y (i.e., the line slopes downward).

The estimated regression equation allows researchers to calculate a predicted value of y for every observed value of x by simple substitution into the prediction equation. For example, if x equals the mother's years of education, and y equals the child's birth weight, an estimated regression line might look like this: $y = 5.75 + (.15)(x)$. For a mother with six years of education ($x = 6$), the predicted birth weight of the child is 6.65 pounds.

When the Pearson correlation coefficient (r) is squared, the resulting number (r^2) can be interpreted as the proportion of variance in y explained by x. For example, if $r^2 = .45$, we would say that the mother's education accounts for or explains 45 percent of the variance in the child's birth weight. Another way to calculate r^2 would be as follows:

Formula 14.21

$$r^2 = \frac{\text{total sum of squares} - \text{error sum of squares}}{\text{total sum of squares}} = \frac{\text{explained variation}}{\text{total variation}}$$

MULTIVARIATE ANALYSIS

Multivariate analysis examines three or more variables at a time. In health services research as in social research, two-variable relationships seldom suffice. Often, instead of one independent variable and one dependent variable, researchers usually need to sort out the effects of several variables on a dependent variable. The inclusion of additional variables is based on both theoretical and practical knowledge, which helps specify the direction of influence and test for spuriousness. A model is properly specified when it correctly reflects the underlying or real-world phenomena. Specification error occurs when the model is not properly stated; that is, when important explanatory variables have been excluded from the model, when unimportant variables have been included, or when the wrong form of the relationship has been assumed. A researcher could introduce many additional variables as control variables, but doing so is unnecessary unless the researcher is guided by theoretical and practical considerations. Moreover, unless the sample size is very large, the investigator rapidly runs out of observations in each cell when many control variables are used simultaneously.

In reporting statistical results, the researcher should not only describe the techniques or models used, but also examine the assumptions of the models and how they are consistent with the nature of the data. Otherwise, the techniques may not be appropriate for the analysis of the data set. In addition to reporting the significance level of the test results (e.g., p values), researchers may also report the confidence intervals of the estimates and the power of statistical tests.

Table 14.9 summarizes some statistical techniques used to analyze three or more variables based on nominal (categorical) or on interval levels of measurement. Ordinal measures may be treated as nominal or interval measures (if equal distance among intervals can be assumed) and the appropriate techniques for those levels may then be used. It should be emphasized that the table is by no means exhaustive. In addition, many multivariate procedures investigate relationships among variables without designating some as independent and others as dependent. For example, principal component and factor analyses examine relationships within a single set of variables. Canonical correlation analysis examines the relationship between two sets of variables. Interested readers should consult both a multivariate and an econometric textbook for detailed discussions

Table 14.9. Level of measurement and analysis involving three or more variables

Dependent Variable	Independent Variable
Nominal /categorical	Nominal /categorical
	Logistic regression (dummy variables)
	Binary segmentation techniques
	Multidimensional contingency table analysis
	Interval-ratio
	Logistic regression
	Logit and probit analysis
	Discriminant analysis
Interval-ratio	Multiple regression (dummy variables)
	ANOVA
	Multivariate analysis of variance (MANOVA)
	Covariance analysis
	Multivariate binary seg=mentation techniques
	Multiple correlation
	Multiple regression
	Multiple curvilinear regression
	Path analysis
	Factor analysis
	Principal component
	Time-series analysis
	Survival analysis
	Cox regression
	Canonical correlation
	Structural models with latent variables

of those and many other multivariate techniques. The following is a partial list of sources:

- *A Guide for Selecting Statistical Techniques for Analyzing Social Science Data* (2nd ed.) by F. M. Andrews et al.

- *Analysis of Categorical Data: Dual Scaling and Its Applications* by S. Nishisato

- *The Foundations of Factor Analysis* by S. A. Mulaik

- *Intermediate Statistics and Econometrics: A Comparative Approach* by D. J. Poirer

- *Multivariate Analysis* by A. M. Kshirsagar

- *Multivariate Analysis* by K. V. Mardia et al.

- *Statistics for Business and Economics: Methods and Applications* (5th ed.) by E. Mansfield

This section discusses some of the more commonly used statistical analysis techniques: multiple regression, logistic regression, and path analysis.

Multiple Regression

Multiple regression is among the most versatile and powerful statistical techniques for analyzing the relationships among variables (Duncan, Knapp, and Miller, 1983). Multiple regression may be used simply to examine the relationships among variables or as an inferential method, to test hypotheses about population parameters.

The general formula for a multiple regression equation may be stated as follows:

Formula 14.22 $y = \beta_0 + \beta_1 x_1 + \beta_2 x_2 + \beta_3 x_3 + \cdots + \beta_i x_i + e$

where y is the dependent variable; each x_i represents an independent variable; β_0 is the y-intercept or the predicted value of y when all values of x are equal to zero; β represents the regression coefficient of each of the associated independent variables, or partial regression coefficient; and e is the error term, or the prediction error.

For example, in addition to the mother's education, empirical evidence indicates that a mother's smoking habit may also affect the child's birth weight. A multiple regression model of the child's birth weight on the mother's education and smoking habit is: $y = 5.37 + .17x_1 - .21x_2$, where y equals weight (pounds), x_1 equals education (years of education), and x_2 equals the mother's smoking habit (packs of cigarettes per day).

β_0 is the predicted birth weight (5.37 pounds) for infants from mothers who have no education and do not smoke. β_1 is the predicted change in weight (.17 pound) for every additional year of the mother's education, holding constant the effect of smoking, and β_2 is the predicted change in weight (−.21 pound) for every additional pack of cigarettes smoked per day, holding constant the effect of education. For a woman with six years of education who smokes two packs of cigarettes a day, then, the predicted birth weight of her child would be 5.97 pounds [(5.37 + .17(6) − .21(2)].

In multiple regression, the multiple correlation coefficient R, which reflects the correlation between the observed values of y and the predicted values of y, is a measure of how well the model fits the data. The square of the multiple correlation coefficient, R^2, is a measure of the proportion of the variance in y explained by all the independent variables in the model. For example, $R^2 = .70$, indicating that 70 percent of the variance in the child's birth weight is explained by the mother's education and smoking habit.

In addition to R^2, the analysis of variance test can be performed for the whole equation. The null hypothesis amounts to all the regression coefficients being zero. The test statistic is an F ratio of the variance explained by the regression equation to the residual or error variance.

In multiple regression, it is sometimes useful to report the standardized coefficients when a researcher is interested in examining the relative effects of the independent variables on the dependent variable. The raw (unstandardized) regression coefficients give the predicted change in y for a unit change in x, but the unit that attaches to each coefficient depends on the metric underlying each variable. Therefore, the magnitudes of the raw coefficients are not directly comparable. The standardized coefficients, on the other hand, are expressed in the standard deviation units and the variables are comparable within a single equation.

So far, the multiple regression model presented assumes an additive effect, that is, y is determined by $x_1 + x_2$. However, this is not a necessary assumption for a regression model. If the presence of an interaction effect (i.e., the impact of one independent variable depends on the value of another independent variable) is suspected, the interaction term of these two variables may be introduced. The model with the interaction term may be specified as follows (Lewis-Beck, 1980):

Formula 14.23 $\qquad y = \beta_0 + \beta_1 x_1 + \beta_2 x_1 x_2 + e$

For example, in examining the impact of education on income, if one wants to test whether the impact of education (x_1) on income (y) varies according to gender (x_2), i.e., sexual discrimination in income determination), an interaction term of *gender and education* ($x_1 x_2$) may be included in the regression model. If the regression coefficient of the interaction term (β_2) is significant, there is evidence that sexual discrimination might exist in income determination.

Assume the following is the result of the regression estimate: $y = 8050 + 630x_1 + 250x_1 x_2$, where y equals annual income (dollars), x_1 equals education (years), and x_2 equals gender (1 = male, 0 = female). Therefore, the regression equation for women is: $y = 8050 + 630x_1 + 250x_1(0)$, or $y = 8050 + 630x_1$. The regression equation for men is: $y = 8050 + 630x_1 + 250x_1(1)$, or $y = 8050 + (630 + 250)x_1$, or $y = 8050 + 880x_1$. According to the model, a woman with 10 years of education will make $14,350 a year [$y = 8050 + 630(10)$], but a man with 10 years of education will make $16,850 a year [$y = 8050 + 880(10)$].

Hierarchical multiple regression may be performed to examine the marginal (additional) impact of certain predictors. In a hierarchical multiple regression, the researcher decides not only how many predictors to enter but also the order in which they are entered. Usually, the order of entry is based on logical or theoretical considerations. For example, if there are three expected predictors (X1, X2, X3) to an outcome, the researcher may decide to enter these separately to examine the marginal impact of the predictors. When the predictor X1 is entered first, it accounts for 25 percent of the variance in Y. The second predictor, X2, accounts for an additional 33 percent of the variance in Y. Then the third predictor, X3, accounts for an extra 25 percent of the variance in Y.

When a multiple regression model includes two or more independent variables that are highly intercorrelated, the results become difficult to interpret. This problem is known as multicollinearity. The problem with collinear variables is that they provide very similar information, and it is difficult to separate out the effects of the individual variables. The tolerance of a variable is one common measure of collinearity. It is defined as $1 - R_i^2$, where R_i is the multiple correlation coefficient when the ith independent variable is predicted from the other independent variables. A small tolerance score indicates the presence of collinearity.

The multiple regression model presented so far is a technique for estimating linear relationships in the data. In many cases, it is necessary to convert the data to forms amenable to analysis by the general linear model by means of mathematical transformations. If a researcher is convinced, based on theoretical or empirical evidence, that relationships among variables are nonlinear, a mathematical specification may be found that is consistent with the type of nonlinearity expected or observed. For example, the researcher can take the logarithm of y. Other arithmetic manipulations include taking a square function (e.g., $y = \beta_0 + \beta_1 x_1 + \beta_2 x_2 + \beta_3 x_2^2 + e$), a cube function ($y = \beta_0 + \beta_1 x_1 + \beta_2 x_2 + \beta_3 x_2^2 + \beta_4 x_2^3 + e$), and so on.

Examples of mathematical transformations include the polynomial model, the exponential model, and the hyperbolic model. The polynomial model may be specified as:

Formula 14.24 $\quad y = \beta_0 + \beta_1 x_1 + \beta_2 x_1^2 + \beta_3 x_1^3 + \cdots + \beta_m x_1^m + e$

This model is appropriate when the slope of the relationship between independent variable x_1 and dependent variable y is expected to change sign as the value of x_1 increases. The exponential model may be specified as:

Formula 14.25 $\qquad\qquad\qquad y = \beta_0 x^{\beta e}$

This model is appropriate when the slope of the curve representing the relationship between x and y does not change sign but increases or decreases in magnitude as the value of x changes. For example, the relationship between health care expenditure and health status in the United States indicates a declining rate of return.

To estimate the coefficients of the exponential model, a researcher could take the logarithm of both sides so that the equation is in linear form and can be estimated by the general linear model:

Formula 14.26 $\qquad\qquad \log y = \log \beta_0 + \beta (\log x) + \log e$

The hyperbolic model may be specified as:

Formula 14.27 $\qquad\qquad\qquad y = \beta_0 + \beta (1/x) + e$

This model may also be called the reciprocal model. It is used when as the value of x gets infinitely large, the value of y approaches β_0. For example, the relationship between marketing expenditure and sales may look like this model. As marketing expenditure is increased indefinitely, sales first increase accordingly but later remain constant when the market is close to saturation.

When independent variables are nominal (e.g., race, gender), the investigator may choose to include these variables in a multiple regression model by creating a set of dummy variables or binary indicators that uniquely code a case into a category of the nominal variable. Dummy variables are typically indexed by the numerical values zero and one. An ordinal-level variable can also be transformed into a set of dummy variables and entered into a regression equation, for example, a variable whose categories are high, medium, and low. Alternatively, ordinal variables may be used as continuous variables if the investigator is willing to assume that the categories are separated by equal intervals.

Table 14.10 reports the raw data about the number of patients visiting emergency rooms and their insurance status for a county general hospital. The

Table 14.10. Raw data on insurance status and number of emergency room visits

Observation	y = Number of E.R. Visits	x = Insurance	d_1 = Public	d_2 = Private	d_3 = None
1	13	1	1	0	0
2	4	1	1	0	0
3	3	1	1	0	0
4	2	2	0	1	0
5	1	2	0	1	0
6	2	2	0	1	0
7	1	2	0	1	0
8	6	3	0	0	1
9	9	3	0	0	1
10	19	3	0	0	1
⋮					
N					

Note: For insurance, the codes are 1 = public (Medicare or Medicaid), 2 = private, and 3 = no insurance or self pay.

variable insurance may be receded into three dummy variables, d_1, d_2, and d_3, as shown. Since any one of the three dummies is a perfect linear function of the other two (i.e., if we know that a patient has neither public nor private insurance, we also know the patient must have no insurance), including all three dummies in the regression model will cause perfect multicollinearity so that the regression coefficients cannot be calculated. Therefore, we have to omit one of the dummy variables from the regression model. Thus, given a variable with k categories, $k - 1$ dummy variables may be created and entered into the regression model.

Estimating the model, that number of emergency room visits is a function of insurance status, requires that the dummy variable representing insurance be used. The results calculated for this model are: $y = 6.25 - 1.22d_1 - 4.95d_2$ and $R^2 = .48$. Specifically, β_0 (the intercept) is the predicted value of y when all independent variables equal zero. The independent variables in this model both equal zero when the patient has neither public ($d_1 = 0$) nor private insurance ($d_2 = 0$), or in other words, when the patient has no insurance. The intercept (6.25) is therefore interpreted as the predicted number of emergency room visits for a patient with no health insurance and is exactly equal to the mean number of emergency room visits for a patient with no health insurance in the sample. Thus, in dummy variable regression involving a single set of dummies, the intercept value is equal to the mean of the dependent variable for the omitted category.

The coefficient β_1 for the dummy variable corresponding to patients with public health insurance represents the change (over the intercept value) in number of emergency room visits for those in the d_2 category. In dummy variable regression involving a single set of dummies, the regression coefficients are interpreted as the difference in means between any one category and the omitted category.

The β_1 coefficient, −1.22, therefore implies that the mean number of emergency room visits by patients with public health insurance is 1.22 times less than the mean number of emergency room visits by patients with no insurance. The predicted number of emergency room visits by patients with public health insurance is 5.03 [or 6.25 − 1.22(1) − 4.95(0)]. Similarly, the predicted number of emergency room visits by patients with private insurance is 1.30 [or 6.25 − 1.22(0) − 4.95(1)], the mean for patients with private insurance. Finally, the R^2 for this model (0.48) means that 48 percent of the variance in number of emergency room visits is explained by patients' insurance status.

Logistic Regression

The distinction between a **logistic regression** model and a linear regression model is that the dependent variable is binary, or dichotomous, in logistic regression (e.g., whether one smokes or not, or has health insurance or not) but continuous in linear regression (Cox and Snell, 1989; Draper and Smith, 1998; Hosmer and Lemeshow, 2001; Kleinbaum, Kupper, Muller, and Nizam, 1997). Logistic regression is based on the assumption that the logarithm of the odds of belonging to one population is a linear function of several predictors (independent variables) in the model. The multiple logistic regression model may be presented as follows:

Formula 14.28 $\ln\left(\dfrac{p}{1 - p}\right) = \beta_0 + \beta_1 x_1 + \beta_2 x_2 + \cdots + \beta_k x_k + e$

When we solve for probability, p, the model can be represented as:

Formula 14.29 $$p = \frac{e^{\beta_0 + \beta_1 x_1 + \beta_2 x_2 + \cdots + \beta_k x_k}}{1 + e^{\beta_0 + \beta_1 x_1 + \beta_2 x_2 + \cdots + \beta_k x_k}}$$

For the multiple logistic regression model in 14.29, the odds ratio relating to the dichotomous independent variable x_i, which is coded as one if present and zero if absent, may be estimated by:

Formula 14.30 Odds ratio $= e^{\beta i}$

Note that when the dependent variable is binary but represents a survival function (e.g., time from receiving treatment until death), survival analysis procedure is used. The survival analysis is then used to make inferences about the effects of treatments, prognostic factors, exposures, and other covariates on the function (see Hosmer, Lemeshow, and Kim, 2002).

As an example of logistic regression, the impact of the financial characteristics of rural primary care programs (PCPs) on the chance of program survival was examined (Shi et al., 1994). A randomly selected national cohort of rural PCPs ($n = 162$) was used to compare financial measures of programs that were continuing and those that were noncontinuing. Financial data were obtained from BCRR forms for the period 1978 to 1987. These Bureau of Common Reporting Requirements forms, which were submitted to the Bureau of Health Care

Table 14.11. Logistic regression of predictors for the continuation of primary care programs

Independent Variable	Dependent Variable			
	Continuing programs = 1	Noncontinuing programs = 0		
	Regression Coefficient	Standard Error	p Value	
(x_i)	(β)	(S_β)		(χ^2)
Intercept	-.306	.275		0.27
Self-sufficiency	.629	.251		0.01
Grant revenue	.438	.221		0.05
Average personnel costs	.00001	.00000		0.02
Patients	.00001	.00000		0.06

Note: n = 162.

Source: Shi, L., Samuels, M. E., Konrad, T. R., Porter, C. Q., Stoskopf, C. H., and Richter, D. L., "Rural Primary Care Program Survival: An Analysis of Financial Variables." *Journal of Rural Health,* 10(3): 173–182, 1994.

Delivery and Assistance of the HHS, are part of the requirement for getting federal grant support for the programs. A stepwise logistic regression procedure was used to calculate the significant predictors of program continuation (see Table 14.11).

The dependent variable is the status of program survival (1 = continuing, 0 = noncontinuing). Independent variables include self-sufficiency (Payments for Services ÷ Total Costs × 100), grant revenue (the percentage of total revenues that come from federal, state, local, or private grants), average personnel costs (Costs of Total Salaried Personnel ÷ Total Number of Salaried Personnel), and patients (the annual number of patients of all ages who have received treatment at the community health centers). Knowing the estimated logistic coefficients (Table 14.11) and using Equation 14.29, we can compute the probability of program survival under different conditions. For example, a program that is 20 percent self-sufficient, receives 20 percent grant revenue, has $15,000 average personnel cost, and\ has an annual patient load of 5,000 has a 29 percent chance of surviving. This probability is obtained by plugging the estimated coefficients from Table 14.11 into Equation 14.29 as follows:

$$p = \frac{e^{[-1.306 + .629(.20) + .438(.20) + .00001(15000) + .00001(5000)]}}{1 + e^{[-1.306 + .629(.20) + .438(.20) + .00001(15000) + .00001(5000)]}}$$

$$p = \frac{e^{-.8926}}{1 + e^{-.8926}}$$

Since $e = 2.71828$, then

$$p = \frac{(2.71828)^{-.8926}}{1 + (2.71828)^{-.8926}} = \frac{.40958968}{1.40958968} = 0.29057369, \text{ or } 29\%$$

The odds ratio (relative risk) of a program noncontinuing given the extent of a specific condition can be computed using the estimated regression coefficients (Table 14.11) and Equation 14.30. For example, the odds ratio of grant revenue is 1.55 ($e_i^\beta = 2.7182^{.438}$), indicating that for a 1 percent increase in grant revenue, the chance of program survival improves by 1.55 times. Similarly, improvement in the self-sufficiency ratio by 1 percent increases the chance of program survival by 1.88 times ($2.71828^{.629}$). Thus, the use of logistic regression provides an efficient way to estimate the probability of the occurrence of an event or condition and the odds ratio (relative risk) of having that event or condition.

Path Analysis

Path analysis is a popular form of multivariate analysis that provides the possibility for causal determination among a set of measured variables (Miller and Salkind, 2002). It is a procedure that gives a quantitative interpretation of an assumed causal system. Path analysis may consist of a series of regression equations, with many variables in the model taking their places respectively as dependent and independent variables (Duncan, 1975). In other words, most of the variables in the model will be dependent in one equation and independent in one or more different equations. A four-variable path model may be delineated as follows:

(1) $x_2 = p_{21}x_1 + p_{2u}R_u$

(2) $x_3 = p_{31}x_1 + p_{32}x_2 + p_{3v}R_v$

(3) $x_4 = p_{41}x_1 + p_{42}x_2 + p_{43}x_3 + p_{4w}R_w$

where p represents the path coefficient, x is the variable, and R is the residual or unexplained variance. The path coefficients (p's) can be derived from the standardized regression coefficients, computed by multiplying an unstandardized coefficient by the ratio of the standard deviation of the independent variable to the standard deviation of the dependent variable (Pindyck and Rubinfeld, 1991). Specifically, path coefficients are identical to partial regression coefficients (β's) when the variables are measured in standard form. With path analysis, both direct and indirect effects of one variable may be computed.

Developing **causal modeling** is the first step in path analysis (Wang, Eddy, and Westerfield, 1992). Causal modeling requires the researcher to think causally about the research question and construct an arrow diagram that reflects causal processes. This type of modeling identifies variables for analysis based on a theoretical framework, literature review, and observations. The resulting models are likely to be theory driven.

Examples of causal structures are provided in Figure 14.4. Panel A depicts a situation where X is causally related to Z but not to Y, and Y is causally related to Z but not to X. Panel B indicates that X is a direct cause of Y and an indirect cause of Z, mediated by Y. Panel C shows X has a cocausal relationship between Y and Z. Finally, panel D demonstrates that Z is causally dependent on both X

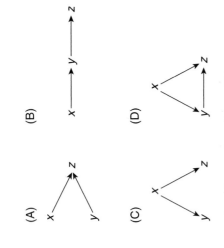

(A)

(B)

(C)

(D)

Figure 14.4. Examples of causal structure diagrams

and Y plus an indirect cause of X via X's impact on Y. The result of causal modeling is the completion of a path diagram that indicates the theoretical or expected relationships among the measured variables in the model.

The second step in path analysis is to compute the path coefficients. Path coefficients reflect the amount of direct contribution of a given variable to another variable when the effects of other related variables are taken into account. Path coefficients may be calculated either through regression programs or zero-order correlations among variables (Loether and McTavish, 1974). The results of the path coefficients may then be entered in the path diagram.

The third step in path analysis is to conduct a "goodness of fit" test. Land (1969) suggests three approaches: (1) examine the amount of variation in the dependent variables that is explained by variables specified in the model; (2) examine the size of path coefficients to see whether they are large enough to warrant the inclusion of a variable or path in the model; and (3) evaluate the ability of the model to predict correlation coefficients that were not used in computation of the path coefficients themselves. The second approach examines the R^2's of the various equations. The first approach entails examining whether the path coefficients are significant. In applying the third approach, the researcher could test an alternative model by substituting factors in the basic model believed to be more important and by adding new factors to the basic model.

The fourth and final step in path analysis is to interpret the results. Both direct and indirect effects of the variables in the causal model may be studied. It should be understood that path analysis does not discover causal relationships but rather gives a quantitative estimate of an assumed causal system based on both theoretical and empirical evidence.

As an example, the relationship between family planning, socioeconomic conditions, and fertility was investigated in six rural villages of China, based on a 1989 random household survey (Shi, 1992). The theoretical model (see Figure 14.5) guiding the analysis concerns the extent to which family planning programs and socioeconomic conditions affect fertility among rural inhabitants. Both family

Figure 14.5. **Theoretical model specifying family planning and socioeconomic conditions as they relate to fertility**

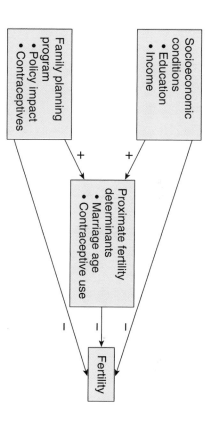

Source: Adapted from the author's study.

planning programs and socioeconomic conditions are hypothesized to have negative direct effects on fertility. The indirect effects of socioeconomic conditions on fertility through family planning and proximate fertility variables are hypothesized to be positive. The indirect effects of family planning programs on fertility through proximate fertility variables are hypothesized to be positive. Finally, the proximate fertility variables are hypothesized to inversely affect fertility.

Table 14.12 displays the path coefficients estimated from regression procedures. All family planning measures and all but one (income level) socioeconomic measure are significantly related to fertility. Further, the family planning measures and female education are significantly related to both proximate fertility measures that are related to fertility. Male education and per capita income

Table 14.12. **Direct, indirect, and total effects of predictor variables on fertility**

| Predictor | Direct Effects | Indirect Effects | | | Total Indirect Effects |
		Marriage Age	Contraception	Total	
	(1)	(2)	(3)	(4)	(5)
Policy impact	−.096	−.006	−.017	−.023	−.119
Male education	.018	−.006	.004	−.002	.016
Female education	−.077	−.007	−.015	−.022	−.099
Per capita income	.0004	.00009	−.00008	.00001	.00041
Income level	−.183	−.026	.020	−.006	−.189
Marriage age	−.043	—	—	—	−.043
Contraception	−.017	—	—	—	−.017
Free contraceptives	−.256	−.021	.020	−.001	−.257

Source: Shi, L., "Determinants of Fertility: Results from a 1989 Rural Household Survey in China." *Social Science Journal,* 29(4): 457–477, 1992.

are both related to contraceptive use. Consistent with the temporally ordered structural model, it is possible for the predictor variables to have sizable effects on fertility decline through indirect paths. These are described in columns 2 through 4 of Table 14.12. When the indirect effects of each variable are added to its direct effects (column 1), we obtain the total effect of that variable on fertility (column 5). Examination of all total effects shows that policy impact, female and male education, free contraceptive provision, and income level assume somewhat greater importance than was implied by consideration of their direct effects alone.

Factor Analysis

Factor analysis is a statistical technique that involves exploring the relationships between variables, determining if related variables can be explained by a smaller number of underlying factors or constructs, and reducing the number of variables in the analysis, if appropriate (Norman and Streiner, 2000). Factor analysis could be applied to any number of health services research topics in which current knowledge is incomplete. One example is measuring depression and anxiety. In order to create an appropriate screening tool that distinguishes between depression and anxiety, a researcher could perform a factor analysis on a pilot screening tool. He or she would screen a sample of patients using the tool, and then perform a factor analysis to see how well (or how poorly) the different types of questions hang together.

There are several distinct steps involved in factor analysis, all of which can be performed using statistical software, such as STATA. First, the researcher chooses relevant variables to be included in the analysis. In the depression and anxiety example, these variables might include "loss of appetite" and "trouble sleeping." Next, using a computer program, the researcher creates a correlation matrix, which standardizes the units of all the variables, and displays how well each of the variables correlates with the other variables meant to measure one factor (e.g., depression or anxiety). Ideally, all of the variables meant to describe depression would correlate strongly with one another, and would not correlate at all with variables meant to describe other factors (e.g., anxiety). The overall adequacy of the correlation matrix is also assessed by the computer program using tests such as the Bartlett Test of Sphericity and the Kaiser-Meyer-Olkin Measure of Sampling Adequacy. The results of these tests will indicate whether particular variables are needed in the analysis (Norman and Streiner, 2000).

The next step in factor analysis involves extracting the factors and deciding which factors to retain. Again, the computer program will run the appropriate tests, which include the Eigenvalue one test and Cattell's scree test. Factors that score above a certain threshold on these tests should be retained, and others may be dropped from the analysis. The next step, rotation of factors, helps simplify the model and spread variability more evenly. Essentially, rotating the factors makes the model easier to interpret; it does not change the fit of the model. After rotating the factors, the researcher can make a final decision about dropping or adding variables, and construct his or her scale for more widespread use (Norman and Streiner, 2000).

Multilevel Analysis

As the name implies, **multilevel analysis** techniques are useful when data exist at several different levels. If data are nested, or if a study has several different units of analysis, multilevel analysis is a valuable tool. For instance, multilevel analysis could be used in: (1) a study comparing quality improvement achievements of departments within several different hospitals, (2) a longitudinal study in which several distinct observations are made on individuals over time, or (3) a meta analysis in which subjects are nested within different studies (Hox, 2002).

In the past, multilevel data would be aggregated or disaggregated to one single level of interest and analyzed using ordinary multiple regression, ANOVA, or another standard statistical method. This strategy for analyzing multilevel data was flawed for two reasons. First, the statistical analysis lost power. In addition, researchers risked committing ecological fallacies by analyzing data at one level and applying the results to data at another level (Hox, 2002; Snijders, 2003).

To avoid these pitfalls, researchers developed multilevel analysis techniques, including multilevel regression models and multilevel models for covariance structures. The multilevel regression model, also called the hierarchical linear model (HLM), is similar to a standard linear regression model. However, in HLM, the probability model for the residuals (i.e., errors) reflects the multilevel structure of the data (Snijders, 2003). Multilevel models for covariance structures are also called structural equation models (SEM). These models can be used for several purposes, including goodness-of-fit estimates, factor analysis, and latent class analysis. SEMs can be estimated using the statistical software package Mplus (Snijders, 2003).

Statistics for Policy Analysis

Chapter 9 discussed several techniques used in health policy analysis, such as decision analysis, cost–benefit analysis, cost-effectiveness analysis, and modeling. Given the broad scope of health policy issues and the diversity of work done by health policy analysts (e.g., program and policy planning, budgeting, evaluation, design, and management), it is often necessary for health policy analysts to use the full range of statistical techniques discussed in this chapter.

An additional statistical tool used by health policy analysts is econometrics. **Econometrics**, simply defined, is statistical methods applied to economic problems (Folland, Goodman, and Stano, 2004). For instance, a basic econometrics method is hypothesis testing. Suppose a policy analyst is interested in determining whether the average cost of hospital care for cardiac bypass surgery differs by region. He or she would formulate a hypothesis (e.g., the average cost of hospital care for cardiac bypass surgery does not differ by region), choose a suitable sample, test the hypothesis by gathering data and calculating the mean cost of hospital care for cardiac bypass surgery in different regions, make the appropriate conclusion regarding the hypothesis, and apply these results to the policy decision at hand.

Regression analysis is another valuable econometric technique for policy analysis. Many health economics issues (e.g., health care costs and utilization) lend themselves to regression analysis. An example of a simple linear econometric regression that could be used by a policy analyst would be an examination of the relationship between the price of diabetic blood testing strips (independent variable) and the quantity of diabetic blood testing strips purchased (dependent variable). If the researcher determined there was a relationship between these two variables using simple regression, he or she could then perform a multiple regression, which would include several variables, in addition to price, that could affect the quantity of diabetic testing strips purchased (e.g., income and education level of the purchaser).

SUMMARY

Before research is formally analyzed, data are first explored to make sure all elements are included in one data file and prepared for hypothesis testing and model building. The choice of appropriate statistics is determined by the level of measurement and the number of variables analyzed. Commonly used descriptive statistics for analyzing one variable at a time include frequency and percentage distributions, measures of central tendency (mean, median, and mode), variability or dispersion (range, standard deviation, variance), shape (frequency or percentage polygon, skewness, kurtosis, leptokurtic, platykurtic), and standard scores (z score, rate, ratio). Commonly used bivariate procedures include cross-tabulation, chi-square (χ^2), phi coefficient (ϕ), coefficient of contingency (C), Cramér's V, Goodman–Kruskal's lambda (λ), relative risk ratio, Kendall's tau (τ), Goodman–Kruskal's gamma (γ), ANOVA, Pearson correlation coefficient (r), and paired t test. Commonly used multivariate statistical procedures include multiple regression, logistic regression, path analysis, factor analysis, and multilevel analysis.

REVIEW QUESTIONS

1. Why do researchers explore and examine data prior to formal analysis?
2. What descriptive statistics have you learned from the chapter? How can they be used (i.e., what level of measurement are they suitable for)?
3. What bivariate statistics have you learned from the chapter? How can they be used (i.e., what level of measurement are they suitable for)?
4. What multivariate analysis procedures have you learned from the chapter? How can they be used (i.e., what level of measurement are they suitable for)?

REFERENCES

Cox, D. R., and Snell, E. J. (1989). *The Analysis of Binary Data* (2nd ed.), London: Methuen.

Draper, N. R., and Smith, H. (1998). *Applied Regression Analysis* (3rd ed.). New York: Wiley.

Duncan, O. D. (1975). *Introduction to Structural Equation Models.* New York: Academic Press.

Duncan, R. C., Knapp, R. G., and Miller, M. C. (1983). *Introductory Biostatistics for the Health Sciences.* Albany, NY: Delmar.

Folland, S., Goodman, A. C., and Stano, M. (2004). *The Economics of Health and Health Care* (4th ed.). Upper Saddle River, NJ: Prentice Hall.

Goodman, L. A., and Kruskal, W. H. (1954). Measures of association for cross-classification. *Journal of the American Statistical Association, 49,* 732–764.

Grady, K. E., and Wallston, B. S. (1988). *Research in Health Care Settings.* Newbury Park, CA: Sage.

Herman, J. L., Morris, L. L., and Fitz-Gibbon, C. T. (1987). *Evaluator's Handbook.* Newbury Park, CA: Sage.

Hosmer, D. W., and Lemeshow, S. (2001). *Applied Logistic Regression: Textbook and Solutions Manual.* New York: Wiley.

Hosmer, D. W., Lemeshow, S., and Kim, S. (2002). *Applied Survival Analysis: Regression Modeling of Time to Event Data.* New York: Wiley.

Hox, J. (2002). *Multilevel Analysis: Techniques and Applications.* Mahwah, NJ: Lawrence Erlbaum Associates.

Kleinbaum, D. G., Kupper, L. L., Muller, K. E., and Nizam, A. (1997). *Applied Regression Analysis and Other Multivariate Methods* (3rd ed.). Belmont, CA: Wadsworth.

Land, K. C. (1969). Principles of path analysis. In E. F. Borgatta (Ed.), *Sociological Methodology.* San Francisco: Jossey-Bass.

Last, J. M. (2001). *A Dictionary of Epidemiology* (4th ed.). New York: Oxford University Press.

Lewis-Beck, M. S. (1980). *Applied Regression.* Beverly Hills, CA: Sage.

Lilienfeld, A. M., and Lilienfeld, D. E. (1994). *Foundations of Epidemiology* (3rd ed.). New York: Oxford University Press.

Loether, H. J., and McTavish, D. C. (1974). *Descriptive Statistics for Sociologists.* Boston: Allyn & Bacon.

Miller, D. C., and Salkind, N. J. (2002). *Handbook of Research Design and Social Measurement* (6th ed.). Thousand Oaks, CA: Sage.

Norman, G. R., and Streiner, D. L. (2000). *Biostatistics: The Bare Essentials.* Hamilton, Ontario: Decker.

Pindyck, R. S., and Rubinfeld, D. L. (1991). *Econometric Models and Economic Forecasts* (3rd ed.). New York: McGraw-Hill.

Shi, L. (1992). Determinants of fertility: Results from a 1989 rural household survey. *Social Science Journal, 29(4),* 457–477.

Shi, L., Samuels, M. E., Konard, R., Porter, C., Stoskopf, C. H., and Richtor, D. (1994). Rural primary care program survival: An analysis of financial variables. *Journal of Rural Health, 10(3),* 173–182.

Singleton, R. A., and Straits, B. C. (2005). *Approaches to Social Research* (4th ed.). New York: Oxford University Press.

Snijders, T. A. B. (2003). Multilevel analysis. In M. Lewis-Beck, A. E. Bryman, and
T. F. Liao (Eds.), *The SAGE Encyclopedia of Social Science Research Methods* (Vol. 2,
pp. 673–677). Newbury Park, CA: Sage.

SPSS Inc. (1997). *SPSS Advanced Statistics.* Chicago: SPSS.

Wang, M., Eddy, J. M., and Westerfield, R. C. (1992). Causal modeling in health survey
studies. *Health Values, 16(4),* 55–57.

CHAPTER 15 ❖

Applying Health Services Research

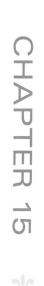

LEARNING OBJECTIVES

- To become aware of the channels for communicating the results of health services research.

- To understand the general format of a research report for refereed journals.

- To appreciate the training needs for a successful health services researcher.

Scientific research is cumulative. Without communicating their research findings, investigators cannot contribute to the cumulative body of knowledge that defines scientific disciplines. Thus, one reason for researchers to publicize their findings is to add to the stock of scientific knowledge so that the research is connected with past inquiry and future investigations can build upon the present.

In addition to the advancement of knowledge, health services researchers are eager to communicate their findings because of the applied nature of their inquiry. Chapter 1 stated that the priorities of HSR are largely established by societal questions and issues surrounding health services for population groups. Much of HSR is conducted to solve health-related problems. Indeed, the products of HSR are often assessed primarily in terms of their usefulness to people with decision-making responsibilities, whether they be clinicians, administrators of health services organizations or government agencies, or politicians and elected officials charged with formulating national health care policy.

This chapter delineates specific communication channels through which research findings can be publicized. The format for writing a scientific report for publication is described. The potential for and constraints of implementing research findings are discussed. The chapter ends with a review of the 10 major stages in HSR covered throughout the book, followed by an examination of the skills needed to become an effective health services researcher.

COMMUNICATING HEALTH SERVICES RESEARCH

Before communicating research findings, investigators must know who their intended audiences are because the types of communication channels vary depending on the audience. Potential audiences may be divided into three groups: the research community, the stakeholders, and the public. The research community includes scientists or would-be scientists who share similar research interests. Stakeholders are those who provide funding for research or have a key role to play in implementing research findings. The public is made up of neither researchers nor stakeholders. Often, the same research can have several different types of audiences, and investigators should adapt their communication styles to specific audiences to maximize comprehension and acceptance. Table 15.1 summarizes the channels of communication commonly used by the different audiences.

Research Community

When the intended audience is part of the research community, certain assumptions can be made as to prior knowledge. Research findings may be summarized rather than explained in great detail. Similarly, more technical terms can be used than would be the case for other audiences.

The most popular means of communicating research results to the scientific community is to write an article for publication in a refereed scientific journal.

Table 15.1. Health services research communication by audience

	Audience		
	Research Community	Stakeholders	Public
Method of communication	Journal articles	Research proposals	Newspapers
	Conference presentations	Reports	Magazines
	Working papers	Symposiums	Television
	Monographs	Testimonies	Radio
	Books	Research notes	Brochures

Appendix 1 lists journals commonly used by health services researchers as well as other social scientists. The length and style of the articles may vary among journals. Before submitting articles for publication, investigators should examine the manuscript preparation guidelines of, and samples of articles previously published by, the journal in question. Since it typically takes months (sometimes even longer) between article submission and publication, researchers often use other means to disseminate their findings.

Another popular means of communicating research findings is through professional conferences. Investigators typically join a number of professional associations related to their research of interest. These associations generally organize periodic (e.g., annual) conferences or meetings to allow members an opportunity to present their research. Since it is usually more difficult to have a paper accepted by a journal than presented at a conference, professional conferences provide an excellent opportunity for a larger number of investigators to communicate their research. Another advantage of conferences over journals is the speed with which researchers can publicize their findings. Refereed journals, particularly the most sought-after ones, usually have a backlog of articles to be published. Investigators may wait many months between submission and request for revision, and formal acceptance and final publication. Most journals allow papers to be presented prior to publication. An added advantage of conferences is that they can be used to invite comments, suggestions, and criticisms. Thus, many researchers use conference presentations as a means of gathering suggestions for revising their papers before formal submission to an academic journal. Since each presentation session has a limited time frame, to achieve maximum feedback, investigators can distribute the draft manuscript and leave their addresses with the audience. Researchers should mark "confidential" on the draft to prevent premature citation.

Working papers and monographs are another form of reporting to the research community. A working paper implies the article is still in progress and not fully polished. It is circulated among colleagues, or those who share the same research interest, with an implicit request for comments and suggestions. Working papers can vary in length and may present only a portion of the research findings. Since researchers' professional reputations are not at stake in a working paper, they can present rather tentative analyses and interpretations, and invite comments on them. While working papers are often the prelude to journal articles, monographs are preparations for books. Monographs are usually written for large and complex projects. Similar to working papers, monographs may be circulated among peers for comments and suggestions. Monographs may also be published internally by some research institutions.

Books generally represent the most comprehensive if not the most prestigious form of research report. They have all the advantages of a monograph—length, detail—but are more polished. Since the publication of research in the form of a book gives the findings an appearance of greater authenticity and worth, and could therefore lead readers to accept the findings uncritically, the researcher has a special obligation to maintain truthfulness.

Stakeholders

When stakeholders are the intended audience, investigators cannot assume any prior knowledge of the research subject and terminology. There are several types of stakeholders, including funders or sponsors, people affected by the results of the research (e.g., clients of an evaluated program, groups interested in the study results for advocacy purposes), and primary users of the research results (e.g., policy makers, program administrators). It is important to consider how to best translate research findings for these different stakeholders (Centers for Disease Control and Prevention, 1999). Introductions and explanations are necessary whenever technical terms and concepts are introduced.

One important group of stakeholders is the funding agency or organization, and the first formal contact with this stakeholder group is through a research proposal. In a research proposal, the investigator tries to convince a prospective sponsor or funder that he or she is qualified to perform the research activities necessary to answer the questions deemed important to the sponsor or funder. Most funding sources require the same basic information for a research proposal, although the details and required format may vary. See Chapter 3 for a review of writing a research proposal.

Perhaps the most common means of communicating with stakeholders is through technical reports. Reports are routinely required by funders and sponsors, and often serve the additional purpose of informing policy makers, program administrators, and other groups interested in the study results. In preparing such a report, researchers should keep in mind the audience for the report—scientific or lay—and their initial reasons for sponsoring the project. The report should be focused and consistent with the purposes of the sponsors or funders for the research. It is usually unwise to include research findings that have no interest or value to the sponsors. At the same time, it may be useful to summarize the ways in which the research has advanced basic scientific knowledge, if it has. In finalizing the funding contract and research protocol, researchers and sponsors should work out an agreement in terms of whether permission is granted to the investigators for publishing research findings in academic journals.

Stakeholders, such as sponsors and policy makers, may be invited to symposiums conducted to discuss the research and its implications for decision makers. Symposiums provide an opportunity not only to communicate research findings, but also to discuss and debate research issues of interest to the stakeholders.

Expert testimony is another means by which researchers can promote awareness and use of their research. Testifying before stakeholders, such as during congressional hearings or state Certificate of Need meetings, requires researchers to be well focused, to speak in nontechnical terms, and to explain fully their findings.

Finally, research notes can be prepared that summarize the basic research design, major findings, and the policy implications. The notes may be adapted from the executive summary portion of the research report, and they can be sent to stakeholders to inform them about a relevant policy issue.

Public

When the intended audience is the general public, investigators can rely on the mass media to publicize significant research findings. Examples include newspapers (both national and local), popular magazines and journals, television programs, and radio talk shows. In addition, special brochures may be prepared that summarize the research and its significant findings. It is critical that presentations use nontechnical language and that any key terms and concepts are defined and explained. No assumptions should be made about the audience's existing knowledge of the research topic. Fact sheets and issue briefs are other ways of synthesizing and communicating research findings to the public. Many government and private research agencies regularly disseminate fact sheets and issue briefs that summarize major studies or analyses. For example, the Henry J. Kaiser Family Foundation has produced periodic issue briefs and fact sheets on such topics as Medicaid/SCHIP (State Children's Health Insurance Program), Medicare, costs, the uninsured, state policy, prescription drugs, HIV/AIDS, minority health, and women's health (http://www.kff.org).

PUBLISHING HEALTH SERVICES RESEARCH

To publish research in a peer-reviewed academic journal, researchers need to be familiar with the journal requirements, follow these requirements in the preparation of the manuscript, and be prepared for rejection and resubmission.

Familiarity with Journal Requirements

Each journal has its own goals, standards of quality, and preferred style. The more accurately these requirements are met, the better an investigator's chances of getting accepted for publication. As a first task, the researcher should become thoroughly familiar with all targeted journals. Manuscript preparation guidelines should be thoroughly studied. If the guidelines cannot be found, the journal office should be contacted and a copy requested. The articles that have been published in the journal should be read and attention paid to the content, writing style, structure and organization, use of tables and charts, and length. The investigator's manuscript, if it is to be published, must be very similar to these. Table 15.2 presents the general format for scholarly papers.

Title

The title of a paper should succinctly and accurately reflect the study contents. Since the title of a paper will be recorded in the investigator's curriculum vitae, preferably it should reflect the area of research the investigator wants to be associated with. Some journals may place a limit on the number of words to be used in a title. If there is such a requirement, it should be adhered to.

Table 15.2. General format for scholarly papers

Title	Succinctly and and accurately reflects study contents
Abstract	Objectives, methods, results, conclusion
Introduction	Problem statement, study purpose, significance
Literature review	Current literature, conceptual framework, research questions or hypotheses
Methods	▪ Design (type of research, implementation procedures)
	▪ Subjects (research population, sample size, sampling procedure, response rate, sample characteristics, biases)
	▪ Measures (operational definitions, observations translated into variables, validity and reliability of measures)
	▪ Analysis (statistical and modeling techniques, data assumptions, testing and control)
Results	▪ Findings that answer the research questions or hypotheses
	▪ Use of subheadings, tables, and figures
Discussion	Key research findings and implications, comparisons with previous research, limitations, future research direction
References	Cited literature
Appendix (optional)	Questionnaire instrument, tables

Abstract

An abstract is a capsule version of the full article that is prepared after the article is written. There is usually a word limit imposed by the journal (e.g., 150 to 200 words). The purpose of an abstract is to help readers decide whether the report is consistent with their interests. An abstract can be prepared by using the same words and phrases in the finished article. Typically, a well-prepared abstract includes a statement of purpose, a description of the design, a description of the setting and research subjects, a statement of intervention (if applicable), a concise summary of the major measures used, a clear and quantified presentation of the results, and a conclusion statement. Some journals require specific ordered content for the abstract. For example, the *Journal of the American Medical Association (JAMA)* requires authors to use the following subheadings for their abstracts: Context, Objective, Design, Setting, Patients (or Participants), Interventions (if there are any), Main Outcome Measures, Results, and Conclusions (http://jama.ama-assn.org). Since titles and abstracts are often the only things researchers have access to in computerized databases, they often decide whether or not to retrieve a paper based solely on its title and abstract.

Introduction

The introduction section lays the groundwork for the rest of the paper. It contains a clear statement of the problem, the major purpose of the study, and its theoretical as well as practical significance. The problem and its significance play an important role in paper acceptance. Studies that are potentially important often address critical questions from either a theoretical or a practical perspective. Articles that use a new methodological approach could also be valuable contributions.

Literature Review

The literature review section focuses on the current literature that clearly frames the study, describes the conceptual framework of the study, and states the research questions or hypotheses. Key studies are reviewed in terms of theoretical and methodological approaches, as well as major findings that document the evolution of the research problem. Such a review provides the framework for the current inquiry, which builds on previous theories and research. The hypotheses or research questions to be addressed fill a gap in the current knowledge and/or research. The theoretical model used by the study can be presented in a figure, such as an arrow diagram. The hypotheses or research questions should be precisely stated and testable. Some journals require literature review to be incorporated in the introduction section. If this is the case, authors need to prepare a concise summary of the literature and a conceptual framework. To allow readers to assess the adequacy and completeness of the literature review, authors should briefly summarize their research methodology, including bibliographic indexes searched; vendor interfaces, strategies, and key terms used; and criteria for inclusion and exclusion of studies.

Methods

The research methods section summarizes how the study was done so that others might replicate it based on the information given. The following subheadings may be used to assist in the preparation of this section: design, subjects, measurement, and analysis. The design of the study tells what type of research was conducted, whether it be experimental, survey, longitudinal, qualitative field study, or a preexisting data model. The procedures for implementing the study should be described in sufficient detail to allow approximate replication. If preexisting data were used, the sources of the data and their completeness, validity, and reliability should be addressed in detail. The design should be appropriate to the research purpose.

The subjects of the study are those who participated in the study. The research population, sample size, sampling procedure, response rate, sample characteristics, and biases, if any, should all be described. Critical evaluation criteria for submitted manuscripts often include appropriate control or comparison groups, proper selection or assignment of subjects, sufficient sample size, sufficient response rate, and appropriate handling of missing data and attrition.

Measurement describes the operational definitions of the variables used in the study, specifies the way in which the observations were translated into variables, and assesses the validity and reliability of the measures. If the study is complicated and lengthy, a complete questionnaire may be attached as an appendix.

The analysis specifies the statistical and modeling techniques used and reviews assumptions made concerning the data. The analysis procedures should be appropriate to the research purpose and data. There should be adequate testing and control for violations of data assumptions (e.g., distribution, linearity, collinearity, and residuals).

Results

The results section presents the findings of the study, which answers the research questions or hypotheses that frame the study. The findings should be presented judiciously but completely. The significance, power, and confidence intervals regarding the findings should also be reported. Tables and figures may be constructed to facilitate the presentation of the results and are placed near the text describing the findings. However, authors should consult the guidelines to see if there is any restriction on the number of tables that can be included in a manuscript. Subheadings may be used to help organize the presentation. They may be phrased to reflect the research questions or hypotheses. In presenting the results it is critical that the research questions or hypotheses be specifically addressed.

Discussion

The discussion section provides a succinct summary of key research findings relevant to the research questions or hypotheses, discusses the implications of the results in terms of theoretical and practical significance, compares the findings to other relevant studies, points out the various limitations of the research and their impact on the results, and suggests directions for future inquiry.

References

The reference section generally includes literature cited in the text of the article. The format of the references varies by journal, and authors should familiarize themselves with the preferred style of the particular journal to which they are submitting before preparing the references.

Appendix

An appendix is usually not required or encouraged by journals. Unless it is a lengthy and complicated study, authors need not use an appendix. An appendix may include such items as the complete research questionnaire and additional tables not already presented in the results section, as well as other items the authors perceive as being relevant to an understanding of the research.

Length

Finally, the length of the paper is usually restricted by journals. Twenty-five typed double-spaced pages, including references and tables, can be used as a rough guide. However, the investigator should check the specific instructions of the journal. If a study is complicated and of great significance, many journals make exceptions in terms of restrictions on the length of the paper or the number of tables included.

Dealing with Rejections

When reports are prepared according to journal guidelines, they have a better chance of being accepted for publication. However, there is no guarantee this will happen. Even experienced researchers receive rejections from time to time. Many factors could influence a rejection decision. The competitiveness of a particular journal is a critical factor. If the acceptance rate is low, say 10 percent of all manuscripts submitted, then, by design, many articles, including those of good quality, will be rejected. Authors may target several journals so that if the paper is rejected by one journal, they may proceed to submit elsewhere. Young scholars may be advised to choose among journals where the competition is less intense. After accumulating some experience and confidence, they can then submit to more competitive journals.

Another factor that affects a paper's acceptance is the review process. Usually, a submitted paper is reviewed by two or more professionals with relevant experience or interests. A good reviewer studies the manuscript carefully, prepares a balanced critique, and points out ways to improve the article. The evaluations are subsequently weighed by the editor, who makes the final decision with regard to acceptance, revision and resubmission, or rejection. Unfortunately, editors do not always know the qualifications of reviewers. Some reviewers could be incompetent themselves. Qualified reviewers may be very busy and so forced to turn down the chance to review. Both reviewers and editors could have their own biases with respect to a particular topic or methodology. Most authors usually have no way of finding out these factors prior to the submission of their papers. However, once a rejection letter is received, the concerns of the editor and reviewers should be studied carefully. If they make sense, these concerns should be addressed prior to resubmitting the paper either to the same journal (if allowed) or elsewhere. If the criticism is irrelevant or off the mark, authors can appeal to the editor and request a reevaluation of the paper.

The most common reason for rejection is an irrelevant (with respect to the journal) or an inferior paper. Sometimes the topic is not relevant to the journal, not significant enough, or the design of the study is flawed. Some concerns are easier to handle than others. If the article is inappropriate for the journal, more relevant journals may be targeted for submission. Usually, a more specialized journal related to the author's area is more likely to accept the paper than a more general journal whose interest merely borders on the author's. If the submitted article is missing certain elements, the missing elements should be included. If the wrong analysis was used, the data should be reanalyzed with the proper approach. However, if the design is flawed or the topic is not significant, there is little an investigator can do other than accept this as a lesson for future reference. After all, not all research is published.

IMPLEMENTING HEALTH SERVICES RESEARCH

Perhaps the ultimate challenge for health services researchers is to see their research findings implemented in policy decisions. The applied nature of HSR indicates that one of its major goals is to apply disciplinary knowledge to solve current and emerging health-related problems so that resources can be better utilized to improve the health status of the population. The synthesis and dissemination of health services research have played and continue to play an important role in health policy formulation and implementation (Ginzberg, 1991). For example, HSR has improved the public's knowledge and understanding of the health care system. Historically, health services research played a major role in early health policy formulation, implementation, and clinical practice with respect to HIV/AIDS-related illness and primary care (Agency for Health Care Policy and Research, 1990; National Center for Health Services Research and Health Care Technology Assessment, 1985).

The analyses made of the effects of alternative RBRVS configurations (i.e., physician payment systems) are a good example of a health services research application. Health services research that has identified disturbingly large gaps in access to needed health care has served as an impetus to policies aimed at health care reform in order to reduce these gaps. The Robert Wood Johnson Foundation's Covering Kids and Families (CKF) initiative represents an elegant integration of health services research and practice (Morgan, Ellis, and Gifford, 2005). The CKF initiative aims to improve states' reenrollment processes for children and families covered by Medicaid and the State Children's Health Insurance Program (SCHIP). An evaluation of the initiative found that it is having a positive impact on reenrollment in 45 states. Specifically, it has allowed states that have succeeded in improving their reenrollment processes to provide valuable advice to struggling states.

However, the application of research knowledge is not always clear-cut, and investigators are often frustrated that their research is not taken seriously or reflected in policies. This section points out some inherent barriers hindering such goal attainment and identifies the requisites to overcoming these barriers.

Relevance

Sometimes a scientifically significant study may not have immediate or obvious policy significance. Another round of investigation may be necessary to make these studies more relevant both clinically and with respect to health policy. Studies that translate scientific discoveries into practical applications are termed *translational research*. Translational research has proven to be a powerful process that drives the clinical research engine. The recent NIH roadmap calls for reengineering the clinical research enterprise by enhancing the discipline of clinical and translational science, issuing institutional clinical and translational science awards, and providing translational research core services (http://nihroad map.nih.gov/clinicalresearch/overview-translational.asp).

Type of Study

The adoption of research findings in policy and practice also depends on the type of study and its likely impact. Research that focuses on clinical practices usually sees quick adoption because clinical policy is more sensitive to research evidence. The advocacy for evidence-based medicine can further enhance this connection. Studies that focus on organizational practices usually see slower adoption because changing organizational practices requires more time; in addition, more entities are involved (e.g., nonclinicians as well as clinicians). The emphasis on continual quality improvement provides a good impetus for organizations to improve.

Research that focuses on national policies takes much longer to influence policy. For example, the extensive studies that demonstrate the health effects of not having insurance have failed so far to achieve universal coverage. This is due to the fact that national policies are formulated through political processes in which stakeholders advocate their own interests through their influence on lawmakers. Research is merely a form of advocacy that competes with other influences. Even though research does not have decisive influence on policy, it does affect policy in the long run. For example, in terms of health insurance, even though the United States still does not have universal coverage, it is moving closer to that goal through a series of incremental approaches by way of Medicare, Medicaid, and SCHIP as well as other state initiatives.

Priorities

There is a potential conflict between policy and research priorities. Decision makers, who choose a course of action in response to a given health problem, are generally concerned about the most pressing problems, those that that hinder the progress of their work. One of the limiting factors in the production of useful HSR is the failure by researchers to study problems that are of most concern to decision makers. Similarly, the failure of decision makers to clearly communicate their problems and concerns to health services investigators often impedes the production of useful and relevant research. The concerns of decision makers may be unknown to researchers or may not coincide with the topics that researchers consider to be of the greatest scientific merit.

To overcome this barrier, the policy and research communities need to have frequent dialogues. Frequent meetings between investigators and decision makers would help in the understanding and appreciating of policy priorities, and research could then be planned to address these priorities. Another possible solution involves ensuring the presence of decision makers in the governing or consultative bodies of research institutions or teams so that needs get expressed and opportunities are identified in current projects.

Timetable

A potential conflict between decision makers and investigators is the different timetables expected of research. Decision makers facing a pressing problem expect the research to be completed immediately. Researchers, on the other hand, are concerned with the validity of the study design and findings. To ensure all phases of the investigation are accomplished properly, they often demand more time than decision makers envision.

One way to reduce this gap is to involve decision makers in the planning phase of the proposed research so that the two sides may come to an agreement as to the timetable for the project. The benefit of such consultation and negotiation is that there will be fewer surprises. Another way to shorten the gap is to create a series of useful progress reports and intermediate results from the study. For example, a review of the current literature on related topics may be provided to decision makers shortly after the research project begins. The results of a pilot test can be forwarded. Analysis of secondary data maintained by the agency may also be presented. During data collection, the participation of respondents and their characteristics can be summarized and reported. Shortly after data collection, descriptive summaries can be shared with decision makers before in-depth analyses are conducted. These intermediate reports can be useful for decision making even before the project has been completed.

Communication

Decision makers and researchers often do not share a common vocabulary. For decision makers, research results must be expressed in understandable vocabulary and free of technical jargon. For investigators, as dictated by the publishing guidelines of scientific journals, results must be communicated in precise scientific terms after a detailed description of the research design and analysis is provided. Many decision makers have trouble understanding the logic of study design or the various statistics used to analyze the data set.

Both researchers and decision makers can contribute to reducing the communication barrier. For investigators, in addition to technical reports for scientific journals, they can write nontechnical reports for decision makers that summarize the most pertinent results. If technical jargon must be used to describe the design or analysis, detailed explanations should be given. In addition, researchers can meet with decision makers to help interpret research findings and answer questions. Also, decision makers can improve their knowledge of scientific research by taking research-related courses and seminars and by reading scientific journals related to their areas.

Scope

Differences between policy and research scopes are another barrier to the implementation of research findings. Since social problems are inherently complicated, involving multiple factors and interconnections, decision makers require useful and relevant research to provide broad, integrated information that assesses all the dimensions of a problem and reflects all the relevant factors. In contrast, investigators are trained to focus on a well-defined, narrow subject matter in order to yield conclusive results.

To reduce the differences between policy and research scopes, it is critical that researchers be knowledgeable about the institution or problem under investigation, fully aware of the dimensions and related issues their research will affect, and able to design an integrated project that takes into account all important policy concerns. Effective research should provide information and analysis that take into account the multiplicity of interests that exist in both the political system and the health care system. If there are research constraints, decision makers need to be informed and their expectations directed accordingly.

Values

Researchers and decision makers may place different values on research. For investigators, the value of research may be to get published in prestigious scientific journals and to contribute to existing literature. For decision makers, the value in a research project is its immediate application to problem solving. While decision makers are concerned with the problems at hand, researchers are likewise concerned with the issues but also with their peers and reputations. In addition, personal values or ideological preferences may influence decision makers' acceptance of research based on scientific evidence.

To narrow the gap in values, decision makers should have a proper and realistic expectation of the value of research. They should be better educated and informed. At a minimum, they need to value the type of contribution scientific inquiry has made toward improved decision making, and to understand the criteria for judging the quality of research. For their part, the scientific community should place a higher premium on efforts toward research applications. Excellence in research should be defined not only as the pursuit of scientific knowledge, but also as the transformation of that knowledge into health policies and problem solving. Also, investigators should recognize their personal biases and predilections and guard against these in the process of research. Only when both sides value each other can research findings be more properly and widely used.

Leadership

Health services research is not a substitute for leadership in implementing research. While investigators can conduct relevant and timely analysis and summarize their research results in understandable reports that can be easily used by decision makers, leadership is required to translate the knowledge derived from HSR into politically acceptable policy. Health services research cannot empower individuals who do not have the necessary authority to implement policies. The development and implementation of health care policy fundamentally depends on the leadership and initiatives of decision makers at various levels and sectors of society.

Rapport

A close rapport needs to be built up between researchers and decision makers. Both sides need each other; they are very much interdependent. Decision makers rely on investigators to assist them in making sound and legitimate decisions that are based on scientific evidence and existing knowledge. Researchers need decision makers to identify, conduct, and implement research, including selecting research problems, obtaining funding, gaining access to research sites and subjects, and implementing research findings. The sooner both sides recognize this interdependency and work toward collaboration, the greater will be the value of health services research to policy formulation and implementation.

TRAINING HEALTH SERVICES RESEARCHERS

In a 1995 report, the Institute of Medicine highlighted four areas that characterize HSR training: the use of a multidisciplinary approach, the focus on basic and applied research, the examination of conceptual and theoretical relationships within and between health systems, and the investigation of both populations and individuals. The report suggested that "a single educational path is neither practical nor desirable" (p. 7) and that HSR needs to offer a range of training opportunities. This perspective is reflected in the variety of National Research Service Award (NRSA) programs (funded by the Agency for Healthcare Research and Quality [AHRQ]) that support HSR training in varied disciplines, including psychology, economics, anthropology, biomedicine, mathematics, political science, sociology, management sciences, and public health. The goal of this typically multidisciplinary training and education program, in addition to providing mentorship to help trainees select and investigate research topics in HSR, is to equip scholars with the necessary knowledge, skills, and experience to conduct research that will meet the evolving needs of patients, providers, health care plans, purchasers, and policy makers.

In September 2005, AHRQ sponsored a Health Services Research Doctoral Training Competencies Conference that defined the knowledge-based and skills-based competencies common to all HSR professionals trained at the doctoral level (see Table 15.3). Further, the conference summarized 21 essential educational domains associated with the 14 competencies (see Table 15.4). Educational domains provide more detailed descriptions of the content of the core competencies and should be reflected in HSR training programs. Near the close of the book is a summary of the knowledge and skills needed to become a competent health services researcher.

Table 15.3. HSR doctoral-level core competencies

No.	Label	Core Competency
1)	Breadth of HSR theoretical and conceptual knowledge	Know how to apply alternative theoretical and conceptual models from a range of relevant disciplines to HSR.
2	In-depth disciplinary knowledge and skills	Apply in-depth disciplinary knowledge and skills relevant to health services research.
3	Application of HSR foundational knowledge to health policy problems	Use knowledge of the structures, performance, quality, policy, and environmental context of health and health care to formulate solutions to health policy problems.
4	Innovative HSR questions	Pose innovative and important research questions, informed by systematic reviews of the literature, stakeholder needs, and relevant theoretical and conceptual models.
5	Interventional and observational study designs	Select appropriate interventional (experimental and quasi-experimental) or observational (qualitative, quantitative, or mixed methods) study designs to address specific health services research questions.
6	Primary data collection methods	Know how to collect primary health and health care data by survey, qualitative, or mixed methods.
7	Secondary data acquisition methods	Know how to assemble secondary data from existing public and private sources.
8	Conceptual models and operational measures	Use a conceptual model to specify study constructs for a health services research question, and then develop variables that reliably and validly measure these constructs.
9	Implementation of research protocols	Implement research protocols with standardized procedures that ensure reproducibility of the science.
10	Responsible conduct of research	Ensure the ethical and responsible conduct of research in the design, implementation, and dissemination of health services research.
11	Multidisciplinary teamwork	Work collaboratively in multidisciplinary teams.

(continues)

Table 15.3. HSR doctoral-level core competencies (continued)

No.	Label	Core Competency
12	*Data analysis*	Use appropriate analytical methods to clarify associations between variables and to delineate causal inferences.
13	*Scientific communication*	Effectively communicate the findings and implications of health services research through multiple modalities to technical and lay audiences.
14	*Stakeholder collaboration and knowledge translation*	Understand the importance of collaborating with policy makers, organizations, and communities to plan, conduct, and translate health services research into policy and practice.

Source: Adapted from *Health Services Research Competencies* (Final Report for Conference Grant R13 HS016070-01), by C. Forrest et al., 2006, November 15, Baltimore, MD: Johns Hopkins University.

Table 15.5 summarizes the major skill areas in which a competent health services researcher must be knowledgeable. They are related to each of the 10 stages in the conduct of HSR described throughout the book. They include knowledge about the subject matter, methodology, statistics, computer application software, writing, and public relations. If investigators lack any of these skills or knowledge, they must make sure others on the research team possess the missing elements, or else outside consultants should be sought. Many of these skills can be acquired in the classroom setting through the integration of theories and practices. However, proficiency in research can be achieved only through the carrying out of numerous research projects that integrate the many phases of health services research. These areas are described in greater detail below. At the end of the chapter is a capstone assignment that synthesizes and integrates the range of concepts covered throughout this book and gives the student an opportunity to demonstrate skills learned.

Subject

The foremost research skill is subject-related knowledge. An in-depth knowledge of the subject matter, available research data, instruments, funding sources, and the design of survey questionnaires is critical for the conceptualization, groundwork, and measurement stages of health services research. The conceptualization phase requires the investigator to understand the general purpose of the research, determine the specific research topic, identify relevant theories and literature, specify the meaning of concepts and variables, and formulate hypotheses

Table 15.4. HSR doctoral level core competencies and their educational domains

No.	Core Competency	Educational Domains
1	Breadth of HSR theoretical and conceptual knowledge	Health, financing of health care, organization of health care, health policy, access and use, quality of care, health informatics, literature review
2	In-depth disciplinary knowledge and skills	(Variable, depending on the discipline or interdisciplinary area of specialization)
3	Application of HSR foundational knowledge to health policy problems	Health, financing of health care, organization of health care, health policy, access and use, quality of care, health informatics, literature review
4	Innovative HSR questions	Scientific method and theory, literature review, proposal development
5	Interventional and Observational Study Designs	Study design, survey research, qualitative research
6	Primary data collection methods	Health informatics, survey research, qualitative research, data acquisition and quality control
7	Secondary data acquisition methods	Health informatics, HSR data sources, data acquisition and quality control
8	Conceptual models and operational measures	Scientific method and theory, measurement and variables
9	Implementation of research protocols	Health informatics, survey research, qualitative research, data acquisition and quality control
10	Responsible conduct of research	Research ethics
11	Multidisciplinary teamwork	Teamwork
12	Data analysis	Advanced HSR analytic methods, economic evaluation and decision sciences
13	Scientific communication	Proposal development, dissemination
14	Stakeholder collaboration and knowledge translation	Health policy, dissemination

Source: Adapted from *Health Services Research Competencies* (Final Report for Conference Grant R13 HS016070-01), by C. Forrest et al., 2006, November 15, Baltimore, MD: Johns Hopkins University.

or research questions. A thorough command of the subject matter with respect to literature and theories is crucial to accomplishing these research requirements.

The groundwork phase of research requires the researcher to identify relevant data sources, explore potential funding sources, develop a research plan or proposal, and prepare organizationally and administratively to carry out the

Table 15.5. Health services research stages and skills

Research Stage	Subject	Methodology	Statistics	Software	Writing	Public Relations
			Knowledge and Skills			
1. Conceptualization	X					
2. Groundwork	X				X	X
3. Research method		X				
4. Research design		X	X			
5. Sampling		X	X			
6. Measurement	X		X			
7. Data collection		X				X
8. Data processing				X		
9. Data analysis			X	X	X	
10. Application					X	X

research. Knowledge of data and funding sources is fundamental to fulfilling these tasks. The measurement, or operationalization, phase is concerned with devising measures linking specific concepts to empirically observable events or variables. Researchers are therefore required to be knowledgeable about the general guidelines and specific techniques in constructing research instruments such as the survey questionnaires.

Methodology

The second research skill is the command of general research methods, or methodology. Understanding the general approaches to research is critical in the selection of research methods, study design, sampling model, and data collection type. Competent investigators should know the pros and cons of the various types of research approaches, including research review, meta analysis, secondary analysis, research analysis of administrative records, qualitative research, case study, experiment, survey research, longitudinal study, and evaluation research; and they should assess their suitability for a given research problem. Investigators should be capable of developing an overall plan or framework for investigation. They must know how to identify the research population, choose the appropriate sampling method, and decide the optimal sample size. They must know the advantages and disadvantages of different data collection methods and select the one that maximizes both response and completion rates.

Statistics

The third important research skill is the command of statistical knowledge, particularly critical in the data analysis, design, sampling, and measurement phases of research. In data analysis, researchers use statistical procedures to analyze collected data and interpret study findings to draw conclusions about hypotheses or research questions. Knowledge about the choice and application of statistical procedures is necessary for conducting research independently and avoiding having to hire a statistician. Statistical knowledge can also enhance research design and sampling, which are based on statistical principles. Measurement decisions are also related to statistical knowledge because different levels of measures are subject to different types of statistical procedures. The design of a research instrument can benefit greatly from statistical knowledge. In finalizing a questionnaire, researchers should think about not only the hypotheses or research questions to be addressed but also the statistical procedures to be used in analyzing the data. Many projects get delayed when data collection is not integrated with analysis. A bad practice is to hire a statistical consultant well after data collection. The consultant is forced to deal with the existing data format, which may restrict the use of more powerful analyses.

Computer Application Software

The fourth research skill particularly critical for large data analyses is knowledge of computer application software. This is especially relevant during the data processing and analysis phases. In data processing, researchers typically transfer the collected raw data to some computer format. In the case of using available data, sorting and merging are often integral parts of the preparation process. In analyzing data, investigators use statistical software to help apply various statistical and modeling protocols.

Writing

The ability to write is another critical research skill. Whether drafting proposals for funding (the groundwork phase) or reports for publication (the application phase), good writing is a required skill and essential for conveying the research to potential funders or users. In many cases, it is a matter of following structured formats (e.g., research proposals, journal articles). However, the ability to write concise and clear sentences and to organize one's thoughts is also important. Excellent references exist that help improve research writing. A few particularly good ones are:

- *A Short Guide to Writing about Social Science* (4th ed.) by L. J. Cuba
- *The Elements of Style* (4th ed.) by W. Strunk and E. B. White
- *Publication Manual of the American Psychological Association* (5th ed.) by the American Psychological Association
- *The Scientist's Handbook for Writing Papers and Dissertations* by A. M. Wilkinson
- *Writing and Thinking in the Social Sciences* by S. Friedman and S. Steinberg
- *Writing for Social Scientists* by H. S. Becker
- *Writing Up Qualitative Research* (2nd ed.) by H. T. Wolcott

Public Relations

Last but not least is public relations skills, which are particularly useful in the groundwork, data collection, and application phases of research, and in project management. In the groundwork phase, seeking funding support for research requires excellent people skills. In data collection, getting access to research sites and subjects necessitates patience and a good rapport. Finally, in the application phase, collaboration with decision makers is vital for policy formulation and implementation based on research findings.

The successful completion of a research project, particularly a large one, requires that the researcher be a capable administrator. Administrative skills are reflected in hiring the research staff, supervising and coordinating research activities, managing time to keep on schedule, and responding to changes and crises. The possession of good human relations skills is a prerequisite for a good project director.

SUMMARY

The audiences for scientific research include the research community, the stakeholders, and the public. For the research community, the common means of communicating research results consist of publications in refereed scientific journals, reading research results in professional conferences, and writing working papers, monographs, and even books. Familiarity with and adherence to journal requirements with regard to content, writing style, structure, organization, use of tables and charts, and length are crucial to publication. When stakeholders are the intended audience, researchers communicate findings through research proposals, technical reports, symposiums, expert testimony, or research notes. To enhance the chances of implementing research findings in policy decisions, both researchers and policy makers should strive to improve communication, mutual understanding, and collaboration and to reduce gaps in research priorities, scope, and timetables. When the intended audience is the general public, researchers may communicate through the mass media or brochures. Health services researchers should continually improve their knowledge of subject matter, methodology, statistics, computer applications, writing, and public relations.

REVIEW QUESTIONS

1. What are the channels for communicating research results?
2. What components are commonly shared by scientific journals when publishing scientific research?
3. How can a person develop the skills necessary to become a capable health services researcher?

CAPSTONE ASSIGNMENT

The capstone project enables you to demonstrate your potential for conducting independent health services research. It focuses on a research topic of your choosing that meets with the approval of your instructor. The completed project, which will be presented to the class, should include:

1. A description of the aim or purpose of the study, its significance, and the research questions/hypotheses.
2. A review of the relevant literature, including both a theoretical framework and the empirical research findings.
3. A detailed discussion of the proposed study methodology, including population and sampling, sample size determination, measurement, data sources and data collection methods, and analysis.
4. An appendix that provides the completed research instrument or questionnaire. If an available data set is used, a codebook should be developed in lieu of a questionnaire.

REFERENCES

Agency for Health Care Policy and Research. (1990). *Health Services Research on HIV/AIDS-Related Illness*. Rockville, MD: Agency for Health Care Policy and Research.

Centers for Disease Control and Prevention. (1999). Framework for program evaluation in public health. *Morbidity and Mortality Weekly Report, 48*, No. RR-11.

Ginzberg, E. (1991). *Health Services Research: Key to Health Policy*. Cambridge, MA: Harvard University Press.

Institute of Medicine. (1995). *Health Services Research: Training and Workforce Issues* (Eds. M. J. Field, R. E. Tranquada, and J. C. Feasley). National Academies Press: Washington, DC.

Morgan, G., Ellis, E., and Gifford, K. (2005). *Covering Kids and Families Evaluation: Areas of CKF Influence on Medicaid and SCHIP Programs*. Robert Wood Johnson Foundation. Retrieved July 16, 2007, from http://www.rwjf.org/files/research/CKFpermanencereport.doc

National Center for Health Services Research and Health Care Technology Assessment. (1985). *Health Services Research on Primary Care*. Rockville, MD: National Center for Health Services Research and Health Care Technology Assessment.

APPENDIX 1

Health Services Research: Selected Journals

Academic Medicine
AIDS Care
American Journal of Epidemiology
American Journal of Hospital Care
American Journal of Law and Medicine
American Journal of Medical Quality
American Journal of Medicine
American Journal of Nursing
American Journal of Preventive Medicine
American Journal of Public Health
American Journal of Public Health
Annual Review of Public Health
Asia-Pacific Journal of Public Health
Australian Journal of Public Health
British Journal of Preventive and Social Medicine
Bulletin of the World Health Organization
Business and Health
Canadian Journal of Public Health
Cancer Research
Carolina Health Services Review
Community Health
Community Health Education
Contemporary Long Term Care
Demography
Ethnicity and Health
Evaluation and the Health Professions
Family and Community Health
Frontiers of Health Services Management
Geriatrics
Gerontologist
Hastings Center Report
Health Administration Education
Health Affairs
Health and Place

Health and Social Work
Health Care Financing Review
Health Care for Women International
Health Care Management Review
Health Care Strategic Management
Health Economics
Health Education
Health Education Quarterly
Health Education Research
Health Legislation and Regulation
Health Management Quarterly
Health Planning and Management
Health Progress
Health Promotion
Health Reports
Health Services Manager
Health Services Research
Health Services Research and Policy
Health Technology Assessment Reports
Health Values
Health, United States
Healthcare Financial Management
Home Health Care Services Quarterly
Hospital and Health Services Administration
Hospital Ethics
Hospital Physician
Hospital Practice
Hospital Progress
Hospital Statistics
Hospital Topics
Hospitals
Human Services in the Rural Environment
Inquiry
International Journal of Health Education
International Journal of Health Services
International Quarterly of Community Health Education
Issues in Law and Medicine
Journal of Aging and Social Policy
Journal of Allied Health
Journal of Ambulatory Care Management
Journal of Community Health
Journal of Epidemiology and Community Health
Journal of Family Practice
Journal of Gerontology
Journal of Health Administration Education
Journal of Health and Human Resources Administration
Journal of Health and Social Behavior
Journal of Health Care for the Poor and Underserved
Journal of Health Care Marketing

Journal of Health Economics
Journal of Health Politics, Policy and Law
Journal of Healthcare Management
Journal of Hospital Marketing
Journal of Human Resources
Journal of Law and Medicine
Journal of Law, Medicine, and Ethics
Journal of Long-Term Care Administration
Journal of Medical Ethics
Journal of Medical Practice Management
Journal of Medicine and Philosophy
Journal of Nurse Midwifery
Journal of Nursing Administration
Journal of Occupational Medicine
Journal of Perinatal and Neonatal Nursing
Journal of Professional Nursing
Journal of Public Health Dentistry
Journal of Public Health Policy
Journal of Rural Health
Journal of Social Issues
Journal of the American Medical Association
Journal of the National Medical Association
Journal of the Society for Health Systems
Journal of the Society for Public Health Education
Journal of Women's Health

Lancet
Managed Health Care Today
Maternal Child Nursing Journal
Medical Care
Medical Care Research and Review
Medical Decision Making
Medical Economics
Medical Group Management Journal
Milbank Quarterly
Modern Healthcare
Monthly Vital Statistics Report
Morbidity and Mortality Weekly Report
Nation's Health
New England Journal of Human Services
New England Journal of Medicine
Nurse Management
Nursing Administration Quarterly
Nursing and Health Care
Nursing Economics
Nursing Outlook
Occupational Health
Patient Care
Perspectives in Healthcare Risk Management
Prevention

Preventive Medicine
Provider
Psychology Health and Medicine
Public Health
Public Health Reports
Public Health Review
Qualitative Health Research
Quality Assurance in Health Care
Quality Review Bulletin
Reports on Health and Social Subjects
Research in Community and Mental Health
Research in Nursing and Health
Scandinavian Journal of Primary Health Care
Science
Social Policy
Social Science and Medicine
Social Work in Health Care
Sociology of Health and Illness
Southern Medical Journal
Topics in Health Care Financing
Vital and Health Statistics. Series 1: Programs and Collection Procedures
Vital and Health Statistics. Series 2: Data Evaluation and Methods Research
Vital and Health Statistics. Series 3: Analytical and Epidemiological Studies
Vital and Health Statistics. Series 4: Documents and Committee Reports
Vital and Health Statistics. Series 5: Comparative International Vital and Health
    Statistics Report
Vital and Health Statistics. Series 10–14: Data from the National Health Survey
Vital and Health Statistics. Series 21: Data on Natality, Marriage, and Divorce
Western Journal of Medicine
Western Journal of Nursing Research

APPENDIX 2

Selected Health Services–Related Professional Associations

Academic Health Science Centers, Group, and Allied Health

American Group Practice Association (AGPA)
American Society of Allied Health Professions (ASAHP)
Association of Academic Health Centers (AAHC)

Administrators

American College of Health Care Administrators (ACHCA)
American College of Health Care Executives (ACHCE)
American Society of Hospital Personnel Administration (ASHPA)
Association of Group Medical Administrators (AGMA)
Association of Mental Health Administrators (AMHA)
Medical Group Management Association (MGMA)

Dentistry

American Association of Dental Schools (AADS)
American Dental Association (ADA)

Health Professionals and Schools of Public Health

American Public Health Association (APHA)
American Rural Health Association (ARHA)

Medical, Hospital, and Pharmaceutical

American Academy of Medical Directors (AAMD)
American Association of Colleges of Pharmacy (AACP)
American College of Physician Executives (ACPE)
American Hospital Association (AHA)
American Medical Association (AMA)
Association of American Medical Colleges (AAMC)

Nursing

American Nurses Association (ANA)
National League of Nursing (NLN)

Programs/Departments of Health Services Policy and Administration

Association for Health Services Research (AHSR)
Association of University Programs in Health Administration (AUPHA)

APPENDIX 3

Funding Sources

Annual Register of Grant Support
A definitive reference book that is published annually. The volume for 1995 has 3,155 entries representing billions of dollars to potential research grant seekers. It is published by National Register Publishing Company, Wilmette, IL 60091.

Aris
Monthly newsletter for the biomedical sciences, social and natural sciences, creative arts, and humanities that lists program guidelines, deadlines, and contacts for research funding, from both governmental and private sources.

Broad Agency Announcements
A source of research funding information from specific federal agencies.

Catalog of Federal Domestic Assistance
A comprehensive catalog of federal programs that includes guidelines, funding amounts, and contact information.

Commerce Business Daily
A resource that provides announcements of sponsored program opportunities through federal contracts.

Contracts and Grants Weekly
A publication that lists the most current deadlines for funding agencies that support a variety of programs.

Directory of Research Grants
A well-indexed source of private and federal programs.

Federal Register
A daily publication that makes available to the public federal agency regulations, proposed regulations, and official deadline notices.

Foundation Directory (and Supplements)
A reference of source materials on all the major national and state foundations and their grant-making activities. It includes basic records filed with the IRS by every private foundation, annual reports, and the Foundation Center's standard reference works. Information is compiled on about 26,000 American foundations. National collections are located at the following two Foundation addresses: The Foundation Center, 888 Seventh

Avenue, New York, NY 10019; and 1001 Connecticut Avenue, Northwest, Washington, DC 20036. See also Donors' Forum, 208 South LaSalle Street, Chicago, IL 60604.

National Institute of Mental Health
The institute supports programs designed to increase the knowledge of and improve the research methods in mental and behavioral disorders.

National Institutes of Health
The NIH offers research and research-training grants and awards in the biomedical and health-related sciences.

Source Book Profiles
A source for the activities, goals, and funding capabilities of most foundations.

Taft Corporate Giving Directory
Offers comprehensive profiles of America's major corporate foundations and charitable giving programs.

APPENDIX 4

Public Health Service Grant Application Forms

Form Pages Only

Application for a

Public Health Service Grant

PHS 398

Includes Research Career Awards
and Institutional National
Research Service Awards

The following form pages are a part of the complete PHS 398 application packet. The packet also includes a booklet with instructions for preparing and submitting your application, as well as definitions, assurances, and other relevant information. Please retain the instructional booklet for future submission of applications.

Department of Health and Human Services
Public Health Services

Grant Application

OMB No. 0925-0001

LEAVE BLANK—FOR PHS USE ONLY.		
Type	Activity	Number
Review Group		Formerly
Council/Board (Month, Year)		Date Received

1. TITLE OF PROJECT (Do not exceed 81 characters, including spaces and punctuation.)

2. RESPONSE TO SPECIFIC REQUEST FOR APPLICATIONS OR PROGRAM ANNOUNCEMENT OR SOLICITATION ☐ NO ☐ YES
(If "Yes," state number and title)
Number: Title:

3. PRINCIPAL INVESTIGATOR/PROGRAM DIRECTOR   New Investigator ☐ No ☐ Yes

3a. NAME (Last, first, middle)	3b. DEGREE(S)	3h. eRA Commons User Name

3c. POSITION TITLE

3d. MAILING ADDRESS (Street, city, state, zip code)

3e. DEPARTMENT, SERVICE, LABORATORY, OR EQUIVALENT

3f. MAJOR SUBDIVISION

3g. TELEPHONE AND FAX (Area code, number and extension)   E-MAIL ADDRESS:
TEL: FAX:

4. HUMAN SUBJECTS RESEARCH	4a. Research Exempt ☐ No ☐ Yes	
☐ No ☐ Yes	If "Yes," Exemption No.	
4b. Human Subjects Assurance No.	4c. Clinical Trial ☐ No ☐ Yes	4d. NIH-defined Phase III Clinical Trial ☐ No ☐ Yes

5. VERTEBRATE ANIMALS ☐ No ☐ Yes	
5a. If "Yes," IACUC approval Date	5b. Animal welfare assurance no.

6. DATES OF PROPOSED PERIOD OF SUPPORT (month, day, year—MM/DD/YY)		7. COSTS REQUESTED FOR INITIAL BUDGET PERIOD		8. COSTS REQUESTED FOR PROPOSED PERIOD OF SUPPORT	
From	Through	7a. Direct Costs ($)	7b. Total Costs ($)	8a. Direct Costs ($)	8b. Total Costs ($)

9. APPLICANT ORGANIZATION
Name
Address

10. TYPE OF ORGANIZATION		
Public: → ☐ Federal ☐ State ☐ Local		
Private: → ☐ Private Nonprofit		
For-profit: → ☐ General ☐ Small Business		
☐ Woman-owned ☐ Socially and Economically Disadvantaged		

11. ENTITY IDENTIFICATION NUMBER

DUNS NO.   Cong. District

12. ADMINISTRATIVE OFFICIAL TO BE NOTIFIED IF AWARD IS MADE
Name
Title
Address
Tel: FAX:
E-Mail:

13. OFFICIAL SIGNING FOR APPLICANT ORGANIZATION
Name
Title
Address
Tel: FAX:
E-Mail:

14. APPLICANT ORGANIZATION CERTIFICATION AND ACCEPTANCE: I certify that the statements herein are true, complete and accurate to the best of my knowledge, and accept the obligation to comply with Public Health Services terms and conditions if a grant is awarded as a result of this application. I am aware that any false, fictitious, or fraudulent statements or claims may subject me to criminal, civil, or administrative penalties.

SIGNATURE OF OFFICIAL NAMED IN 13.   DATE
(In ink. "Per" signature not acceptable.)

Use only if responding to a Multiple PI pilot initiative. See http://grants.nih.gov/grants/multi_pi/index.htm for details.

Contact Principal Investigator/Program Director (Last, First, Middle):

3. PRINCIPAL INVESTIGATOR

3a. NAME (Last, first, middle)	3b. DEGREE(S)	3h. NIH Commons User Name
3c. POSITION TITLE	3d. MAILING ADDRESS (Street, city, state, zip code)	
3e. DEPARTMENT, SERVICE, LABORATORY, OR EQUIVALENT		
3f. MAJOR SUBDIVISION		
3g. TELEPHONE AND FAX (Area code, number and extension) TEL: FAX:	E-MAIL ADDRESS:	

3. PRINCIPAL INVESTIGATOR

3a. NAME (Last, first, middle)	3b. DEGREE(S)	3h. NIH Commons User Name
3c. POSITION TITLE	3d. MAILING ADDRESS (Street, city, state, zip code)	
3e. DEPARTMENT, SERVICE, LABORATORY, OR EQUIVALENT		
3f. MAJOR SUBDIVISION		
3g. TELEPHONE AND FAX (Area code, number and extension) TEL: FAX:	E-MAIL ADDRESS:	

3. PRINCIPAL INVESTIGATOR

3a. NAME (Last, first, middle)	3b. DEGREE(S)	3h. NIH Commons User Name
3c. POSITION TITLE	3d. MAILING ADDRESS (Street, city, state, zip code)	
3e. DEPARTMENT, SERVICE, LABORATORY, OR EQUIVALENT		
3f. MAJOR SUBDIVISION		
3g. TELEPHONE AND FAX (Area code, number and extension) TEL: FAX:	E-MAIL ADDRESS:	

3. PRINCIPAL INVESTIGATOR

3a. NAME (Last, first, middle)	3b. DEGREE(S)	3h. NIH Commons User Name
3c. POSITION TITLE	3d. MAILING ADDRESS (Street, city, state, zip code)	
3e. DEPARTMENT, SERVICE, LABORATORY, OR EQUIVALENT		
3f. MAJOR SUBDIVISION		
3g. TELEPHONE AND FAX (Area code, number and extension) TEL: FAX:	E-MAIL ADDRESS:	

Principal Investigator/Program Director (Last, First, Middle):

DESCRIPTION: See instructions. State the application's broad, long-term objectives and specific aims, making reference to the health relatedness of the project (i.e., relevance to the **mission of the agency**). Describe concisely the research design and methods for achieving these goals. Describe the rationale and techniques you will use to pursue these goals.

In addition, in two or three sentences, describe in plain, lay language the relevance of this research to **public** health. If the application is funded, this description, as is, will become public information. Therefore, do not include proprietary/confidential information. **DO NOT EXCEED THE SPACE PROVIDED.**

PERFORMANCE SITE(S) (organization, city, state)

Principal Investigator/Program Director (Last, First, Middle):

KEY PERSONNEL. See instructions. *Use continuation pages as needed* to provide the required information in the format shown below.
Start with Principal Investigator(s). List all other key personnel in alphabetical order, last name first.

Name	eRA Commons User Name	Organization	Role on Project

OTHER SIGNIFICANT CONTRIBUTORS

Name		Organization	Role on Project

Human Embryonic Stem Cells ☐ No ☐ Yes

If the proposed project involves human embryonic stem cells, list below the registration number of the specific cell line(s) from the following list:
http://stemcells.nih.gov/registry/index.asp. *Use continuation pages as needed.*

If a specific line cannot be referenced at this time, include a statement that one from the Registry will be used.

Cell Line

Number the *following* pages consecutively throughout
the application. Do not use suffixes such as 4a, 4b.

Form Page 2-continued

Principal Investigator/Program Director (Last, First, Middle):

The name of the principal investigator/program director must be provided at the top of each printed page and each continuation page.

RESEARCH GRANT
TABLE OF CONTENTS

Principal Investigator/Program Director (Last, First, Middle):

DETAILED BUDGET FOR INITIAL BUDGET PERIOD
DIRECT COSTS ONLY

FROM | THROUGH

PERSONNEL (Applicant organization only)		Months Devoted to Project				DOLLAR AMOUNT REQUESTED (omit cents)		
NAME	ROLE ON PROJECT	Cal. Mnths	Acad. Mnths	Summer Mnths	INST BASE SALARY	SALARY REQUESTED	FRINGE BENEFITS	TOTAL
	Principal Investigator							
SUBTOTALS →								

CONSULTANT COSTS

EQUIPMENT (Itemize)

SUPPLIES (Itemize by category)

TRAVEL

PATIENT CARE COSTS — INPATIENT
PATIENT CARE COSTS — OUTPATIENT

ALTERATIONS AND RENOVATIONS (Itemize by category)

OTHER EXPENSES (Itemize by category)

CONSORTIUM/CONTRACTUAL COSTS | DIRECT COSTS

SUBTOTAL DIRECT COSTS FOR INITIAL BUDGET PERIOD (Item 7a, Face Page) | $

CONSORTIUM/CONTRACTUAL COSTS | FACILITIES AND ADMINISTRATIVE COSTS

TOTAL DIRECT COSTS FOR INITIAL BUDGET PERIOD | $

PHS 398 (Rev. 04/06) | Page____ | Form Page 4

Principal Investigator/Program Director (Last, First, Middle): _____

BUDGET FOR ENTIRE PROPOSED PROJECT PERIOD
DIRECT COSTS ONLY

BUDGET CATEGORY TOTALS		INITIAL BUDGET PERIOD (from Form Page 4)	ADDITIONAL YEARS OF SUPPORT REQUESTED			
			2nd	3rd	4th	5th
PERSONNEL: Salary and fringe benefits. Applicant organization only.						
CONSULTANT COSTS						
EQUIPMENT						
SUPPLIES						
TRAVEL						
PATIENT CARE COSTS	INPATIENT					
	OUTPATIENT					
ALTERATIONS AND RENOVATIONS						
OTHER EXPENSES						
CONSORTIUM/ CONTRACTUAL COSTS	DIRECT					
SUBTOTAL DIRECT COSTS (Sum = Item 8a, Face Page)						
CONSORTIUM/ CONTRACTUAL COSTS	F&A					
TOTAL DIRECT COSTS						

TOTAL DIRECT COSTS FOR ENTIRE PROPOSED PROJECT PERIOD	$

JUSTIFICATION. Follow the budget justification instructions exactly. Use continuation pages as needed.

Principal Investigator/Program Director (Last, First, Middle):

BUDGET JUSTIFICATION PAGE
MODULAR RESEARCH GRANT APPLICATION

	Initial Period	2nd	3rd	4th	5th	Sum Total (For Entire Project Period)
	(Item 7a, Face Page)					*(Item 8a, Face Page)*
DC less Consortium F&A						
Consortium F&A						
Total Direct Costs						$

Personnel

Consortium

Principal Investigator/Program Director (Last, first, middle):

RESOURCES

FACILITIES: Specify the facilities to be used for the conduct of the proposed research. Indicate the performance sites and describe capacities, pertinent capabilities, relative proximity, and extent of availability to the project. If research involving Select Agent(s) will occur at any performance site(s), the biocontainment resources available at each site should be described. Under "Other," identify support services such as machine shop, electronics shop, and specify the extent to which they will be available to the project. Use continuation pages if necessary.

Laboratory:

Clinical:

Animal:

Computer:

Office:

Other:

MAJOR EQUIPMENT: List the most important equipment items already available for this project, noting the location and pertinent capabilities of each.

Principal Investigator/Program Director (last, First, Middle):

CHECKLIST

TYPE OF APPLICATION *(Check all that apply.)*

☐ NEW application. *(This application is being submitted to the PHS for the first time.)*

☐ REVISION/RESUBMISSION of application number: _____
(This application replaces a prior unfunded version of a new, competing continuation/renewal, or supplemental/revision application.)

☐ COMPETING CONTINUATION/RENEWAL of grant number: _____
(This application is to extend a funded grant beyond its current project period.)

☐ SUPPLEMENT/REVISION to grant number: _____
(This application is for additional funds to supplement a currently funded grant.)

☐ CHANGE of principal investigator/program director.

Name of former principal investigator/program director:

☐ CHANGE of Grantee Institution.   Name of former institution:

☐ FOREIGN application   ☐ Domestic Grant with foreign involvement   List Country(ies) Involved:

INVENTIONS AND PATENTS
(Competing continuation/renewal appl. only)

☐ No

☐ Yes. If "Yes,"   ☐ Previously reported
                    ☐ Not previously reported

1. PROGRAM INCOME *(See instructions.)*

All applications must indicate whether program income is anticipated during the period(s) for which grant support is request. If program income is anticipated, use the format below to reflect the amount and source(s).

Budget Period	Anticipated Amount	Source(s)

2. ASSURANCES/CERTIFICATIONS *(See instructions.)*

In signing the application Face Page, the authorized organizational representative agrees to comply with the following policies, assurances and/or certifications when applicable. Descriptions of individual assurances/certifications are provided in Part III. If unable to certify compliance, where applicable, provide an explanation and place it after this page.
•Human Subjects Research •Research Using Human Embryonic Stem Cells •Research on Transplantation of Human Fetal Tissue •Women and Minority Inclusion Policy •Inclusion of Children Policy •Vertebrate Animals•

•Debarment and Suspension •Drug-Free Workplace *(applicable to new [Type 1] or revised/resubmission [Type 1] applications only)* •Lobbying •Non-Delinquency on Federal Debt •Research Misconduct •Civil Rights (Form HHS 441 or HHS 690) •Handicapped Individuals (Form HHS 641 or HHS 690) •Sex Discrimination (Form HHS 639-A or HHS 690) •Age Discrimination (Form HHS 680 or HHS 690) •Recombinant DNA Research, Including Human Gene Transfer Research •Financial Conflict of Interest •Smoke Free Workplace •Prohibited Research •Select Agent Research •PI Assurance

3. FACILITIES AND ADMINSTRATIVE COSTS (F&A)/ INDIRECT COSTS. See specific instructions.

☐ DHHS Agreement dated: _____   ☐ No Facilities And Administrative Costs Requested.

☐ DHHS Agreement being negotiated with _____ Regional Office.

☐ No DHHS Agreement, but rate established with _____ Date _____

CALCULATION* *(The entire grant application, including the Checklist, will be reproduced and provided to peer reviewers as confidential information.)*

a. Initial budget period:	Amount of base $ _____	x Rate applied _____	0.00%	% = F&A costs	$ _____
b. 02 year	Amount of base $ _____	x Rate applied _____	0.00%	% = F&A costs	$ _____
c. 03 year	Amount of base $ _____	x Rate applied _____	0.00%	% = F&A costs	$ _____
d. 04 year	Amount of base $ _____	x Rate applied _____	0.00%	% = F&A costs	$ _____
e. 05 year	Amount of base $ _____	x Rate applied _____	0.00%	% = F&A costs	$ _____

TOTAL F&A Costs $ _____

*Check appropriate box(es):

☐ Salary and wages base   ☐ Modified total direct cost base

☐ Off-site, other special rate, or more than one rate involved *(Explain)*   ☐ Other base *(Explain)*

Explanation *(Attach separate sheet, if necessary.)*:

Principal Investigator/Program Director (Last, First, Middle):

Place this form at the end of the signed original copy of the application.
Do not duplicate.

PERSONAL DATA ON
PRINCIPAL INVESTIGATOR(S)/PROGRAM DIRECTOR(S)

The Public Health Service has a continuing commitment to monitor the operation of its review and award processes to detect—and deal appropriately with—any instances of real or apparent inequities with respect to age, sex, race, or ethnicity of the proposed principal investigator(s)/program director(s).

To provide the PHS with the information it needs for this important task, complete the form below and attach it to the signed original of the application after the Checklist. When multiple PIs/PDs are proposed, complete a form for each. **Do not attach copies of this form to the duplicated copies of the application.**

Upon receipt of the application by the PHS, this form will be separated from the application. This form will **not** be duplicated, and it will **not** be a part of the review process. Data will be confidential, and will be maintained in Privacy Act record system 09-25-0036, "Grants: IMPAC (Grant/Contract Information)." The PHS requests the last four digits of the Social Security Number for accurate identification, referral, and review of applications and for management of PHS grant programs. Although the provision of this portion of the Social Security Number is voluntary, providing this information may improve both the accuracy and speed of processing the application. Please be aware that no individual will be denied any right, benefit, or privilege provided by law because of refusal to disclose this section of the Social Security Number. The PHS requests the last four digits of the Social Security Number under Sections 301(a) and 487 of the PHS Acts as amended (42 U.S.C. 241a and U.S.C. 288). All analyses conducted on the date of birth, gender, race and/or ethnic origin data will report aggregate statistical findings only and will not identify individuals. If you decline to provide this information, it will in no way affect consideration of your application. Your cooperation will be appreciated.

DATE OF BIRTH (MM/DD/YY)		SEX/GENDER
SOCIAL SECURITY NUMBER (last 4 digits only)	XXX-XX-	☐ Female ☐ Male

ETHNICITY

1. Do you consider yourself to be Hispanic or Latino? (See definition below.) Select one.

☐ **Hispanic or Latino.** A person of Mexican, Puerto Rican, Cuban, South or Central American, or other Spanish culture or origin, regardless of race. The term, "Spanish origin," can be used in addition to "Hispanic or Latino."

☐ **Not Hispanic or Latino**

RACE

2. What race do you consider yourself to be? Select one or more of the following.

☐ **American Indian or Alaska Native.** A person having origins in any of the original peoples of North, Central, or South America, and who maintains tribal affiliation or community attachment.

☐ **Asian.** A person having origins in any of the original peoples of the Far East, Southeast Asia, or the Indian **subcontinent**, including, for example, Cambodia, China, India, Japan, Korea, Malaysia, Pakistan, the Philippine Islands, Thailand, and Vietnam. (Note: Individuals from the Philippine Islands have been recorded as Pacific Islanders in previous data collection strategies.)

☐ **Black or African American.** A person having origins in any of the black racial groups of Africa. Terms such as "Haitian" or "Negro" can be used in addition to "Black or African American."

☐ **Native Hawaiian or Other Pacific Islander.** A person having origins in any of the original peoples of Hawaii, Guam, Samoa, or **other** Pacific Islands.

☐ **White.** A **person** having origins in any of the original peoples of Europe, the Middle East, or North Africa.

☐ Check here if you do not wish to provide some or all of the above information.

Principal Investigator/Program Director (Last, First, Middle): _____

Targeted/Planned Enrollment Table

This report format should NOT be used for data collection from study participants.

Study Title: _____

Total Planned Enrollment: _____

TARGETED/PLANNED ENROLLMENT: Number of Subjects			
Ethnic Category	**Sex/Gender**		
	Females	**Males**	**Total**
Hispanic or Latino			
Not Hispanic or Latino			
Ethnic Category: Total of All Subjects *			
Racial Categories			
American Indian/Alaska Native			
Asian			
Native Hawaiian or Other Pacific Islander			
Black or African American			
White			
Racial Categories: Total of All Subjects *			

* The "Ethnic Category: Total of All Subjects" must be equal to the "Racial Categories: Total of All Subjects."

Principal Investigator/Program Director (Last, First, Middle): _____

Inclusion Enrollment Report

This report format should NOT be used for data collection from study participants.

Study Title: _____

Total Enrollment: _____   **Protocol Number:** _____

Grant Number: _____

PART A. TOTAL ENROLLMENT REPORT: Number of Subjects Enrolled to Date (Cumulative) by Ethnicity and Race

Ethnic Category	Sex/Gender		
	Females	Males	Unknown or Not Reported	Total
Hispanic or Latino				
Not Hispanic or Latino				
Unknown (individuals not reporting ethnicity)				
Ethnic Category: Total of All Subjects*				*

Racial Categories			
American Indian/Alaska Native				
Asian				
Native Hawaiian or Other Pacific Islander				
Black or African American				
White				
More Than One Race				
Unknown or Not Reported				
Racial Categories: Total of All Subjects*				*

PART B. HISPANIC ENROLLMENT REPORT: Number of Hispanics or Latinos Enrolled to Date (Cumulative)

Racial Categories	Females	Males	Unknown or Not Reported	Total
American Indian or Alaska Native				
Asian				
Native Hawaiian or Other Pacific Islander				
Black or African American				
White				
More Than One Race				
Unknown or Not Reported				
Racial Categories: Total of Hispanics or Latinos**				**

* These totals must agree.
** These totals must agree.

CDA TOC Substitute Page

Candidate (Last, first, middle): _____

Use this substitute page for the Table of Contents of Research Career Development Awards. Type the name of the candidate at the top of each printed page and each continuation page.

RESEARCH CAREER DEVELOPMENT AWARD
TABLE OF CONTENTS (Substitute Page)

Page Numbers

Letters of Reference* *(attach unopened references to the Face Page)*

Section I: Basic Administrative Data

Face Page (Form Page 1) 1

Description, Performance Sites, Key Personnel, Other Significant Contributors, and Human Embryonic Stem Cells (Form Page 2) 2

Table of Contents (this CDA Substitute Form Page 3) .... ____

Budget for Entire Proposed Period of Support (Form Page 5) .... ____

Biographical Sketches *(Candidate, Sponsor[s],* Key Personnel and Other Significant Contributors**
   —Biographical Sketch Format page) (Not to exceed four pages) .... ____

Other Support Pages (not for the candidate) .... ____

Resources (Resources Format page) .... ____

Section II: Specialized Information

Introduction to Revised/Resubmission Application* *(Not to exceed 3 pages)* .... ____

1. The Candidate

A. Candidate's Background .... ____

B. Career Goals and Objectives: Scientific Biography .... ____   *(Items A-D included in 25 page limit)*

C. Career Development/Training Activities during Award Period .... ____

D. Training in the Responsible Conduct of Research .... ____

2. Statements by Sponsor, Co-Sponsor(s),* Consultant(s),* and Contributor(s)* .... ____

3. Environment and Institutional Commitment to Candidate

A. Description of Institutional Environment .... ____

B. Institutional Commitment to Candidate's Research Career Development .... ____

4. Research Plan

A. Specific Aims .... ____

B. Background and Significance .... ____   *(Items A-D included in 25 page limit)*

C. Preliminary Studies/Progress Report .... ____

D. Research Design and Methods .... ____

E. Human Subjects Research .... ____

   Targeted/Planned Enrollment Table (for new and continuing clinical research studies) ... ____

F. Vertebrate Animals .... ____

G. Select Agent Research .... ____

H. Literature Cited .... ____

I. Consortium/Contractual Arrangements* .... ____

J. Resource Sharing .... ____

Checklist .... ____

Appendix (Five collated sets. No page numbering necessary.) .... ☐ Check if Appendix is included

Number of publications and manuscripts accepted for publication *(not to exceed 5)* _____

Note: Font and margin requirements must conform to limits provided in the Specific Instructions.

*Include these items only when applicable.

CITIZENSHIP

☐ U.S. citizen or noncitizen national   ☐ Permanent resident of U.S. (If a permanent resident of the U.S., a notarized statement must be provided by the time of award.)

CAREER DEVELOPMENT AWARD REFERENCE REPORT GUIDELINES
(Series K)

Title of Award:

Type of Award: **Application Submission Deadline:** _____

Name of Candidate (Last, first, middle):

Name of Respondent (Last, first, middle):

The candidate is applying to the National Institutes of Health for a Career Development Award (CDA). The purpose of this award is to develop the research capabilities and career of the applicant. These awards provide up to five years of salary support and guarantee them the ability to devote at least 75–80 percent of their time to research for the duration of the award. Many of these awards also provide funds for research and career development costs. The award is available to persons who have demonstrated considerable potential to become independent researchers, but who need additional supervised research experience in a productive scientific setting.

We would appreciate receiving your evaluation of the above candidate with special reference to:

- potential for conducting research;
- evidence of originality;
- adequacy of scientific background;
- quality of research endeavors or publications to date, if any;
- commitment to health-oriented research; and
- need for further research experience and training.

Any related comments that you may wish to provide would be welcomed. These references will be used by PHS committees of consultants in assessing candidates.

Complete the report in English on 8-1/2 x 11" sheets of paper. Return your reference report to the candidate sealed in the envelope as soon as possible and in sufficient time so that the candidate can meet the application submission deadline. References must be submitted with the application.

We have asked the candidate to provide you with a self-addressed envelope with the following words in the front bottom corner: "DO NOT OPEN—PHS USE ONLY." Candidates are not to open the references. Under the Privacy Act of 1974, CDA candidates may request personal information contained in their records, including this reference. Thank you for your assistance.

436

Kirschstein-NRSA TOC
Substitute Page

Principal Investigator/Program Director
(Last, first, middle): _____

Type the name of the principal investigator/program director at the top of each printed page and each continuation page. (For type specifications, see PHS 398 Instructions.)

INSTITUTIONAL RUTH L. KIRSCHSTEIN NATIONAL RESEARCH SERVICE AWARD
TABLE OF CONTENTS (Substitute Page)

Page Numbers

Face Page (*Form Page 1*) 1

Description, Performance Sites, Key Personnel, Other Significant Contributors, and Human Embryonic Stem Cells (*Form Page 2, Form Page 2-continued, and additional continuation page, if necessary*) 2

Table of Contents (*this Kirschstein-NRSA Substitute Form Page 3*) ....

Detailed Budget for Initial Budget Period (*Kirschstein-NRSA Substitute Form Page 4*) ....

Budget for Entire Proposed Period of Support (*Kirschstein-NRSA Substitute Form Page 5*) ....

Biographical Sketch—Principal Investigator/Program Director *(Not to exceed four pages)* ....

Other Biographical Sketches *(Not to exceed four pages for each)* ....

Resources ....

Research Training Program Plan

Introduction to Revised/Resubmission Application, *if applicable* *(Not to exceed 3 pages)* ....

Introduction to Supplemental/Revision Application, *if applicable* *(Not to exceed one page)* ....

  A. Background ....
  B. Program Plan ....
    1. Program Administration ....
    2. Program Faculty .... *(Items A-D: not to exceed 25 pages,*
    3. Proposed Training .... *excluding tables*)*
    4. Training Program Evaluation ....
    5. Trainee Candidates ....
  C. Minority Recruitment and Retention Plan ....
  D. Plan for Instruction in the Responsible Conduct of Research ....
  E. Progress Report (Competing Continuation Applications Only) ....
  F. Human Subjects ....
  G. Vertebrate Animals ....
  H. Select Agent Research ....
  I. Multiple PI Leadership Plan (if applicable) ....
  J. Consortium/Contractual Arrangements ....

Checklist ....

Appendix *(Five collated sets. No page numbering necessary for Appendix.)*

☐ Check if Appendix is included

* Font and margin requirements must conform to limits provided in PHS 398 Specific Instructions.

Kirschstein-NRSA Initial Budget
Period Substitute Page

Principal Investigator/Program Director:
(Last, first, middle)

DETAILED BUDGET FOR INITIAL BUDGET PERIOD
DIRECT COSTS ONLY (Kirschstein-NRSA Substitute Page)

	FROM	THROUGH
		DOLLAR TOTAL

STIPENDS

PREDOCTORAL

POSTDOCTORAL *(Itemize)* — No. Requested:

OTHER *(Specify)* — No. Requested:

TOTAL STIPENDS

TUITION and FEES *(Itemize)* — No. Requested:

TRAINEE TRAVEL *(Describe)*

TRAINEE RELATED EXPENSES (including Health Insurance)

TOTAL DIRECT COSTS FOR INITIAL BUDGET PERIOD *(Also enter on Face Page, Item 7)* $

**Kirschstein-NRSA Entire Budget
Period Substitute Page**

Principal Investigator/Program Director:
(Last, first, middle)

BUDGET FOR ENTIRE PROPOSED PERIOD OF SUPPORT
DIRECT COSTS ONLY (Kirschstein-NRSA Substitute Page)

BUDGET CATEGORY TOTALS	INITIAL BUDGET PERIOD (from Form Page 4)	ADDITIONAL YEARS OF SUPPORT REQUESTED			
		2nd	3rd	4th	5th
	No.	No.	No.	No.	No.
PREDOCTORAL STIPENDS					
POSTDOCTORAL STIPENDS					
OTHER STIPENDS					
TOTAL STIPENDS					
TUITION AND FEES					
TRAINEE TRAVEL					
TRAINEE RELATED EXPENSES (including Health Insurance)					
TOTAL DIRECT COSTS					

TOTAL DIRECT COSTS FOR ENTIRE PROPOSED PROJECT PERIOD *(Item 8a, Face Page)* $

JUSTIFICATION. For all years, explain the basis for the budget categories requested. Follow the instructions for the Initial Budget Period and include anticipated postdoctoral levels.

Principal Investigator/Program Director (Last, First, Middle):

DO NOT SUBMIT UNLESS REQUESTED
Competing Continuation Applications
KEY PERSONNEL REPORT

All Key Personnel for the Current Budget Period

Name	Degree(s)	SSN (last 4 digits)	Role on Project (e.g. PI, Res. Assoc.)	Date of Birth (MM/DD/YY)	Months Devoted to Project		
					Cal	Acad	Summer

Mailing address for application

Use this label or a facsimile

All applications and other deliveries to the Center for Scientific Review must come either via courier delivery or via the United States Postal Service (USPS.) Applications delivered by individuals to the Center for Scientific Review will no longer be accepted.

Applications sent via the USPS EXPRESS or REGULAR MAIL should be sent to the following address:

> **CENTER FOR SCIENTIFIC REVIEW**
> **NATIONAL INSTITUTES OF HEALTH**
> **6701 ROCKLEDGE DRIVE**
> **ROOM 1040 ñ MSC 7710**
> **BETHESDA, MD 20892-7710**

NOTE: All applications sent via a courier delivery service (non–USPS) should use this address, but CHANGE THE ZIP CODE TO 20817.

The telephone number is 301-435-0715. C.O.D. applications will *not* be accepted.

For application in response to RFA

Use this label or a facsimile

IF THIS APPLICATION IS IN RESPONSE TO AN RFA, be sure to put the RFA number in line 2 of the application face page. In addition, after duplicating copies of the application, cut along the dotted line below and staple the RFA label to the bottom of the face page of the original and place the original on top of your entire package. Failure to use this RFA label could result in delayed processing of your application such that it may not reach the review committee on time for review. ***Do not use*** the label unless the application is in response to a specific RFA. Also, applicants responding to a specific RFA should be sure to follow all special mailing instructions published in the RFA.

RFA No.

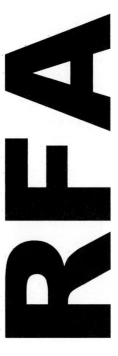

Mailing address for application
Use this label or a facsimile

All applications and other deliveries to the Center for Scientific Review must come either via courier delivery or via the USPS. Applications delivered by individuals to the Center for Scientific Review will no longer be accepted.

Applications sent via the USPS EXPRESS or REGULAR MAIL should be sent to the following address:

```
┌ ─ ─ ─ ─ ─ ─ ─ ─ ─ ─ ─ ─ ─ ─ ─ ─ ┐
│   CENTER FOR SCIENTIFIC REVIEW   │
│  NATIONAL INSTITUTES OF HEALTH   │
│      6701 ROCKLEDGE DRIVE        │
│      ROOM 1040 – MSC 7710         │
│     BETHESDA, MD 20892-7710       │
└ ─ ─ ─ ─ ─ ─ ─ ─ ─ ─ ─ ─ ─ ─ ─ ─ ┘
```

NOTE: All applications sent via a courier delivery service (non-USPS) should use this address, but CHANGE THE ZIP CODE TO 20817

The telephone number is 301-435-0715. C.O.D. applications will *not* be accepted.

For application in response to SBIR/STTR
Use this label or a facsimile

IF THIS APPLICATION IS IN RESPONSE TO AN SBIR/STTR Solicitation, be sure to put the SBIR/STTR Solicitation number in line 2 of the application face page. In addition, after duplicating copies of the application, cut along the dotted line below and staple the appropriate SBIR or STTR label to the bottom of the face page of the original and place the original on top of your entire package. If this SBIR or STTR application is in response to an RFA, be sure to also include the RFA No. in the space provided below.

SBIR
RFA No. _____ (if applicable)

STTR
RFA No. _____ (if applicable)

APPENDIX 5

Table of random numbers

Random Numbers

10097	32533	76520	13586	34673	54876	80959	09117	39292	74945
37542	04805	64894	74296	24805	24037	20636	10402	00822	91665
08422	68953	19645	09303	23209	02560	15953	34764	35080	33606
99019	02529	09376	70715	38311	31165	88676	74397	04436	27659
12807	99970	80157	36147	64032	36653	98951	16877	12171	76833
66065	74717	34072	76850	36697	36170	65813	39885	11199	29170
31060	10805	45571	82406	35303	42614	86799	07439	23403	09732
85269	77602	02051	65692	68665	74818	73053	85247	18623	88579
63573	32135	05325	47048	90553	57548	28468	28709	83491	25624
73796	45753	03529	64778	35808	34282	60935	20344	35273	88435
98520	17767	14905	68607	22109	40558	60970	93433	50500	73998
11805	05431	39808	27732	50725	68248	29405	24201	52775	67851
83452	99634	06288	98083	13746	70078	18475	40610	68711	77817
88685	40200	86507	58401	36766	67951	90364	76493	29609	11062
99594	67348	87517	64969	91826	08928	93785	61368	23478	34113
65481	17674	17468	50950	58047	76974	73039	57186	40218	16544
80124	35635	17727	08015	45318	22374	21115	78253	14385	53763
74350	99817	77402	77214	43236	00210	45521	64237	96286	02655
69916	26803	66252	29148	36936	87203	76621	13990	94400	56418
09893	20505	14225	68514	46427	56788	96297	78822	54382	14598
91499	14523	68479	27686	46162	83554	94750	89923	37089	20048
80336	94598	26940	36858	70297	34135	53140	33340	42050	82341
44104	81949	85157	47954	32979	26575	57600	40881	22222	06413
12550	73742	11100	02040	12860	74697	96644	89439	28707	25815
63606	49329	16505	34484	40219	52563	43651	77082	07207	31790
61196	90446	26457	47774	51924	33729	65394	59593	42582	60527
15474	45266	95270	79953	59367	83848	82396	10118	33211	59466
94557	28573	67897	54387	54622	44431	91190	42592	92927	45973
42481	16213	97344	08721	16868	48767	03071	12059	25701	46670
23523	78317	73208	89837	68935	91416	26252	29663	05522	82562
04493	52494	75246	33824	45862	51025	61962	79335	65337	12472
00549	97654	64051	88159	96119	63896	54692	82391	23287	29529
35963	15307	26898	09354	33351	35462	77974	50024	90103	39333
59808	08391	45427	26842	83609	49700	13021	24892	78565	20106
46058	85236	01390	92286	77281	44077	93910	83647	70617	42941
32179	00597	87379	25241	05567	07007	86743	17157	85394	11838
69234	61406	20117	45204	15956	60000	18743	92423	97118	96338
19565	41430	01758	75379	40419	21585	66674	36806	84962	85207
45155	14938	19476	07246	43667	94543	59047	90033	20826	69541
94864	31994	36168	10851	34888	81553	01540	35456	05014	51176
98086	24826	45240	28404	44999	08896	39094	73407	35441	31880
33185	16232	41941	50949	89435	48581	88695	41994	37548	73043
80951	00406	96382	70774	20151	23387	25016	25298	94624	61171
79752	49140	71961	28296	69861	02591	74852	20539	00387	59579
18633	32537	98145	06571	31010	24674	05455	61427	77938	91936
74029	43902	77557	32270	97790	17119	52527	58021	80814	51748
54178	45611	80993	37143	05335	12969	56127	19255	36040	90324
11664	49883	52079	84827	59381	71539	09973	33440	88461	23356
48324	77928	31249	64710	02295	36870	32307	57546	15020	09994
69074	94138	87637	91976	35584	04401	10518	21615	01848	76938
09188	20097	32825	39527	04220	86304	83389	87374	64278	58044
90045	85497	51981	50654	94938	81997	91870	76150	68476	64659
73189	50207	47677	26269	62290	64464	27124	67018	41361	82760
75768	76490	20971	87749	90429	12272	95375	05871	93823	43178
54016	44056	66281	31003	00682	27398	20714	53295	07706	17813

Source: RAND Corporation, 1955. *A Million Random Digits with 100,000 Normal Deviates.* Copyright 1955 and 1983 by the RAND Corporation. Used by permission.

GLOSSARY

The numbers in parentheses refer to chapters in the book.

Accuracy (10) Proximity of the estimates derived from a sample to the true population value. This is a function of systematic sampling error.

Acquiescence (13) Responses to questions based on the respondent's perception of what would be desirable to the interviewer.

Activities of daily living (ADL) (2) These are instruments that are often used to measure functional activity limitations of the elderly and the chronically ill. They include the ability of a person to function independently or with assistance in activities such as bathing, dressing, toileting, transferring into and out of a bed or chair, continence, and eating. See also *instrumental activities of daily living (IADL)*.

Agency relationship (2) Physicians make medical decisions on behalf of patients because of patients' relative ignorance. However, physician decisions typically reflect not only the preferences of their patients but also their own self-interest, the pressures from professional colleagues and institutions, a sense of medical ethics, and a desire to make good use of available resources.

Analytic/causal research (2) See *explanatory research*.

Anonymity (1) The situation in which the identity of the research subjects remains unknown, even to the researchers.

Applied (1) Involves using established principles to solve specific problems. Health services research is an applied field. See also *applied research*.

Applied research (2) This type of research is almost always defined by its practical, problem-solving orientation and is determined as much by what one wants to do, is paid to do, and can do as by the needs of theory development.

Area Resource File (3) The file pools data from various sources to facilitate health analysis both cross-sectionally and longitudinally. It is prepared by the Department of Health and Human Services' Bureau of Health Professions, Health Resources and Services Administration, and Public Health Service.

Assumptions (1) Suppositions that are considered to be true but have not been tested.

Asymmetrical relationship (1) A form of relationship between two variables in which change in one variable is accompanied by change in the other, but not vice versa.

Attrition (7) A threat to internal validity, attrition refers to the loss of subjects in an experiment. Attrition poses the greatest threat to internal validity when there is differential attrition, that is, when the experimental and control groups have different dropout rates. Invariably, those subjects who drop out differ in important ways from those who remain so that the experimental conditions are no longer equivalent in composition.

Auspices (13) Responses to questions dictated by an opinion or image of the sponsor, rather than the actual questions.

Basic/pure research (2) See *theoretical research*.

Behavioral Risk Factor Surveillance System (3) A program that provides state health agencies with the funding, training, and consultation necessary to collect behavioral risk factor data.

Behavioral risk factors (2) Certain lifestyles deemed harmful to a person's health and predictive of increased risk of certain diseases and mortality. Examples are cigarette smoking, alcohol abuse, lack of exercise, unsafe driving, poor dietary habits, and uncontrolled hypertension.

Biomedical research (1) Research primarily concerned with the conditions, processes, and mechanisms of health and illness at the sub-individual level.

Bivariate analysis (14) Bivariate analysis examines the relationship between two variables at a time. Bivariate analysis may be conducted to determine whether a relationship exists between two variables (i.e., effect), and, if a relationship exists, how much influence one variable has on the other (i.e., magnitude).

Burden of illness (2) Direct and indirect economic costs associated with the use of health care resources and functional restrictions imposed by illness.

Case study (6) A popular qualitative research method, a case study may be defined as an empirical inquiry that uses multiple sources of evidence to investigate a real-life social entity or phenomenon. It is particularly valuable when the research aims to capture individual differences or unique variations from one program setting to another, or from one program experience to another. A case can be a person, an event, a program, an organization, a time period, a critical incident, or a community. Regardless of the unit of analysis, a case study seeks to describe that unit in depth and detail, in context, and holistically.

Causal modeling (14) An integral step in path analysis, causal modeling requires the researcher to think causally about the research question and construct an arrow diagram that reflects causal processes. This type of modeling identifies variables for analysis based on a theoretical framework, literature review, and observations. The resulting models are likely to be theory driven.

Causal relationship (1) A form of relationship between two or more variables in which change in one variable causes change in other variables.

Causal research (2) See *explanatory research*.

Certificate of Need (CON) (2) A state-based regulatory measure responsible for the planning and diffusion of expensive medical technology. It is a process by which hospitals or other health care providers seeking a substantial expansion of their scope of services or physical facilities pursue prior approval from a government-endorsed entity.

Chi-square (14) A common test for independence. Chi-square (χ^2) is based on a comparison between an observed frequency table and an expected frequency table, that is, the table the researcher would expect to find if the two variables were statistically independent, or unrelated to each other.

Chi-square-based measures (14) These measures are used to assess the extent of the relationship between two nominal-level variables. They modify the chi-square statistics to reduce the influence of sample size and degrees of freedom and to restrict the values between zero and one. Examples include the phi coefficient (ϕ), Pearson's coefficient of contingency (C), and Cramér's V.

Clinical research (1) Research focusing primarily on studying the efficacy of the preventive, diagnostic, and therapeutic services applied to individual patients.

Cluster sampling (11) A probability sampling method that first breaks a population into groups or clusters and then randomly selects a sample of the clusters.

Code sheet (13) A code sheet may be called a "data transfer sheet" because responses from the instrument are recorded or transferred onto the code sheet before being entered into the computer. Code sheets are usually necessary for questionnaires with open-ended questions in which precoding is impossible.

Codebook (13) A document that describes the locations allocated to different variables and lists the numerical codes assigned to represent different attributes of variables.

Coding (13) The assignment of numbers to questionnaire answer categories and the indication of column locations for these numbers in the computer data file.

Cohort study (5) A cohort study examines specific subpopulations (cohorts) as they change over time. A cohort consists of persons (or other units, such as organizations) who experience the same significant life event within a specified period of time (e.g., a particular illness) or have some characteristic in common (e.g., same date of birth or marriage, membership in the same organization, and so on).

Cold-deck imputation (8) A method for minimizing the effect of missing values on data analysis. Cold-deck imputation applies group estimates (e.g., means) to individuals with missing values. The group estimate applied to individuals with missing values can be an overall group estimate or a subgroup estimate for the subgroup to which the individuals with the missing values belong.

Comparison group (7) A control group selected by a nonrandom method. The comparison group should be as similar as possible to the experimental group.

Complexity (10) The amount of information to be gathered and the number of sampling stages.

Computer-aided personal interviewing (CAPI) (13) Rather than a paper questionnaire, this interviewing method is used when the interview is conducted face-to-face on a computer, usually a laptop. The interviewer is prompted with the questions by the computer, and response codes are keyed in directly according to the respondent's answers.

Computer-assisted telephone interview (CATI) (13) This interviewing method involves a system in which survey questionnaires are displayed on computer terminals for telephone interviewers, who type respondents' answers directly into the computer.

Concept (1) Mental image or perception. Concepts may be impossible to observe directly, such as equity or ethics, or they may have referents that are readily observable, such as a hospital or a clinic.

Conceptual framework (1) The philosophical concerns, theories, and methodological approaches to scientific inquiry that characterize a particular discipline.

Conceptualization (2) The refinement and specification of abstract concepts into concrete terms.

Concurrent validity (12) A measure of validity, concurrent validity may be tested by comparing the results of one measurement with those of a similar measurement administered to the same population at approximately the same time. If both measurements yield similar results, then concurrent validity can be established.

Confidentiality (1) Where information identifying a research subject is not made available to anyone involved in the study.

Constant (1) A concept whose value is fixed.

Constant comparative analysis (6) This type of analysis is the process by which one piece of data (such as one interview or one statement) is compared to others to develop an understanding of the relationship among the different pieces. Through this process, the researcher develops a better understanding of a human phenomenon within a particular context.

Construct (1) An intangible or nonconcrete characteristic or quality with respect to which individuals or populations differ.

Construct validity (12) A measure of validity, construct validity refers to the fact that the measure captures the major dimensions of the concept under study.

Contamination (7) Occurs when the methods or materials of the intervention program are used to some extent by the supposed control group.

Content analysis (5) A research method appropriate for studying human communication and aspects of social or health behavior. The basic goal is to take a verbal, nonquantitative document and transform it into quantitative data. The usual units of analysis in content analysis are words, paragraphs, books, pictures, advertisements, television episodes, and the like.

Content validity (12) A measure of validity, content validity refers to the representativeness of the response categories related to each of the dimensions of a concept.

Control group (7) Includes those individuals or other units of analysis that do not receive the treatment or program, or receive an alternative treatment or program.

Controlled experiment (7) See *laboratory experiment.*

Convenience sampling (11) A nonprobability sampling method, convenience sampling relies on available subjects for inclusion in a sample.

Cost–benefit analysis (CBA) (9) This type of analysis compares the benefits of a program with its costs. Both direct and indirect benefits and costs are identified, quantified, translated into a common measurement unit (usually a monetary unit), and projected into the future to reflect the lifetime of a program. The net benefits may be used to judge the efficiency level of the program, or they may be compared with those of other competing programs.

Cost-effectiveness analysis (CEA) (9) This type of analysis compares the benefits of a program with its costs but requires monetizing only the costs. CEA expresses program benefits in outcome units. The efficacy of a program in attaining its goals or in achieving certain outcomes is assessed in relation to the monetary value of the resources or costs put into the program.

Cross-section data (3) Data collected at one point in time. The principal advantage is the relative inexpensiveness when a large sample size is used. The principal disadvantage is their transitory nature, which makes causal association difficult. See also *panel data, time-series data.*

Cross-sectional survey (8) In this type of survey, data on a sample or cross-section of respondents chosen to represent a particular target population are gathered at essentially one point in time, or within a short period of time.

Data cleaning (13) The process of checking for and correcting errors related to data coding, transfer, and entry.

Data dictionary (13) A data dictionary is used when data are assembled from multiple places. It contains a list of all files in the database, the number of records in each file, and the names and descriptions of each field.

Deductive imputation (8) A method for minimizing the effect of missing values on data analysis. Deductive imputation uses information from other parts of the questionnaire to fill in the missing pieces. For example, one can use the respondent's name to fill in missing information on gender.

Deductive process (1) A process of scientific inquiry that emphasizes theory as guidance for research. Hypotheses are derived from existing theories and serve as guidance for further research.

Demonstration (7) Interventions carried out primarily to extend or test the applicability of already existing knowledge rather than to add to scientific knowledge.

Dependent variable (1) The variable whose value is dependent upon other variables but which cannot itself affect other variables. In a causal relationship, the effect is a dependent variable.

Descriptive research (2) One of the general purposes of research. Descriptive research is undertaken to describe or portray the characteristics of some phenomenon, such as an individual, group, organization, community, event, or situation, with the purpose of formulating these descriptions as conceptual categories.

Deviant case sampling (6) See *extreme case sampling*.

Diagnostic-related groups (DRGs) (2) A prospective payment system for hospital care used by Medicare or other insurers. DRG criteria typically include the patient's age, sex, principal and secondary diagnoses, procedures performed, and discharge status.

Dimension (2) A specifiable aspect or facet of a concept.

Direct relationship (1) See *positive relationship*.

Discounting (9) Discounting is the technique to reduce costs and benefits that are spread out over time to their present values or to their common future values.

Distribution (14) A distribution organizes the values of a variable into categories. A frequency distribution, also known as a marginal distribution, shows the number of cases that fall into each category. A percentage distribution may be obtained by dividing the number or frequency of cases in the category by the total N.

Double-barreled questions (12) Double-barreled questions really ask two separate questions in one statement. They are biased because respondents may have different answers for each of the questions.

Double-blind experiment (7) Experiment in which neither the subjects nor the experimenters know which is the experimental group and which is the control group.

Ecological fallacy (5) Refers to the possibility that patterns found at a group level differ from those that would be found at an individual level. Thus, it may not be appropriate to draw conclusions at the individual level based on analyzing aggregate data. See also *individualistic fallacy*.

Ecological validity (7) The degree to which study results can be generalized across settings. A study has high ecological validity if it generalizes beyond the laboratory to more realistic field settings.

Econometrics (14) The application of statistical methods to economic problems.

Effect size (4) The size or strength of the impact of one factor on another.

Efficiency (10) The attainment of the most accurate and precise estimates at the lowest possible cost.

Empiricism (1) An approach used in scientific inquiry to discover the patterns of regularity in life. Such an approach relies on what humans experience through their senses: sight, hearing, taste, smell, and touch.

Environment (2) Events external to the body over which the individual has little or no control. Environment includes physical and social (political, economic, cultural, psychological, and demographic) dimensions.

Environmental health research (1) Research that concentrates on services that attempt to promote the health of populations by treating their environments rather than by treating specific individuals.

Environmental theory (2) An environment-focused theory of disease causation that identifies environmental risk factors to account for the occurrence of diseases. Traditional environmental risk factors include poor sanitation, filth, and pollutants. With increasing industrialization, recent environmental risk factors include overcrowding, workplace safety and stress, housing, and others.

Epidemiological research (1) Research that focuses on the population level by studying the frequency, distribution, and determinants of health and diseases.

Ethical standards (1) Standards for conducting research that take into account all relevant ethical issues so as to assure the safety and rights of study participants.

Ethnographic (6) A type of qualitative inquiry that describes a culture after extensive field research. The primary method of ethnographers is participant observation through immersion in the culture under study. See also *qualitative research.*

Evaluation research (9) The systematic application of scientific research methods for assessing the conceptualization, design, implementation, impact, and/or generalizability of organizational or social (including health services) programs.

Experimental group (7) Those individuals or other units of analysis that receive the treatment or program.

Experimental research (7) Involves planned interventions carried out so that explicit comparisons can be made between or across different intervention conditions to test a scientific hypothesis.

Explanatory research (2) One of the general purposes of research. Explanatory research is conducted to explain factors associated with a particular phenomenon, examine the relationships among variables, answer cause–effect questions, or make projections into the future. It attempts to seek answers to research hypotheses or problems. Explanatory research may also be called "analytic" or "causal research."

Exploratory research (2) One of the general purposes of research. Exploratory research is undertaken when relatively little is known about the phenomenon under investigation. Such an approach often results in meaningful hypotheses about the research problem.

External validity (7, 10) Related to the generalizability of the experimental results. An experiment is considered externally valid if its results can be generalized to the population, setting, treatment, and measurement variables of interest.

Extreme case sampling (6) A qualitative research sampling method. extreme case sampling focuses on cases that are unusual or special in some way. It may distort the manifestation of the phenomenon of interest. It is also called "deviant case sampling."

Face validity (12) If a measure has face validity, it appears to be appropriate for its intended purpose. On its "face," the measure seems valid.

Factor analysis (14) A statistical technique that involves exploring the relationships between variables, determining if related variables can be explained by a smaller number of underlying factors or constructs, and reducing the number of variables in the analysis, if appropriate.

Field experiment (7) A study that meets all the requirements of a true experiment but is conducted in a natural setting. The experiment takes place as subjects are going about a common activity, and the manipulations and observations are so subtle and unobtrusive that subjects' normal behavior is not disrupted.

Field research (6) A term frequently used to denote qualitative research. In field research, qualitative investigators observe, describe, and analyze events happening in a natural social setting (i.e., the field). Field research implies having direct and personal contact with people under study in their own environments. See also *qualitative research*.

Financing (health services) (1) Financing is concerned with the magnitude, trend, and sources of medical care spending and consists of both public- and private-sector funding sources.

Fixed-column format (13) The process of storing information, in the computer data file, for each variable in the same column for all respondents.

Focus group study (6) A type of in-depth interview, focus group study is an interview with a small group of people on a specific topic. A focus group typically consists of six to twelve people who are brought together in a room to engage in a guided discussion of some topic for one to two hours. Participants in the focus group are selected on the basis of relevancy to the topic under study. See also *in-depth interview*.

Focused interview (6) See *in-depth interview*.

Germ theory (2) A popular disease-focused theory that provides the foundation for biomedical research. With germ theory, microorganisms are the causal agent. The source of disease is at the individual level and the disease is communicated from one person to another (referred to as contagion). Strategies to address disease focus on identification of those people with problems and on follow-up medical treatment.

Grounded theory (1) Theories created on the basis of observation rather than deduction from existing theories. A grounded theory may be developed by: (a) entering the fieldwork phase without a hypothesis, (b) describing what happens, and (c) formulating explanations as to why it happens on the basis of observation.

Hawthorne effect (1) The reactive effect of research on the social phenomena being studied, that is, the attention from the researchers alters the very behavior that the researchers wish to study. See also *reactive effect, reactivity*.

Health and Retirement Study (3) A source of longitudinal data on the elderly population maintained by the University of Michigan and supported by the National Institute on Aging.

Health Insurance Portability and Accountability Act (HIPAA) (13) Enacted by the U.S. Congress in 1996, HIPAA requires the establishment of national standards for electronic health care transactions and national identifiers for providers, health insurance plans, and employers. HIPAA provisions address the security and privacy of health data, establishing minimum federal standards for protecting the privacy of individually identifiable health information

Health maintenance organization (HMO) (2) An organization that receives a fixed payment per subscriber to provide all medical care. Employees may pay the premium directly to the HMO, or the employer may pay a portion of the premium for its employees as part of the benefits package.

Health services (2) The total societal effort, whether private or public, to provide, organize, and finance services that promote the health status of individuals and the community.

Health services research (1) An applied multidisciplinary field that uses scientific inquiry to produce knowledge about the resources, provisions, organizing, financing, and policies of health services at the population level.

Health status (2) The state of physical health, mental health, and social well-being.

Heuristics (6) A form of phenomenological inquiry focusing on intense human experience from the point of view of the investigator and co-researchers. It is through the intense personal experience that a sense of connectedness develops between researchers and subjects in their mutual efforts to elucidate the nature, meaning, and essence of a significant human experience. See also *phenomenological inquiry, qualitative research.*

Historical analysis (5) The attempt to reconstruct past events (descriptive history) and the use of historical evidence to generate and test theories (analytical history).

History (7) A threat to internal validity, history consists of events in the subjects' environment, other than the manipulated independent variable, that occur during the course of the experiment and may affect the outcome of the experiment.

Hot-deck imputation (8) A method for minimizing the effect of missing values on data analysis. Hot-deck imputation uses the actual responses of individuals with similar characteristics and assigns those responses to individuals with missing values.

Hypothesis (1) A proposition stated in a testable form and predicting a particular relationship between two or more variables.

Incidence (2) The number of new cases of a disease in a defined population within a specified period of time.

Independent variable (1) The variable capable of effecting change in another variable. In a causal relationship, the cause is the independent variable.

In-depth interview (6) A qualitative research method consisting of three types of interviews: the informal conversational interview, the standardized open-ended interview, and the general interview guide approach. In-depth interviews (sometimes called "focused interviews") may be conducted with an individual or a group.

Individualistic fallacy (5) In analyzing individual data, researchers should guard against committing this type of fallacy, which attributes the study outcome to individual measures only and ignores community and area effects on the study outcome. See also *ecological fallacy.*

Inductive process (1) A process of scientific inquiry that emphasizes research as impetus for theory. Existing theories are corroborated and modified and new theories are developed based on the analysis of research data. The resulting corroborated, modified, or reconstructed theories serve as guidance for future research along similar lines of inquiry.

Informed consent (1) The understanding that prospective research subjects must be made fully aware of the procedures and risks involved in the research prior to agreeing to participate.

Institutional Review Board (IRB) (1, 10) A panel of persons that reviews research plans with respect to ethical implications and makes recommendations for compliance with appropriate standards.

Instrumental activities of daily living (IADL) (2) IADL scales are used to measure less severe functional impairments and to distinguish between more subtle levels of functioning. Compared with ADL, they require a finer level of motor coordination. IADL include the ability to walk a quarter mile, ascend or descend a flight of stairs, stand or sit for long periods, use fingers to grasp or handle, and lift or carry a moderately heavy or heavy object. See also *activities of daily living (ADL).*

Instrumentation (7) A threat to internal validity, instrumentation refers to unwanted changes in the characteristics of the measuring instrument or in the measurement procedure. This threat is most likely to occur in experiments when the instrument is a human observer, who may become more skilled, more bored, or more or less observant during the course of the study. Instrumentation effects also may occur when different observers are used to obtain measurements in different conditions or parts of an experiment.

Integrative research review (4) Integrative research review summarizes past research by drawing conclusions from many separate studies addressing similar or related hypotheses or research questions. The integrative reviewer aims to accomplish the following objectives: present the state of the knowledge concerning the topic under review, highlight issues previous researchers have left unresolved or unstudied, and direct future research so that it is built on cumulative inquiry. See also *methodological review, policy-oriented review, research review, theoretical review.*

Intensity sampling (6) A qualitative research sampling method, intensity sampling involves the same logic as extreme case sampling but with less emphasis on the extremes. It samples information-rich although not unusual cases that manifest the phenomenon of interest intensely but not extremely. See also *extreme case sampling.*

Interaction between selection bias and the intervention (7) A factor that might affect representativeness or external validity of research, interaction between selection bias and intervention occurs when subjects selected are not representative of the population and may respond better or worse than the general population to the intervention.

Interaction effect of testing (7) A factor that might affect representativeness or external validity of research, the interaction effect of testing occurs when a pretest increases or decreases the subjects' sensitivity or responsiveness to the experimental variable, thus making the results unrepresentative of the population who have not received any pretest.

Internal consistency reliability (12) This measure of the reliability of the items in a test can be determined in several ways. Split-half reliability, as the name implies, involves splitting the test into two halves and correlating one half to the other half. If each item on a test is scored dichotomously (i.e., yes–no, pass–fail, true–false), the proper method for determining internal consistency reliability is the Kuder–Richardson 20. By contrast, if each item on a test has multiple choices, Cronbach's alpha is the appropriate method.

Internal validity (7, 10) An experiment is internally valid to the extent that it rules out the possibility that extraneous variables, rather than the manipulated independent variable, are responsible for the observed outcome of the study.

International Classification of Functioning, Disability, and Health (ICF) (2) A system approved by the World Health Organization that provides a comprehensive, holistic framework for classifying health and disability focused on functionality.

Interrater reliability (12) A measure of reliability, involving the use of different people to conduct the same procedure, such as an interview, observation, coding, rating, and so on, and comparing the results of their work. To the extent that the results are highly similar, interrater reliability has been established.

Interval measures (12) Those variables whose attributes are not only rank-ordered but are separated by equal distances.

Intervening variable (1) A variable between the independent and dependent variables. Its identification strengthens the causal inference.

Interview survey (8) In interview surveys, researchers or interviewers ask the questions, provide the response categories (if applicable) orally, and then record the respondents' choices or answers. These can be conducted face-to-face—either in person or via web camera—or by phone.

Inverse relationship (1) See *negative/inverse relationship.*

Kurtosis (14) The extent to which cases or observations cluster around a central point.

Laboratory experiment (7) Experiments conducted in artificial settings where researchers have complete control over the random allocation of subjects to treatment and control groups and the degree of well-defined intervention.

Leading questions (12) Leading questions use particular wording to suggest a particular answer. They are biased because they hint at a desired answer rather than eliciting what the respondent feels.

Leptokurtic (14) When cases cluster around a central point more than they would in a normal distribution.

Lifestyle theory (2) A popular individual behavior-focused theory of disease causation that tries to isolate specific behaviors (e.g., smoking or lack of exercise) as causes of many health problems. These behaviors are deemed risky and unhealthy. The strategy for improving health status is through changing these behaviors.

Lifestyles (2) See *behavioral risk factors.*

Linear relationship (1) A form of relationship between two variables in which the two variables vary at the same rate regardless of whether the values of the variables are low, high, or intermediate.

Loaded questions (12) Loaded questions use words and phrases that reflect the investigator's perception of a particular issue or event. They are biased because they suggest certain beliefs that could influence the respondent's answers.

Logistic regression (14) Logistic regression is based on the assumption that the logarithm of the odds of belonging to one population is a linear function of several predictors (independent variables) in the model. In logistic regression, the dependent variable is binary, or dichotomous (e.g., whether one smokes or not, whether one has health insurance or not).

Longitudinal survey (8) The longitudinal survey takes a single sample and follows it or another similar sample with repeated (at least two) surveys, over a period of time.

Matching (7) A commonly used nonrandom assignment method, matching is the attempt to make the control group as similar to the experimental group as possible.

Maturation (7) A threat to internal validity, maturation refers to any psychological or physical changes taking place within subjects as a result of the passing of time regardless of the experimental intervention.

Mean (14) As a measure of central tendency, the mean is the arithmetic average computed by adding up all the values and dividing by the total number of cases.

Measurement (12) The process of specifying and operationalizing a given concept.

Measurement errors (12) The sources of differences observed in elements that are not caused by true differences among elements.

Measurement reliability (10, 12) The extent to which consistent results are obtained when a particular measure is applied to similar elements. A reliable measure will yield the same or a very similar outcome when it is reapplied to the same subject or subjects sharing the same characteristics being measured.

Measurement validity (10, 12) The extent to which important dimensions of a concept and their categories have been taken into account and appropriately operationalized. A valid measure has response categories truly reflecting all important meanings of the concept under consideration.

Measures of central tendency (14) Summaries of the information about the average value of a variable: a typical value around which all the values cluster. See also the three commonly used measures of central tendency: *mean, median,* and *mode.*

Measures of dispersion (14) See *measures of variability/dispersion*.

Measures of variability/dispersion (14) The spread or variation of the distribution. See also the commonly used measures of variability: *range, standard deviation,* and *variance.*

Median (14) As a measure of central tendency, the median is the middle position, or midpoint, of a distribution. It is computed by first ordering the values of a distribution and then dividing the distribution in half, that is, half the cases fall below the median and the other half above it.

Medicaid (2) Joint federal-state medical insurance for the following categories: (a) Aid to Families with Dependent Children (AFDC) families; (b) those covered by Supplemental Security Income (SSI), including the aged, the blind, and the disabled; and (c) state-designated "categorically needy" and/or "medically needy" groups. Every state Medicaid program provides specific basic health services. States may determine the scope of services offered (e.g., limit the days of hospital care or the number of physician visits covered). Payments are made directly to providers of services for care rendered to eligible individuals. Providers must accept the Medicaid reimbursement level as payment in full.

Medical chart review (13) This process abstracts critical patient and treatment information based on the medical records of the patients. Medical chart review helps identify the answers to "What happened?" in regard to a patient's care.

Medical Expenditure Panel Survey (3) A series of surveys conducted by the Agency for Healthcare Research and Quality on financing and use of medical services in the United States.

Medicare (2) Medical insurance that covers hospital, physician, and other medical services for: (a) persons 65 and over, (b) disabled individuals who are entitled to Social Security benefits, and (c) end-stage renal disease victims. Part A of Medicare covers hospital insurance. Part B is a supplementary medical insurance, providing payments for physicians, physician-ordered supplies and services, outpatient hospital services, rural health clinic visits, and the like. Until 1992, Medicare operated primarily on a fee-for-service basis for physicians and related services and, until 1983, on a cost-based retrospective basis for hospital services. Since 1983, the Medicare hospital prospective payment system (PPS) has used diagnosis-related groups (DRGs) to classify cases for payment. Since 1992, the Medicare physician payment system has adopted a resource-based relative value system (RBRVS).

Medicare Current Beneficiary Survey (3) Medicare data collected from a representative national sample of the Medicare population.

Medicare Enrollment and Claims Data (3) A population-based administrative data set providing Medicare utilization and enrollment data.

MEDLINE (4) The world's leading bibliographic database of medical information, covering more than 3,500 journals since 1966 and containing information found in the publications *Index Medicus, International Nursing Index,* and *Index to Dental Literature.* MEDLINE contains abstracts of articles published by the most common U.S. and international journals on medicine and health services.

Mental set (13) The responses to later items of the questionnaire influenced by perceptions based on previous items.

Meta analysis (4) A statistical analysis that combines and interprets the results of independent studies of a given scientific issue for the purpose of integrating the findings. It allows the reviewer to synthesize the results of numerous tests so that an overall conclusion can be drawn.

Methodological review (4) Methodological review summarizes different research designs used to study a particular topic and compares studies with different designs in terms of their findings. The purpose is to identify the strengths and weaknesses of different designs for a particular topic and separate fact from artifact in research results. See also *integrative research review, policy-oriented review, research review, theoretical review.*

Methodology (10) See *research method.*

Midtests (7) Measurements made during the time the intervention or program is being implemented; short for mid-program or mid-experiment tests.

Mode (14) As a measure of central tendency, the mode is the value (or category) of a distribution that occurs most frequently.

Model (7) A representation of a system that specifies its components and the relationships among the components.

Multidisciplinary (1) An area of research incorporating aspects or expertise from multiple scientific disciplines.

Multilevel analysis (14) Techniques useful when data exist at several different levels. If data are nested, or if a study has several different units of analysis, multilevel analysis is a valuable tool.

Multiple imputation (8) A method for minimizing the effect of missing values on data analysis. Multiple imputation generates multiple simulated values for each incomplete datum, then iteratively analyzes data sets with each simulated value substituted in turn. Multiple imputation methods yield multiple imputed replicate data sets, each of which is analyzed in turn. The results are combined and the average is reported as the estimate.

Multiple regression (14) An examination of the impact of two or more independent variables on a dependent variable. Generally, the variables are measured at the interval-ratio level. Multiple regression may be used to examine the relationships among variables or as an inferential method to test hypotheses about population parameters.

Multiple-treatment interference (7) This phenomenon occurs when multiple treatments are applied to the same subjects, largely because the effects of prior treatments are often not erasable. It then becomes difficult to determine the true cause of the outcomes.

Multivariate analysis (14) An examination of the relationship among three or more variables at a time. The inclusion of additional variables is based on both theoretical and practical knowledge, which helps specify the direction of influence and test for spuriousness.

Narrative analysis (6) This type of analysis involves generating, interpreting, and representing the stories of study subjects. A narrative can be a long life story, a short anecdote, or a description of a particular event or time in a person's life. In health services research, narrative analysis can help improve knowledge in areas such as patients' personal experiences with disease.

National Ambulatory Medical Care Survey (3) A data set obtained through a national sample of office-based physicians and a systematic random sample of physician office visits during a seven-day period.

National Center for Health Statistics (3) Founded in 1960, the National Center for Health Statistics is the principal federal agency that collects, analyzes, and disseminates health statistics.

National Health and Nutrition Examination Survey (3) A series of surveys conducted by the National Center for Health Statistics that is an excellent source of data on health and nutrition.

National Health Interview Survey (3) This survey, conducted by the National Center for Health Statistics, is the principal source of information on the general health status of the civilian, noninstitutionalized population of the United States.

National Hospital Discharge Survey (3) A continuous nationwide survey of inpatient utilization of short-stay hospitals, conducted by the National Center for Health Statistics, that allows sampling at the census division level.

National Nursing Home Survey (3) This survey provides a series of national samples of nursing homes, their residents, and their staff, facilitating research on the general health status of the nursing home population and the characteristics of nursing home facilities.

National Vital Statistics System (3) Annual databases, which were started in 1968, that provide the most detailed picture of vital statistics information.

Natural experiment (7) Experiments conducted in real-life settings rather than in laboratories or the controlled environment. Researchers rely on truly naturally occurring events in which people have different exposures that resemble an actual experiment.

Natural science (1) The rational study of the universe via rules or laws of natural order.

Needs assessment (9) A type of evaluation with the purpose of identifying weaknesses or deficiency areas (i.e., needs) in the current situation that can be remedied or of projecting future conditions to which the program will need to adjust.

Negative/inverse relationship (1) A form of relationship between two variables in which increase (decrease) in one variable is accompanied by decrease (increase) in the other variable.

Nominal definition (2) A specification of concepts that is built on the consensus or norm concerning what a particular term should mean.

Nominal measures (12) Nominal measures classify elements into categories of a variable that are exhaustive and mutually exclusive. There is no rank-order relationship among categories and one cannot measure the distance between categories.

Nonlinear relationship (1) A form of relationship between two variables in which the rate at which one variable changes in value is different for different values of the second variable.

Nonprobability sampling (11) In this type of sampling, the probability of selecting any sampling unit is not known because units are selected through a nonrandom process. A nonprobability sample may be biased because certain units may be more or less likely to be included in the sample.

Normal curve/bell curve (14) A graph representing the density function of the normal probability distribution.

Objectivity (1) A basic characteristic of scientific inquiry that requires researchers to carry out research-related activities unaffected by their emotions, conjectures, or personal biases.

Observation unit (11) A term used in sampling. The observation unit is the unit from which data are actually collected.

Observational research (6) A term frequently used to denote qualitative research because observation is a primary method of qualitative research. Qualitative researchers observe for the purpose of seeing the world from the subject's own perspective.

Qualitative observation emphasizes direct observation, usually with the naked eye, and takes place in the natural setting. Also called "participant observation." See also *participant observation, qualitative research.*

Odds ratio (14) The ratio of two odds, that is, the ratio of the probability of occurrence of an event to that of nonoccurrence. See also *relative risk ratio.*

Operational definition (2) The specification of concepts that is built on a particular observational or data collection strategy. An operational definition spells out precisely how the concept will be measured.

Operationalization (1) A process that translates general concepts into specific indicators and specifies how a researcher goes about measuring and identifying the variables.

Opportunity costs (9) A concept used to value costs, opportunity costs reflect alternative ways resources can be utilized.

Ordinal measures (12) Those indicators or variables whose attributes may be logically rank-ordered along some progression.

Outcome evaluation (9) A type of evaluation concerned with the accomplishments and impact of the program and its effectiveness in attaining the intended results.

Outcomes research (1) Research that seeks to understand the end result of particular health care practices and interventions.

Panel data (3) A combination of cross-section and time-series data, surveying the same groups over time. Its principal advantage is its ability to capture trends and causal associations. Its main disadvantages are attrition rates and its relative expensiveness. See also *cross-section data, time-series data.*

Panel study (5, 8) A panel study takes as its basis a representative sample of the group of interest, which may be individuals, households, organizations, or any other social unit, and follows the same unit over time with a series of surveys.

Paradigm (1) A general perspective; a fundamental model or scheme that breaks down the complexity of the real world and organizes our views. Often, a paradigm directs researchers to look for answers and provides them with concepts that are the building blocks of theories.

Parallel forms reliability (12) To avoid potential testing effects associated with test–retest reliability measures, one may create a parallel (or alternative) form of the test. To establish parallel forms reliability (i.e., the level of correlation between the original test and the parallel test), a group of participants completes both tests with little time in between. Similar to test–retest reliability, parallel forms reliability is established when the correlation coefficient for the two sets of scores is at least 0.80.

Parameters (11) The summary numerical description of variables about the population of interest.

Participant observation (6) A popular qualitative research method in which the researcher is fully engaged in experiencing the setting under study while at the same time trying to understand that setting through personal experience, observation, and talking with other participants about what is happening. Through direct experience with and observation of programs, the researcher can gain information that otherwise would not become available. See also *observational research.*

Path analysis (14) A procedure that provides the possibility for causal determination among a set of measured variables. It gives a quantitative interpretation of an assumed causal system. Path analysis may consist of a series of regression equations, with many variables in the model taking their places respectively as dependent and independent variables. In other words, most of the variables in the model will be dependent in one equation and independent in one or more other equations.

Pearson product–moment correlation coefficient (14) The Pearson product–moment correlation coefficient (*r*) is a measure of association between two interval-ratio-level variables.

Peer review (1) A process for the review of research findings by independent scientists in order to objectively assess the validity of the research in question.

Phenomenological inquiry (6) A type of qualitative inquiry focusing on the experience of a phenomenon for particular people. The phenomenon being experienced may be an emotion (e.g., loneliness, satisfaction, anger), a relationship, a marriage, a job, a program, an organization, or a culture. In terms of subject matter, phenomenological inquiry holds that what is important to know is what people experience and how they interpret the world. In terms of research methodology, phenomenological inquiry believes the only way for researchers to really know what another person experiences is to experience it for themselves through participant observation. See also *heuristics, participant observation, qualitative research.*

Placebo (1) An inert substance or neutral condition used as a control in a research study.

Platykurtic (14) When cases cluster around a central point less than they would in a normal distribution.

Policy (2) Planning and decision making conducted at various levels, ranging from health service practices to state legislation to congressional action.

Policy analysis (9) A type of evaluation with the purpose of laying out goals, using logical processes to evaluate identified alternatives, and exploring the best way to reach these goals.

Policy-oriented review (4) Review summarizing current knowledge of a topic so as to draw out policy implications of study findings. Such review requires knowledge of the major policy issues and debates as well as common research expertise. See also *integrative research review, methodological review, research review, theoretical review.*

Population (11) The target for which investigators generate the study results.

Population validity (7) Refers to the representativeness of the sample of the population and the generalizability of the findings. A study has high population validity if the sample closely represents the population and the study findings work across different kinds of people.

Positive/direct relationship (1) A form of relationship between two variables in which both variables vary in the same direction, that is, an increase in the value of one variable is accompanied by an increase in the value of the second variable, or a decrease in the value of one variable is accompanied by a decrease in the value of the second variable.

Positivism (1) A fundamental assumption of scientific inquiry that holds that life is not totally chaotic or random but has logical and persistent patterns of regularity.

Posttests (7) Tests given at the end of a program or an experiment; short for "post-program" or "post-experiment tests."

Power (11) Closely linked to sample size, the power of a research study is that study's probability of rejecting a null hypothesis (i.e., the probability of making a correct decision). The higher the power of a study, the better.

Precision (10) Precision refers to the degree to which further measurements will produce the same or similar results. This is a function of random sampling error.

457

Predictive validity (12) A measure of validity that may be examined by comparing the results obtained from the measurement with some actual later occurring evidence that the measurement aims at predicting. When there is a high degree of correspondence between the prediction and actual event—the predicted event actually takes place—then predictive validity is established.

Prestige (13) Responses to questions intended to improve the image of the respondent in the eyes of the interviewer.

Pretests (7) Tests given before a program or an experiment starts; short for "preprogram," or "preexperiment tests."

Prevalence (2) The number of instances of a given disease in a given population at a designated time.

Primary data source (3) The collection of data by researchers themselves. See also *secondary data source*.

Primary research (5) The analysis of data collected by the researcher firsthand. The data originate with the research; they are not there before the research is undertaken. See also *secondary research*.

Probability sampling (11) In probability sampling, all sampling units in the study population have a known, nonzero probability of being selected in the sample, typically through a random selection process.

Process (1) A series of activities that bring about an end result or product.

Process evaluation (9) A type of evaluation that focuses on how a particular program operates. It is concerned with the activities, services, materials, staffing, and administrative arrangements of the program.

Proportional reduction in error (PRE) (14) A broad framework that helps organize a large number of measures for levels of data known as nominal, ordinal, and even interval-ratio. PRE-based measures are typically ratios of a measure of error in predicting the values of one variable based on that variable alone and the same measure of error based on knowledge of an additional variable. The logic behind this framework is that if prior knowledge about another variable improves the knowledge of this variable, then these two variables are related.

Proposition (1) A statement about one or more concepts or variables. Propositions are the building blocks of theories.

Pure research (2) See *theoretical research*.

Purposive sampling (11) A nonprobability sampling method that selects sampling elements based on expert judgment in terms of the representativeness or typical nature of population elements and the purpose of the study.

Qualitative research (6) Research methods employed to find out what people do, know, think, and feel by observing, interviewing, and analyzing documents. Specifically, it attempts to gain individuals' own accounts of their attitudes, motivations, and behavior. See also *case study, ethnographic, field research, heuristics, observational research, participant observation, phenomenological inquiry, symbolic interactionism*.

Quality of life (2) Factors that enhance or reduce the meaningfulness of life, including independent functioning, family circumstances, finances, housing, job satisfaction, and so forth.

Quality-adjusted life year (QALY) (9) An outcome unit that incorporates changes in survival and changes in health-related well-being by weighting years of life to reflect the value of health-related quality of life during each year.

Quasi-experimental (7) Experimentation that lacks the random assignment to conditions, which is essential for true scientific investigation.

Quota sampling (11) A nonprobability sampling method that specifies desired characteristics in the population elements and selects appropriate ratios of population elements that fit the characteristics of the sample.

Random digit dialing (RDD) (8) A method for reducing potential selection bias caused by the increasing use of unlisted telephone numbers. In RDD, known residential prefixes are sampled and the last four digits of the telephone number are selected by means of a table of random numbers.

Random error (11) See *sampling error*.

Random number generator (RNG) (11) A computational device designed to generate a sequence of numbers that lacks any pattern.

Random sampling (7) The process of selecting units in an unbiased manner to form a representative sample from a population of interest.

Randomization (7) The process of taking a set of units and allocating them to an experimental or control group by means of some randomizing procedure.

Randomized clinical trial (1) A medical experiment in which subjects in a population are randomly allocated into groups, usually called "experiment" and "control" groups, to receive or not receive an experimental procedure. The results are assessed by comparison of outcome measures in the experiment and control groups.

Range (14) A measure of dispersion, range is the difference between the highest (maximum) and lowest (minimum) values in a distribution.

Rate (14) A rate is computed by dividing the number of cases or events in a given category by the total number of observations. The resulting proportion is then expressed as any multiple of 10 that clears the decimal, usually 100 or 1,000.

Ratio (14) A ratio is one number divided by another: the frequency of observations in one category is divided by the frequency in another category of a distribution.

Ratio measures (12) Measurements similar to interval measures except that ratio measures are based on a nonarbitrary or true-zero point. The true-zero property of ratio measures makes it possible to divide and multiply numbers meaningfully and thereby form ratios. See also *interval measures, ratio*.

Reactive effect (5) Changes in behavior that occur because subjects are aware they are being studied or observed. This is a potential bias in data collection. See also *Hawthorne effect, reactivity*.

Reactive effects of the experimental arrangements (7) A factor that might affect representativeness or external validity of research, the reactive effects of the experimental arrangements refer to control group subjects getting exposed to part of the experimental intervention, thus limiting the generalizability of the true experimental effect.

Reactivity (1) See *Hawthorne effect, reactive effect*.

Records (5) Systematic accounts of regular occurrences.

Regression toward the mean (7) See *statistical regression*.

Relative risk ratio (14) A measurement of the strength of association between the presence of a factor (x) and the occurrence of an event (y). For example, it is the ratio of the incidence of a disease (e.g., lung cancer) among the exposed (e.g., those who smoke) to the incidence of a disease among the unexposed (e.g., those who don't smoke).

Reliability (12) A reflection of the extent to which the same result occurs from repeated applications of a measure to the same subject. See also *validity*.

Replication (1) The ability to repeat research and replicate findings, which is a necessary aspect of validating scientific knowledge.

459

Research design (10) The planning of research, research design specifies the questions to be studied, the data to be collected, and the methods of data collection and analysis.

Research method (10) A body of knowledge that reflects the general philosophy and purpose of the research process, the assumptions and values that serve as a rationale for research, the general approach of data collection and analysis, and the standards used for interpreting data and reaching conclusions.

Research proposal (3) A description of the specific study a researcher intends to accomplish and how. The components of a research proposal generally include the following elements: a title page, a table of contents, an abstract, a detailed project description, references, a detailed budget, a human subjects review, and appendices.

Research review (4) Research review provides a synthesis of existing knowledge on a specific question, based on an assessment of all relevant empirical research that can be found. See also *integrative research review, methodological review, policy-oriented review, theoretical review.*

Research/study population (10) The target group to which study results are generalized.

Resources (health services) (1) Human and nonhuman resources required for the provision of health services. Human resources consist of both physician and nonphysician providers. A major nonhuman health services resource is medical technology.

Right to service (1) The right of research subjects assigned to a no-treatment control to later receive the experimental treatment if it offers beneficial effects.

Sample size (11) The magnitude of the sample of a given population, sample size is determined by a number of factors including the characteristics of the population, the nature of the analysis to be conducted, the desired precision of the estimates, the resources available, the study design, and the anticipated response rate.

Sampling (11) The process of selecting a subset of observations from an entire population of interest so that characteristics from the subset can be used to draw conclusions or make inferences about the entire population of interest.

Sampling bias (11) A tendency to favor the selection of units that have particular characteristics. It describes deviations that are not a consequence of chance alone. Sampling bias is also known as systematic error.

Sampling design (11) The method used to select the sampling units. It may be classified into probability and nonprobability sampling methods. See also *nonprobability sampling, probability sampling.*

Sampling element (11) A term used in sampling. Sampling element refers to the unit of the sample to be collected and provides the information base for analysis.

Sampling error (11) When a sample does not represent the population well because of chance, sampling error occurs. Sampling error comprises the differences between the sample and the population that are due solely to the particular units that happen to have been selected. Sampling error is also known as random error.

Sampling fraction (11) The sampling fraction reflects the proportion of subjects to be sampled for the study.

Sampling frame (11) A list of sampling units from which the sample is actually selected.

Sampling unit (11) The actual unit that is considered for selection.

Saturation (6) The point during an in-depth interview at which the interviewer starts to hear the same ideas repeated and no new information being shared.

Scientific inquiry (1) Research by scientists that produces knowledge and improves understanding of particular aspects of the world.

Scientific method (1) A procedure that uses observation and experimentation to distinguish between competing scientific theories.

Scientific theory (1) The logical aspect of science. It is used as a framework to guide the understanding and explanation of patterns of regularity in life.

Secondary analysis (5) The reanalysis of data collected by another researcher or organization, including the analysis of data sets collated from a variety of sources to create time-series or area-based data sets. See also *primary research.*

Secondary data source (3) The use of data collected by others. See also *primary data source.*

Selection (7) A threat to internal validity, selection is present whenever there are systematic differences in the selection and composition of the experimental and control groups.

Self-administered questionnaire survey (8) Questionnaires completed by the respondents themselves in which they read the questions and enter their own answers.

SF-36 (2) A widely used multipurpose short-form health survey.

Simple random sampling (11) A probability sampling method, simple random sampling means that every unit in a population has an equal probability of being included in a sample.

Simple regression (14) An examination of the impact of one independent variable on another, dependent variable. Generally, both variables are measured at the interval-ratio level.

Simulation (7) A special kind of model: a model in motion and operating over a period of time to show, not only the structure of the system (what position each variable or component occupies in the system and the way the components are related or connected), but also the way change in one variable or component affects changes in the values of the other variables or components. See also *model.*

Skewed (14) Also referred to as skewness, a distribution of cases that is not symmetric, that is, when more cases are found at one end of the distribution than the other.

Skewness (14) See *skewed.*

Small area analysis (1) The use of large administrative databases to obtain population-based measures of utilization and resource allocation.

Snowball sampling (11) A nonprobability sampling method, snowball sampling relies on informants to identify other relevant subjects for study inclusion.

Social contacts (2) The number of social activities a person performs within a specified time period. Examples include visits with friends and relatives and participation in social events, such as conferences and workshops. See also *social well-being.*

Social desirability (13) Responses to questions based on what is perceived as being socially acceptable or respectable, positive or negative.

Social resources (2) The extent that social contacts such as close friends and relatives can be relied on for tangible and intangible support. Social resources represent personal evaluations of the adequacy of interpersonal relationships. See also *social well-being.*

Social science (1) The study of human behavior and social phenomena.

Social well-being (2) Social well-being extends beyond the individual to encompass the quantity and quality of social contacts and resources across distinct domains of life, including community, family, and work. See also *social contacts, social resources.*

Socioeconomic status (SES) (2) An important social measure and a strong and consistent predictor of health status. The major components of SES include income, education, and occupational status.

Sociography (6) A type of case study, sociography denotes the social mapping of a community's structure, institutions, and patterns of relationships. This type of case study is heavily used in social anthropology for research on nonindustrialized societies, but it is also used to study towns and communities in industrialized societies. See also *case study*.

Spearman rank correlation coefficient (14) This coefficient of rank correlation (r_s) is a measure of association between two ordinal-level variables.

Split-half reliability (12) A measure of reliability, split-half reliability involves preparing two sets (or two halves) of a measurement of the same concept, applying them to research subjects at one setting, and comparing the correlation between the two sets of measurements. To the extent that the correlation is high, the measurement is reliable.

Spurious relationship (1) A spurious relationship exists when two variables appear to be related only because both are caused by a third variable. The variable that causes a spurious relationship is an antecedent variable, which occurs first and is causally related to both the independent and dependent variables.

Standard deviation (14) A measure of dispersion, the standard deviation is defined as the square root of the variance.

Standard scores (14) Descriptions of the relative position of an observation within a distribution. For example, the z score uses both the mean and standard deviation to indicate how many standard deviations above or below the mean an observation falls.

Statistical imputation (8) A method for minimizing the effect of missing values on data analysis. Statistical imputation uses statistical procedures for the assignment of missing values. For example, multiple regression may be used for data imputation by using nonmissing data to predict the values of missing data.

Statistical regression (7) A threat to internal validity, statistical regression is the tendency for extreme subjects to move (regress) closer to the mean or average with the passing of time. This phenomenon is likely to affect experimental results when subjects are selected for an experimental condition because of their extreme conditions or scores. The more deviant the score, the larger the error of measurement it probably contains. On a posttest, an investigator expects the high scorers to decline somewhat on the average and the low scorers to improve their relative standing regardless of the intervention. Also called "regression toward the mean."

Statistics (11) The summary numerical description of variables about a sample.

Straight-line relationship (1) See *linear relationship*.

Stratified purposeful sampling (6) A qualitative research sampling method, stratified purposeful sampling is carried out to combine a typical case sampling strategy with others, essentially taking a stratified purposeful sample of above-average, average, and below-average cases.

Stratified sampling (11) A probability sampling method, stratified sampling divides the population into nonoverlapping groups or categories, called strata, and then conducts independent simple random sampling for each stratum.

Suppressor variable (1) A variable that suppresses the relationship by being positively correlated with one of the variables in the relationship and negatively correlated with the other, with the result that the two variables in the relationship appear to be unrelated. The true relationship between the two variables will reappear when the suppressor variable is controlled for.

Survey of Mental Health Organizations (3) Introduced in 1998, the survey provides valuable information on the sociodemographic, clinical, and treatment characteristics of patients served by mental health facilities.

Survey research (8) The use of a systematic method to collect data directly from respondents regarding facts, knowledge, attitudes, beliefs, and behaviors of interest to the researcher, and the analysis of these data using quantitative methods.

Symbolic interactionism (6) A method of qualitative analysis focusing on a common set of symbols and understanding that have emerged to give meaning to people's interactions. The importance of symbolic interactionism to qualitative research is its distinct emphasis on the importance of symbols and the interpretative processes that undergird interactions as fundamental to understanding human behavior. See also *qualitative research*.

Symmetrical relationship (1) A form of relationship between two variables in which change in either variable is accompanied by change in the other variable.

Systematic error (11) See *sampling bias*.

Systematic sampling (11) A probability sampling method, systematic sampling selects every *k*th element from the sampling frame after a random start.

Term (2) Names that represent a collection of apparently related, observed phenomena.

Testing (7) A threat to internal validity, testing refers to changes in what is being measured brought about by reactions to the process of measurement. Typically, people will score better or give more socially desirable or psychologically healthier responses the second time a test or scale is administered to them.

Test–retest reliability (12) A measure of reliability that involves administering the same measurement to the same individuals at two different times. If the correlation between the same measures is high (usually greater than 0.80), then the measurement is believed to be reliable.

Theoretical research (2) Scientific study involving the testing of hypotheses developed from theories that are intellectually interesting to the researcher. Theoretical research is also called "basic" or "pure research."

Theoretical review (4) This type of review summarizes the relevant theories used to explain a particular topic and compares them with regard to accuracy of prediction, consistency, and breadth. Theoretical review contains a description of major findings, assesses which theory is most powerful and consistent with known findings, and refines a theory by reformulating or integrating concepts from existing theories. See also *integrative research review, methodological review, policy-oriented review, research review*.

Time sampling (6) A qualitative research sampling method that samples periods (e.g., months of the year) or units of time (e.g., hours of the day). It is used when programs are believed to function in different ways at different time periods or units.

Time-series data (3) Data that follow the same unit of observation over time. Its principal advantage is its ability to capture historical trends and changes. Its principal disadvantages are limited observations and the relative expensiveness when a large sample size is used. See also *cross-section data, panel data*.

Time-series tests (7) A series of tests or measurements, usually given at equal intervals before and after the program or experiment.

Trend study (5, 8) A study with a repeated cross-sectional design in which each survey collects data on the same items or variables with independently selected samples of the same general population of interest.

Triangulation (6) The combination of several methodologies in the study of the same phenomenon or program.

Typical case sampling (6) A qualitative research sampling method that provides a qualitative profile of one or more typical cases. It is helpful to those not familiar with the program in question.

Unit of analysis (11) The object about which investigators wish to draw conclusions based on their study.

Unit of observation (3) The level from which data are actually collected or recorded.

Univariate analysis (14) An examination of the characteristics of one variable at a time. Descriptive statistics are produced in univariate analysis.

Validity (12) The validity of a measure is the extent to which it actually assesses what it purports to measure. If a measure is supposed to reflect the quality of care, a researcher would expect improvements in quality to affect the measure positively. See also *reliability*.

Variable (1, 11) A concept that has more than one measurable value.

Variance (14) A measure of dispersion that indicates the extent to which each of the values of a distribution differs from the mean. It is defined as the average squared deviation from the mean.

Voluntary participation (1) The principle that "captive audiences" (e.g., those in prisons, universities, and workplaces) are not to be coerced into participating in research.

INDEX